Mental Health Across the Lifespan

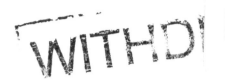

Mental wellbeing is an integral part of being, and feeling, healthy, and it is estimated that one in four people will suffer from some form of mental illness during their lifetime. In spite of this, it is often overlooked in mainstream healthcare. The overall aim of this book is to provide knowledge and understanding of how mental health affects human beings from conception through to end-of-life, and the challenges that society as a whole has to address in the treatment of mental health.

Beginning with an exploration of historical, social and cultural contexts, the book then goes on to discuss mental health care, and mental health promotion, during pregnancy and early parenthood, childhood, adolescence and young adulthood, adulthood for both men and women, and in older people. Containing reflective exercises, the chapters are designed to provide an easily accessible and engagingly written introduction to mental health.

Containing chapters that can be read and reviewed in isolation, or used as an entire text, *Mental Health Across the Lifespan: A handbook* provides a solid introduction to mental health for students. The book will also act as a useful reference for doctors, nurses, midwives, health visitors, allied health professionals, and health and social care support workers who have no specialist mental health training but often work in partnership with, and care for, people suffering from mental health issues.

Mary Steen is the Professor of Midwifery at the School of Nursing and Midwifery, Division of Health Sciences, University of South Australia (UniSA). She is the Chair of the Mothers, Babies & Families Research Group and facilitates the promotion of research and scholarly activities both nationally and internationally. She has previously been a Professor of Midwifery in the UK and holds visiting professorships at the University of Chester, UK and Port Harcourt University, Nigeria. She has a vast amount of nursing and midwifery clinical experience in both hospital and community settings, and has a special interest in maternal mental health and wellbeing.

Michael Thomas is the interim Vice-Chancellor and Professor of Organizational Leadership at the University of Central Lancashire, Preston, UK. He was previously the Pro Vice-Chancellor and Professor of Eating Disorders at the University of Chester and has held professorships in eating disorders and mental health at two previous universities. Mike has over thirty-three years' experience of c   un his own community-based clinic for severe and enduring e   list in mental health trauma and general mental health conditio

Mental Health Across the Lifespan

A handbook

Edited by Mary Steen and Michael Thomas

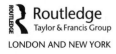

Routledge
Taylor & Francis Group

LONDON AND NEW YORK

First published 2016
by Routledge

2 Park Square, Milton Park, Abingdon, Oxon OX 14 4RN
and by Routledge

711 Third Avenue, New York, NY 10017

Routledge is an imprint of the Taylor & Francis Group, an informa business

British Library Cataloguing-in-Publication Data
A catalogue record for this book is available from the British Library

Library of Congress Cataloging-in-Publication Data
Mental health across the lifespan : a handbook / edited by Mary Steen and
Michael Thomas.
  p. ; cm.
Includes bibliographical references and index.
I. Steen, Mary, editor. II. Thomas, Mike, PhD, editor.
[DNLM: 1. Mental Disorders—prevention & control—Great Britain.
2. Mental Health Services—Great Britain. WM 140]
RA790.5
362.19689—dc23
2015016575

ISBN: 978-1-138-02168-6 (hbk)
ISBN: 978-1-138-02170-9 (pbk)
ISBN: 978-1-315-77757-3 (ebk)

Typeset in Times New Roman
by Swales & Willis Ltd, Exeter, Devon, UK

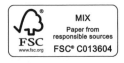

Printed and bound by CPI Group (UK) Ltd, Croydon, CR0 4YY

During our lives every one of us will either suffer from or have a relative or a close family friend that suffers from a mental health problem.

(Norman Lamb, former Minister of State for Care and Support, UK)

This book is dedicated to all the people in the world who are suffering from a mental health problem and their relatives or close friends and the professionals/ support workers who are providing care and support.

Contents

Figures, tables and boxes

Figures

Tables

Boxes

Contributors

Amy Baker, Lecturer, University of South Australia, Australia.

Kirsty Baker, Lecturer in Mental Health Nursing, University of South Australia, Australia.

Mandy Drake, Senior Lecturer, Faculty of Health and Social Care, University of Chester, UK.

Monika Ferguson, Research Associate, University of South Australia, Australia.

Brendan Gough, Institute of Health and Wellbeing, Leeds Beckett University, UK.

Ben Green, Director at the Institute of Medicine, University of Chester, UK.

Vijaya Kurmandas, Dean RAKMHSU, Ras al-Khaimah Medical and Health Sciences University, United Arab Emirates.

Andrew Lovell, Professor of Learning Disabilites, University of Chester, UK.

Thomas Moncur, Staff Nurse, Cornwall Partnership NHS Foundation Trust, UK.

Richard Mottershead, Senior Lecturer in Mental Health Nursing, University of Chester, UK.

Charles Masulani Mwale, Director of Services, St John of God Hospitaller Services, Malawi.

Elizabeth Newnham, Senior Lecturer and PhD candidate, School of Nursing and Midwifery, University of South Australia, Australia.

Nicholas Procter, Chair, Mental Health Nursing, University of South Australia, Australia.

Gary Raine, Institute of Health and Wellbeing, Leeds Beckett University, UK.

Steve Robertson, Institute of Health and Wellbeing, Leeds Beckett University, UK.

Mark Robinson, Institute of Health and Wellbeing, Leeds Beckett University, UK.

Mary Steen, Chair of the Mothers, Babies and Families Research Group, University of South Australia, Australia.

Scott Steen, PhD student, Centre of Psychological Therapies in Primary Care, University of Chester, UK.

Michael Thomas, Interim Vice Chancellor, University of Central Lancashire, UK.

Alison Owen Traynor, Lecturer in Nursing, Bangor University, UK.

Preface

Mental health is an integral part of health. The World Health Organization states:

> Mental health is a state of wellbeing in which the individual realizes his or her own abilities, can cope with the normal stresses of life, can work productively and fruitfully and is able to make a contribution to his or her community.
>
> (WHO, 2010)

It is vitally important that preventative methods to remain mentally well are promoted and that when mental health problems occur these are recognised as being as important as physical health problems. This preventative approach needs to be adopted throughout a person's life to ensure that support and services are readily available. Recently, there has been an increase in online mental health services which offer an alternative way to access help and support, and this approach can also work alongside mental health services to reach many more people who have mild to moderate mental health problems.

There is a wide variation in attitudes, beliefs, cultures, services and care throughout the world and how this influences population health. Therefore, the editors of this textbook identified a need to publish a book that would provide an insight into the multi-complexities and challenges that encompass mental health.

This textbook is aimed at the reader who is interested in mental health and wellbeing from a professional and general perspective. The overall aim of the book is to provide some knowledge and understanding of how mental health affects human beings from conception to the end of the life cycle and the challenges that society as a whole have to address. This is brought to life with the inclusion of case studies, a practitioner's reflective account and the recognition that mental health should be taken as seriously as physical health throughout life's journey.

The reader will find that the book commences with a historical overview of mental health care and then subsequent chapters examining mental health across the lifespan from pregnancy to childhood, adolescence, adulthood and ending with older age. Each chapter will highlight the objectives and focus of the topic considered and where relevant provide case studies to illustrate main points. Chapters also have reflective exercises to help the reader consider further about what they have read.

As editors, we could have requested that the expert authors followed the same exact chapter format and provide the same perspectives and approaches to mental health across the lifespan and following the same page format and layout. This is commonly found in many textbooks with the objective of providing text familiarity and consistency, but we know from our own experiences that a general scrutiny of mental health approaches indicates that there are several different views and opinions. We therefore rejected the usual uniformity approach to collating chapters and instead asked our contributors to give us their unique insights into mental health, which could be supported by evidence. We also gave them freedom to write in their own style and we have resisted the temptation to provide uniformity in our editing. You will therefore find that the chapters provide 'essays' which reflect the thinking and interests of our contributors. By allowing stylistic and, to a degree, content freedom (within the constraints of the book's aims and objectives), we have attempted to provide a diversity of views and opinion which reflects the reality of approaches to mental health wellbeing. As Thomas outlines in his chapter on the historical developments in mental health care, many of the advances in care and treatment were outcomes of heated debates and professional opinions. Mistakes have been made and opportunities missed due to the continuous struggle between different viewpoints and the drive for one approach or another to have dominance, control and power over the way mental health care is delivered. We are not comfortable with these traditional approaches and have tried to provide a platform whereby there is a commonality of shared values, for example the rights of service users and families to have priority in planning care, the need to show compassion to those experiencing mental health conditions and the need to understand and translate evidence into care that is dignified and supportive of an individual's life choices. We also wanted our contributors to give the reader different perspectives and approaches to the commonality of mental health and wellbeing. The differences would reflect their own individual thinking, views and experiences. We, therefore, chose contributors who could provide diverse and interesting thinking across the lifespan on the subject of mental health within this text book. Furthermore, approaches to mental health care and delivery demonstrate global differences in culture, ethnicity, gender, age and the way service users influence professionals. We have tried to capture these various differences in the way we have collated the chapters within this book. The authors were given freedom to express their own approaches and opinions supported by evidence, and consequently the reader will find chapters that take sociological perspectives alongside others that take medical, clinical, psychological or political approaches. The same applies to the authors themselves who variously have backgrounds in academia, research, clinical practice or professional organisations. We believe that it is more helpful for the reader to be exposed to these different views so that they can gain further understanding of the variety of models, schools and approaches to mental health care and how they differ in application across different cultures and societies.

For example Drake and Steen M, both active university-based clinicians and practitioners in psychotherapy and midwifery respectively, take a practice-based approach, as does Moncur. Steen, S is a full-time mental health researcher and gives an epidemiological account of adolescence. Lovell, also a university-based clinician with expertise within the areas of mental health and learning disabilities, takes a sociological perspective. Green is a practising psychiatrist and provides a medical perspective. Thomas, a university leader and practising psychotherapist, provides a historical overview of power, economics and professional status. Newnham writes from a feminist perspective. Procter and his colleagues give a global epidemiological account of societies, and Ferguson and colleagues utilise a family-focussed theory practice approach for the child chapter. Mottershead and his co-authors provide a mix of psychological and clinical aspects, whilst Robertson and colleagues take more of a sociological stance.

Each contributor therefore applies their own experiences and insights into the sometimes shocking statistics, studies and research findings found in global mental health care and provides the reader with more diversity and depth not only on specific mental health conditions but also on cultural approaches and societal differences. The advantage of providing differences of perspectives is somewhat self-evident for us as editors. This does mean that some chapters cover similar ground, for example common mental health conditions such as anxiety or depression are frequently presented across all age groups, and it is reasonable to therefore find they are covered in most chapters. However, they are covered in different ways, some in more depth than others, some taking a specific approach such as diagnosis, others a sociological slant and still others providing epidemiological perspectives. Equally, some authors take a trans-international overview, some concentrate on geographical regions and others look at cultural diversity within the same societies and countries. We take the view that these reflect the differences found in contemporary mental health care and enrich the reader's understanding of mental health. To give one example, the reader can find a number of approaches in relation to depression, from biomedical to familial or societal causes of the condition to medical and cultural diagnosis, symptom presentations, prevalence across countries, its acceptance as a mental health or existential condition and care and treatment approaches from prevention, self-help, public health, medication and meditation.

The book can be very helpful in different ways. The chapters can be taken in isolation, as individual and unique essays focusing on the subject itself, or they can be taken as a whole, contributing and enriching the totality of the book to provide differences in insights and perspectives regarding mental wellbeing and health across the lifespan. The teacher, lecturer or service user may wish to concentrate on the case presentations as study aids or to provide a focus for discussion in groups, whilst the reflective exercises can lead to further exploration of personal attitudes, evidence-based care and societal attitudes towards mental health and wellbeing. There is a helpful glossary adapted from a number of acknowledged sources which can aid understanding whilst the references provide both further reading and access to evidence-based data sets.

So whether you are a service user or carer, a health clinician or practitioner, an academic, a politician, a student of mental health, a student studying care or social science, someone interested in people and the human condition or just a curious browser we hope you enjoy the book, that it stimulates thinking and most importantly, that it changes or enriches your own perspective regarding mental health and wellbeing.

About the book

The textbook contains nine chapters:

This textbook will be introduced by an exploration of the history of mental health. It will describe and discuss available literature relating to historical evidence on how people with mental health illnesses were managed and treated. This will set the scene for the book to then focus upon mental health within societies and cover different aspects relating to ethnicity, age groups and gender in the following two chapters.

Further chapters will then cover mental health through the spectrum of life 'from the cradle to the grave'. Chapters will focus on mental health during pregnancy and early parenthood, childhood, adolescence and young adults, adult men, adult women and the aged population.

A helpful **glossary of mental health terms** is included to help readers define mental health.

Chapter 1: A historical review of mental health care

This chapter will set the scene and review the historical evidence surrounding mental health over the centuries. It will explore and discuss what influenced the transition from local parish and community care to institutionalised care. Issues and factors influencing mental health care and services and the implications this has for mental health care and practice today will be covered and debated. This chapter will help a range of healthcare professionals, students and support workers to understanding how mental health has been managed through the ages. It will also help readers to reflect on their own attitudes, beliefs and approaches towards mental health and how these personal attributes can have an impact on the care and the support they give and how it is received by members of the public.

Chapter 2: Mental health within society and societies

This chapter will focus on mental health within society and highlight differences and similarities within other societies throughout the world. It will inform and guide the reader as to how superstition and cultural beliefs can still have an impact upon the treatment of people within society. It will review the important role that society as a whole and within local communities can play in helping or hindering resilience or relapse of a mental health illness in individuals. Social capital benefits will be further explored.

This chapter will also discuss the best available evidence to promote positive mental health status in individuals and how society and the government needs to play its part in promoting a mentally as well as a physically healthier nation. In addition, the risks associated with a poor mental health status such as rapid social change, work related stress, gender and race discrimination, stigma and shame, social exclusion, unhealthy lifestyle, risks of personal safety and violence, physical illness and violations of human rights will be discussed to enable the reader to put societal influences into context.

Chapter 3: Mental health within different ethnic groups and minorities

This chapter will explore barriers and cultural beliefs that interfere with seeking help and the utilisation of mental health services by different ethnic groups and minorities. Intolerance towards mental ill-health, the power of stigma and shame and religious beliefs within different ethnic groups and minorities will be discussed. This chapter will specifically cover four main themes, cultural barriers, religion, stigma and fear. The experiences of health professionals and people with mental health issues will be explored in order to create an understanding of the idioms of distress, cultural constructions and explanatory health beliefs within the ethnic minorities.

Chapter 4: Mental health during pregnancy and early parenthood

This chapter will focus on highlighting the needs of pregnant women and newly birthed mothers who either have an on-going mental health problem or are at risk of developing one during pregnancy, childbirth and following birth. The recognition of mild to moderate mental health issues will be covered: issues such as anxiety and stress, panic symptoms, phobias, baby blues, antenatal depression, postnatal depression (including paternal), eating disorders, substance misuse and then more severe mental health conditions such as puerperal psychosis, schizophrenia and bipolar disorder.

This chapter will briefly discuss how health professionals can offer support to pregnant women, partners and their families and when becoming a parent so they can make informed decisions about their health and wellbeing and their newborn. Case scenarios will be included to give the reader an insight into some mothers' experiences with mental health issues and the care and support needed for these mothers.

Chapter 5: Mental health during childhood

This chapter will focus on how some children can become mentally unwell. However, it will commence by looking at promoting positive mental health in children and how this can positively influence them to have confidence and believe in their ability to cope when growing up. Family, friends and peer influences will be explored, along with how these can affect a child's mental health both positively and negatively. There will be further discussion and exploration of how poor mental health in childhood can be associated with mental health problems later on in one's life.

This chapter will briefly examine how professionals can offer support to parents so they can make informed decisions about their children's health and wellbeing. Case scenarios will be presented to assist the reader to understand some of the mental health problems discussed.

Chapter 6: Adolescence and young adult mental health

This chapter will focus specifically on how adolescents and young adults can be emotionally and mentally healthy. It will commence by looking at promoting positive mental health in this age group and how this can positively influence them to have confidence and believe in their ability to cope during puberty and the transition to adulthood. Family, friends and peer influences will be explored and how these can affect a young person's mental health both positively and negatively will be covered. There will be further discussion of how poor mental health in adolescence and young adulthood can be associated with mental health problems later on in life.

This chapter will briefly discuss how professionals and support workers can offer support to parents who have children reaching puberty, so they can make informed decisions about their health and wellbeing. Case scenarios will be presented to assist the reader to understand some of the mental health problems discussed in relation to this age group.

Chapter 7: Mental health in adult men

This chapter will start by looking at ways of promoting positive mental health in men and how this can positively influence them to have confidence and believe in their ability to cope with life and social stressors. It will explore what the support family, friends and peer can offer and how these different groups can affect a man's mental health both positively and negatively. There will be further discussion of how poor mental health during the early stages of a man's life can be associated with mental health problems later on.

This chapter will briefly discuss how health professionals can work closely with families and local communities to offer men support so they can make informed decisions about their mental health and wellbeing. Case scenarios will be presented to assist the reader to understand some of the mental health problems men encounter.

Chapter 8: Mental health in adult women

This chapter will be introduced by looking at ways of promoting positive mental health in women and how this can positively influence them to have confidence and believe in their ability to cope with life and social stressors. What it means to be a woman and what the support family, friends and peer group can offer will be explored. There will be further discussion of how poor mental health during the early stages of a woman's life can be associated with mental health problems later on.

This chapter will briefly discuss how professionals can work closely with families and local communities to offer women support so they can make informed decisions about their mental health and wellbeing. Case scenarios will be presented to assist the reader to understand some of the mental health problems women encounter.

Chapter 9: Mental health in the aged population

This final chapter will focus on mental health in the aged population. Many older people have a positive outlook when approaching the final stage of their life cycle, but some are at risk of developing mental health problems due to several health and social stressors. One of the most common mental health problems the aged population are at risk of is depression, which often goes unrecognised. Coping with health, social and financial issues can have an impact on mental health status and the death of a partner, family members and friends can take their toll.

Mental health problems in an older person can vary in severity and may be obvious or subtle. A depressive state, sudden changes in attitude or lack of concern in addressing daily living activities may well be signs of an older person experiencing poor mental health. Disturbed sleep patterns, poor eating habits, decline in personal appearance or hygiene and withdrawal from social contact may alert family members to seek help and advice from health services and support networks. A practitioner's reflective account and two case scenarios give insights into some of the mental health problems an older person can encounter and the challenges carers can face.

Glossary of terms

Term	Definition
adaptive behaviour[2]	Behaviour that enhances an individual's chances of development and survival.
addiction[3]	A compulsive use of substances or repetitive behavioural pattern which leads to a form of psychological dependency with poor control.
affect[3]	Refers to a person's feelings or mood.
agitation[3]	Refers to a disturbance in either mental or motor activity in a mental health context.
Alzheimer's disease[3]	One of the several dementia diseases characterised by progressive loss of memory, intellectual functioning, language, judgement and impulse control.
anorexia nervosa[3]	One of the diagnostic eating disorders usually referred to as self-induced starvation despite the abundance of food. The word anorexia refers to its mental health basis.
anti-psychotic[3]	Refers to psychotropic medication prescribed for severe chronic or enduring mental health conditions.
anxiety[3]	A wide-spread cognitive emotional and physical mental health problem where the individual is preoccupied with specific issues and which has a detrimental effect on a person's lifestyle. Its physical characteristics include increased heart rate, increased gastric problems, high blood pressure and frequency of micturition as well as either diarrhoea or constipation. Psychologically it can manifest itself as feelings of fear particularly over a sustained period of time, sadness, unrest and general agitation. Although anxiety is considered a diagnostic criteria in itself, there are many anxiety related mental health conditions and it is hard to think of any mental health diagnosis that does not present with some or all aspects of anxiety.

anxiolytic[2]

Anxiety reducing properties usually referring to psycho-pharmaceutical products.

attachment[3]

The term is used in psychology to refer to the primary link between a child and main care giver. Seen as critical to emotional and cognitive development.

autism[3]

Refers to impaired development in social and communications skills, first demonstrated in infancy.

avoidance[1]

Refraining from situations or experiences which may cause distress

biopsychosocial[2]

The interaction between an individual's physical, psychological and social processes and environment.

bipolar[3]

Refers to the two sides of extreme mood continuum with one side being mania and the other depression. Bipolar is occasionally referred to as manic depressive disorder or diurnal disorder.

bulimia nervosa[3]

One of the eating disorder diagnoses. Characterised by binge eating copious amount of food to the point of feeling over filled, sometimes but not always followed by self-induced vomiting or aperient use. Some individuals will exhibit patterns of bulimia nervosa following previous presentation of anorexia nervosa.

chronicity[1]

The length of time a person has a presenting medical condition. Sometimes used to describe severity, i.e. chronic and severe medical conditions.

cognition[2]

Concerned with mental processes.

Cognitive Behaviour Therapy (CBT)[3]

One of the talking therapies that provides a problem-based approach and can be seen as a treatment intervention over a short, medium or long term.

comorbidity[1]

An individual presenting with signs and symptoms that would meet the diagnostic criteria for both physical and mental health conditions.

complementary therapies[3]

Often seen as non-medical therapies that encompass certain practices and interventions such as herbalism, acupuncture, chiropractice. Complementary therapies have benefits for the individual and are often fully accepted by the medical establishment. The term is often used interactively with alternative therapies which do not have the same acceptance in medical circles. Alternative therapies include practices such as crystal therapy, spiritual healing and aromatherapy.

complex presentation[1]

An individual presenting with symptoms that would meet the diagnostic criteria for one or more dominant conditions but with additional factors which complicate daily life. For example depression, alcoholism and anxiety.

compulsion[3]

Repetitive and ritualistic behaviours often used to avoid stressful events or recurrent thoughts or impulses.

Creutzfeldt-Jakob Disease (CJD)[3]	One of the dementia diseases, the main presentations are motor and sensory as well as mental disturbances.
crisis intervention[3]	Short-term, usually immediate focussed intervention to manage with an immediate cause of stress.
culture[3]	Refers to either an individual, a group of individuals or a population and the way that they internalise and externalise the expression of their beliefs, values and social norms.
delusion[2]	A persistent belief held despite strong evidence to the contrary and sometimes out of synch with the person's cultural, social and faith background.
demographic[2]	Relating to human populations.
depression[3]	One of the most common mental disorders presented through a number of mood behavioural and thinking symptoms. The main characteristic of depression is a marked and sustained lowering of mood with a loss of interest, accompanied usually by loss of concentration, energy and judgement.
derealisation[3]	Often one of the dissociative symptoms and refers to the sense that the person believes that their immediate environment or the world is unreal.
diagnostic criteria[1]	A validated or an agreed formula which outlines symptoms and presentations and leads to a diagnosis of a condition.
discrimination[3]	Treating others on the basis of prejudice.
dissociation[3]	A mental defence mechanism often related to post traumatic stress disorder in which the person feels separated from their world and sometimes their body and in severe cases conscious awareness.
eating disorders[3]	A term used to describe a number of clinical conditions including anorexia nervosa, bulimia nervosa, binge eating disorders and fad eating disorders. Most of the eating disorders relate to a person's psychological adaption and eating behaviours as well as excessive exercising of purging. Usually, there is a disturbance in a person's normal eating habits in an environment where there is an abundance of food.
Foetal Alcohol Syndrome (FAS)[3]	Presentation of developmental deficits seen in the children of women who have consumed alcohol during pregnancy.
functional mental health disorders[3]	Used to describe mental health conditions which are separated from those that have clearly defined physical causes. Most mental health conditions come under functional headings, i.e. depression, anxiety, obsessive compulsive disorders, phobias, eating disorders, mood disorders and severe psychosis.
hallucination[2]	A false perception through any of the five senses and related to a strong awareness and reaction to a stimulus that does not exist.

HIV/AIDS related dementia[3]	A form of dementia due to reduced immunity or viral damage to the brain.
holistic[2]	Usually considered to mean the totality of an individual's physical, psychological, social, spiritual and environmental aspects.
hopelessness[3]	A state of despair often also related to loss of hope and one of the characteristics of depression.
hyperactivity[3]	Excessive activity out of proportion to a person's environment or age or context.
hypochondriasis[3]	A persistent fear of having a serious disorder often based on an exaggerated misinterpretation of normal physical and mental functions.
hypomania[3]	A syndrome, often referring to an elated mood state, but less severe than mania. Hypomania is generally considered to have a short active phase.
illusion[3]	A cognitive misinterpretation of an external stimulus. The external stimulus exists but the interpretation of it is wrong.
insight[3]	A person's cognitive awareness and level of understanding regarding the rationale and meaning of their interaction with the world.
insomnia[3]	Refers to disturbed sleep, in particular the inability to fall asleep or difficulty staying asleep or early morning awakening. Often symptomatic of mental conditions.
intervention[2]	An act or product with the aim of improving outcomes, for example providing psychological therapies, prescribing pharmaceutical products or changing a person's living environment.
Korsakoff's syndrome[3]	One of the dementias usually based on chronic alcohol consumption and usually presented by the creation of clearly false memories, sometimes hallucinations and disorientation.
maladaptive behaviour[2]	Behaviour that reduces an individual's potential to overcome the stimulus or stressor. For example drinking large amounts of alcohol as a form of self-medication when dealing with post-traumatic stress disorder would be considered a maladaptive behaviour.
mania[3]	A mental health disorder presented by extreme levels of elated feelings, often delusions of grandeur and physical over-activity.
mental health[3]	A relative term related to an individual's overall wellbeing usually referring to how they interact with others and their communities in an adaptive way that is considered culturally and socially normal.
mental illness[3]	A term used to cover a medical approach to mental health conditions.
mental state examination[1]	An assessment of an individual's mental health status using a variety of validated measuring instruments.

mindfulness[1]	A technique close to a type of meditation which encourages the individual to focus less on their thoughts and moods or bodily sensations or to also focus on potential change and/or acceptance of a chronic condition.
NICE[2]	The acronym for the National Institute for Health and Clinical Excellence. It was formerly known as the National Institute for Clinical Excellence, hence NICE, but has continued to use these four letters despite the addition of the work 'Health' in the title.
obsessions[3]	Repetitive and ritualistic and recurrent thoughts.
obsessive compulsive disorders[3]	A mental health condition with high levels of anxiety where the person experiences persistent and obtrusive negative thoughts accompanied by strong urges to carry out specific behavioural actions. Obsessive compulsive disordered behaviour and thinking is often an attempt by the individual to prevent a potential and feared outcome from occurring.
organic mental health conditions[3]	Refer to those mental health symptoms and presentations which can be related back to a physical condition. Most often these are of the dementia disorders.
panic[3]	Extreme state of anxiety from acute to severe panic attacks which are highly disturbing to the individual as they include severe palpitations, hyperventilation, chest pain, nausea and somatic pain due to muscle tension.
pathological[2]	Relating to a disease or a disorder.
personality disorder[3]	The term used to describe an individual whose thinking, feeling and often behaviour differ significantly from those expected in the person's environment, culture or context. However, there are several different diagnostic personality disordered criteria and debate has continued amongst mental health professions for over a hundred years about the extent to which a level of personality disorder actually exists in a person's interaction with the world and people.
phobia[3]	An exaggerated or irrational fear of an event or an object.
polypharmacy[2]	Multiple medication approaches to treat a disorder.
precipitating factors[1]	Events or incidents of perceptions that are the catalyst for the onset of a mental health condition.
predisposing factors[1]	Historical factors which have the potential to influence the onset of mental health conditions. Can also be seen as a resilience level in the influence on precipitating factors.
prevalence[1]	A presentation of conditions in a population in a ratio of number per thousand.

psychoanalysis[3]	A form of talking psychotherapy in which both the therapist and the client explore the client's conscious and unconscious patterns of thinking and feeling.
psychomotor[2]	Voluntary muscle activity often triggered by mental activity.
psychophysiological[1]	A term used to describe both psychological and physical presentation or to describe the impact that a psychological condition has on the body.
psychosis[3]	A term often used in the medical fraternity to describe a chronic or acute episode where the individual loses touch with reality and exhibits a number of behavioural and psychological symptoms which are out of touch with reality or the context in which they operate.
psychosocial[2]	The interaction between an individual and their social environment, particularly how a person perceives or is affected cognitively by their social environment.
remission[1]	A period in time when symptoms of a mental health or physical disorder are not presented.
resilience[2]	The capacity to cope with stresses for a period of time. The longer the period of time, the more resilient the person is.
schizophrenia[3]	An increasingly archaic word referring to a type of psychosis where the individual begins to suffer from a chronic mental health condition and a loss of their links in mood, thinking and behaviour with reality, the world and context.
self-harm[3]	Referring to physical acts that damage the body, often used to relieve emotions or feelings or tensions that have built up to an unacceptable level.
self-consciousness[1]	The term used to describe a person's perception of their self-image in a specific situation.
self-focus[1]	Hyper awareness of the self at the expense of the awareness of other factors.
somatic[1]	Referring to the physical body.
stigma[3]	Where the individual is devalued or discredited based on a mistake, a misconception or an exaggeration characteristic with no support in reality. Stigma is a severe form of mental distress that can lead to social exclusion and precipitate mental disorders.
stress[3/1]	In biological and chemical terms referring to a stimulus or a demand that generates or has the potential to generate a reaction. In mental health terms it refers to a chronic habitual condition leading to emotional and physical discomfort. Some authors interchange stress with anxiety but many mental health practitioners see them as two separate conditions. Some cultures and societies do not recognise stress as a mental health condition but as a natural reaction to living in the world.

substance misuse[3]	A term used to describe dependence on a substance which alters a person's functioning or impairs their judgement on a day-to-day basis.
suicide[3]	The act of killing oneself.
symptom[2]	Observable presentations of signs of a disorder that meet or could meet a diagnostic criteria.
syndrome[2]	A collection of signs and symptoms that do not necessarily meet a criteria for a disease disorder but nevertheless form a unique and usually observable pattern. For example many psychotic type disorders could be viewed as a syndrome disorder.
third sector[2]	Refers to the voluntary, charitable or social enterprise sector of care.
thought disorder[3]	The term used to describe people who present with impaired thought processes or disorganised thought processes demonstrated through incoherent speech, use of unintelligible words or sometimes not being able to provide a verbal response to questions. Most often found in individuals with severe and enduring psychosis.
trauma[3]	Often refers to an event or series of events that leads to physical and mental damage. Trauma can be acute or chronic.

Notes

1 Thomas, M & Drake, M (2012) Cognitive Behaviour Case Studies, Publisher Sage, London.
2 Pryj Machuks (2011) Mental Health Nursing, an evidence based introduction, Sage, London
3 Wrycraft, N (2009) An Introduction to Mental Health Nursing, McGraw-Hill, Open University Press, Berkshire, England. Also Antai-Otong, D (2008) Psychiatric Nursing, Biological and Behavioural Concepts, 2nd Edition, Thomson, Elmar Learning, Canada.

Acknowledgements

A special thanks to all the authors who have given their valuable time to write the chapters of this book. Their individual contributions have enriched the text and given meaningful insights for mental health across the lifespan. We are very grateful to Leeanne Ralston, Francesca Sweeting, Paul Holgate, Scott Steen, Ashlee Wells Jackson and Jamie McCartney for giving their permission to use photographs. We are also grateful to the people who gave consent to use their personal stories at disguised case studies for educational purposes.

We would also like to personally thank Louisa Vahtrick at Taylor and Francis/Routledge Publishing Ltd and Jane Olorenshaw and Thomas Newman at Swales and Willis Ltd for their copy-editing/publishing support.

Thank you

Mary Steen and Michael Thomas

1 A historical review of mental health care

Michael Thomas

Introduction

For mental health professions and care service users there have been, and continue to be, many viewpoints and attitudinal positions, which has led to theoretical 'schools' and perspectives, adversarial positions regarding treatment, debates about the nature of mental health itself and whether 'illness' factually exists. These debates have been influenced by social trends, advancements in technology, theoretical 'leaders' and more latterly by the voices of individuals who experience mental health issues. Sometimes the decisions made have been at great cost, for example long-term incarceration genuinely perceived as 'good' for the individual and treatments which, with the gift of hindsight, look positively bizarre and tortuous.

Such disagreements and debates are held within the constraints of the narrative and discourse that societal norms and cultures deem appropriate for the time, and care must be used to ensure that past practices and languages are not compared against current social norms. After all history will judge whether the practices of today were appropriate and relevant and whether the language used to discuss mental health reflects care and compassion or benefits the individual service user. Historically individuals have variously been labelled, sometimes as euphemisms, as patients, residents, guests, clients, service users and more recently, individuals with lived experience, whilst over time mental health experiences have been stigmatised and derided as madness, lunacy, idiocy, melancholy, psychopathy, shell-shock, neurosis, hysteria or the worried well. Medical dominance has led to 'diagnostic' conditions such as schizophrenia, psychosis, depression, mania, dysthymia, anxiety, personality disorders or post-traumatic stress conditions and a demarcation line was drawn between 'conditions' defined as neurosis and psychosis and more recently between 'common' and 'severe' mental health conditions. The word 'stress' has become more prominent and socially accepted with its blurring of physical and psychological symptoms and is currently used to cover a wide range of presentations, whilst the phrase 'personality disorder' remains stigmatising.

Such language is not timeless and words change in their definitions, contexts and application as they lose discursive value and meaning within that particular timeframe. The language used evolves to mirror cultural and social mores and has an impact on other social systems, and so the history of mental health is one of flux, of constant cultural, societal, legal, linguistic, attitudinal and knowledge evolution which impacts on care interventions. Profound questions of humanity constantly need to be answered and today is little different from the last century. Ultimately, society has not been good at meeting the needs of individuals who sit at the heart of all the systems and interventions; as history shows, time and again they sit there alone.

Mental health care can best be viewed as developments in areas which interweave and which rely on small advances in the one to push advances in the others. The developments of mental health professions and care interventions were often in response to social and political advances which reacted to technical and economic developments, and studying the historical course of care often requires an understanding of when and where these different areas nudge each other along. The voices of the individual, families or service users are usually heard only as passive responses to the ebb and flow of these phenomena, floating in the eddies and swirls of historical advances: sometimes sinking beneath it all. In the history of mental health care you can hear their voices and learn of their experiences, but it is rare to find examples where they have influenced mental health interventions and they are more often the focus for, rather than the agent of, change. In this chapter the development of mental health care attempts to demonstrate how the social, political and economic forces impact on each other to influence the experiences of the person seeking mental health support and intervention.

Historical overview

This chapter will review the historical development of mental health and explore the influences which led to the transformation of care from the local parish and community to institutionalised hospitals and, more recently, to a mix of NHS community and hospital care. The chapter will examine factors facing mental health care and practice in the present day by examining mental health care through the past three centuries. This perspective will help the reader to reflect on their own attitudes, beliefs and approaches to mental health care and how these personal attributes can have an impact on the care and support they give and how this may be received by members of the public.

This chapter will consider:

- The history of mental health services and how this has impacted upon contemporary mental health care;
- How health services for mental health have evolved;
- How care and support services for mental health have evolved;
- In particular, how health professionals' specialities within mental health and community support have evolved;
- The historical mental health challenges and then relate these to contemporary issues.

The early years

Prior to the fifteenth century the level of knowledge was crude, with little understanding of how to alleviate the distress of symptoms, and the reality for the vast majority of Europeans with a mental health condition was an early death due to neglect. A very small, wealthy minority could buy care through individual contracts or by donating money to one of the church organisations who would provide shelter and comfort as long as the money lasted. A small number were classed as 'holy fools', blessed because they had been touched at birth by the hand of God which no human mind could comprehend, and protected in part by the church and the local community, although it is unclear whether any survived if they demonstrated deteriorating mental health symptoms. There is little evidence to indicate what life may been like for the ordinary individual experiencing poor mental health before the sixteenth century but we know life was hard, with small population groups surviving diseases, poor crops, war and servitude and seeking pleasures when and where it was sanctioned (Burke, 2009). Based on what is known about the life of the person neither rich nor famous, it is probably fair to assume that deteriorating mental health meant misery, decline and a lonely death. There was no real concept of a 'state' except for the kingdom, the church and feudal lords, which brought power and compliance but no real sense of community responsibility. Instead, personal responsibility and accountability was socially esteemed, working to support the family was the norm whilst helping others was seen as virtuous only if one could afford the time or money. For most people work was through family contacts and if none could be found then the individual left their community in search of a living; care or lack of it was not an issue for the authorities but for the individual and the family. The situation has improved in many ways but, fundamentally, this core debate continues to dominate social policy over four hundred years later with neoconservatives still arguing with democratic liberals about the balance between state and individual responsibility for those in need.

Income could buy relief and potential 'cures' which meant that the entrepreneurial person could make a living, honestly or not as there were no regulations to discriminate between either. As Burke (2009) highlights, the charlatan grew in popularity during the sixteenth and seventeenth centuries, only gaining the reputation for pretentions and quackery later in the next century. Originally an individual who travelled from town to town selling 'medicines' and using comedy and jesting to attract the crowds, the charlatan was perceived as a peripatetic healer, and whilst some may have held knowledge and skills many merely acted the part to get what money they could. Burke (2009) suggests that the drama and comedic element of the physician's role (imagine how important humour must have been as relief for the ordinary person in the fifteenth and sixteenth centuries) played a part in the rising social status when compared to the growing resentment against lawyers, bankers and tax collectors during this period, a resentment which continues to this day. In popular songs and plays of the time the travelling charlatan practising his, always male, quackery is usually portrayed as a fool, an eccentric or a comedian, which in itself may be an earlier reference to having been touched by God. Gradually, originally in the towns and cities, the charlatan disappeared, even the name becoming stigmatising, replaced by a more respectable presentation of a scholar-physician, more thoughtful and serious in their deliberations and who also happened to receive higher fees. They began to separate from the herbalists and the barbers who in turn evolved their professions into pharmacy and surgery, although knowledge remained rudimentary; a high level of excitement was brought about in medical circles by the discovery of the body's circulatory blood, for example, but this had been known to the farmer, butcher and chef for several centuries without comment.

General medicine continued to develop into a 'serious' profession with the physician now performing comedy routines for the rich within their warm and inviting houses and the future pharmacist settling into a lower social role, selling medicines in the streets and villages. But the charlatan had to compete with the growing number of travelling 'players' attracting the crowds, often working as families or small tightly knit groups, and the roads of Europe began to be busier and state intervention began to stir. The charlatans had to start seeking permission to ply their trade and often, in return for such grants, had to lead community singing or carry news around the towns as they tried to sell their wares. Their status began to suffer as general medicine went indoors and plied to the rich and as street entertainers began to appear, juggling and singing and doing routines previously done by the charlatan who gained a reputation for selling 'quack' goods. As work became harder to find many took on activities that would bring them food, warmth or shelter and adopted (badly) the practices of selling sham interventions or being poorly convincing minstrels, musicians, singers or other types of entertainers. There were many wanderers fighting for the same food and warmth, many were disabled through accidents or disease, some would have presented with severe mental health conditions and most would receive nothing but derision and mockery from a public seeking their own relief from daily pressures. Yet to seek alms or charity was still perceived as socially unacceptable, a lowering of status, basically begging for scraps of food and living on the barest necessities. It was difficult but more acceptable to move on, go to the next town or village and seek some solace there with further performances. By 1572 the roads in England became so crowded that the Restraining of Vagabonds Act was put in force requiring entertainers to gain permission from two Justices of the Peace before they could travel (Burke, 2009).

The authorities had intervened earlier when the state had tried to deal with the growing number of individuals and groups who differentiated themselves deliberately from charlatan-physicians and the myriad street entertainers. As the roads grew busier those sorts of traveller were not yet problematic but what did concern those in power was the rising number of groups of itinerant preachers, prophets or diviners who began to preach a different sort of healing, one more related to changes in social structures and an end to the power of local gentry and challenged the church, one aligned to the economics of sharing resources more fairly amid claims that God was on their side. In the early part of the fifteenth century such heresy provoked the implementation of the Inquisition and later the witch-finding trials which did not take into account any mental health issues, and many were caught in their net. More alert souls adopted different guises to continue their work, some continuing as charlatans, some known as 'cunning men' or 'wise women' (often a midwife) and in central Europe as 'wise ones' or 'knowers'. They kept a low profile and were sometimes protected by leaders within local communities, more so if they were raised there, who would help them to avoid trials altogether by naming them 'white witches or sorcerers' or a 'practitioner in physic'. After all, an individual who knew how to use herbs, tonics, fumes and oils alongside prayers, meditations, songs and rituals had some social worth; particularly when they could provide solace to both physical and psychological symptoms (Burke, 2009). This was no short historical event but went on for over a century with periodic convulsions of witch-hunting and seeking out those deemed to practise or espouse dark magic; in reality those viewed as potentially disruptive to the work of the church and the government.

Still, avoiding the attention of those seeking evidence of witchcraft was difficult, and if practitioners had an observable mental health condition they would often be the focus of verbal and physical assaults and, at worst, executed for practising magic. If they had objects or property of value they were ripe for being brought to the attention of the witch-finders with the accuser having opportunities to take their possessions if the vulnerable was taken into care or prison (Dolan, 1994).

'Taken in' by the authorities was itself a euphemism, as prisons and hospitals did not really exist and detention was often no more than a chain attached to a wall away from main thoroughfares. Neither the community nor the authorities accepted any responsibility if an individual was detained, and the family had to provide food and clothing. This could be difficult enough if family members had to travel a distance, but even locally there was precious little space in a day. Life was hard, often brutal, and surviving the day was paramount, most people filling their daylight hours with chores and little, if any, time for unplanned events. For the itinerant traveller it was even worse as there was not even the possibility of family support. Many with mental health conditions wasted away, their cries for comfort ignored and weakening as the combination of distress, ill health and the elements ended in a pauper's grave, unmarked and unknown. No action was taken by the authorities because most people neither sanctioned ill-treatment nor rewarded good deeds; indifference would be the nearest modern approach.

This social acceptance of individual or familial responsibility for care was actively pursued by government until the late seventeenth century partly because it was considered the social norm, partly because there was no concept of state care and partly because tax-raising to boost the royal coffers was more often to do with military matters than social concerns. Compliance regarding social behaviour was left to local courts and, in the main, local practices. Early death and sickness rates were high, and into this space moved the physicians, welcomed as they provided a more scientific basis for treating physical illness. The rise of philosophical and scientific knowledge also provided new career opportunities for the children of the wealthy that had previously entered the royal courts, the law or the church. However, in the mental health field, society remained less tolerant and care remained a family issue; there was no status for physicians who wanted to work with the 'mentally ill' and no voices to speak up for their needs. When the state and legislature did interfere they were punitive; for example, the high rates of infanticide in the latter part of the sixteenth and early seventeenth centuries led to a 1624 Act which made it a crime for unmarried mothers to kill their own (illegitimate) child, the courts basing their decision on the view that women were temperamentally more likely to kill their offspring whilst ignoring the fact that men may have encouraged the infanticide or that the women were subjected to abuse, suffered depression or experienced other mental health conditions (Dolan, 1994). Following the enactment of the legislation there grew a number of prosecutions against vagrant wet-nurses and wise women (midwives) who would have illegitimate infants passed to them and who were then accused of killing the child, often through abandonment. This also had the social consequence for future developments of female professions as consequently women carers found it much harder to move in the social circles enjoyed by male barbers, herbalists and physicians.

Depression (melancholy) and suicide amongst men were seen as more a religious issue than a health one and melancholy was viewed as a weak family trait. Amongst middle class males it could have a devastating effect on other family members, as a wife and children could be killed because the husband knew well that his suicide would lead to destitution for the family; in a melancholic state it may be seen as preferable if the whole family died rather than suffer such indignity. In Southern England alone 75 per cent of marital murders committed over sixty years between the mid-sixteenth to the first quarter of the seventeenth century were by men against their wives (Dolan, 1994). The law began to take more of an interest as the number of cases grew, particularly if the man survived and could be charged with murder, but, in the main, if a suicide succeeded the issue was left as a church matter. The law was on the side of men, for example, the 1632 Act of Coverture legislated for a woman, once legally married and given the title of a 'wife', to surrender her behaviour, actions and worldly goods to her husband's control, although legal self-responsibility could be returned to the woman if she became a widow, was deserted or if she committed a criminal act. Not surprisingly, it was therefore easier for the husband to coerce his wife to commit infanticide or other crimes as, once they were committed and she was caught, he could argue that she had been responsible for her own actions and, as such, her behaviour was clearly illegal; the crimes were therefore committed outside of his control. For women with mental health problems a marriage to an unsympathetic husband could be ruinous, as her behaviour could be construed as outside of his responsibility and he could present a case suggesting she had broken coverture, allowing him to legally leave the marriage whilst keeping all her worldly goods as she fell into destitution. Such legislation remained in force for the next two centuries and it was not uncommon, as the social status of mental health doctors rose and mental health institutions were built, for husbands to pay such doctors to 'certify' their wives as 'insane' and place them in a secure environment whilst in the process releasing the husband from any responsibility for her or the marriage in the eyes of the law.

One can see, by the beginning of the seventeenth century, a rising number of husbands murdered by anxious wives who lacked any legal or state protection. This came after another intense period of witch-finding in the 1580s against vulnerable women and those with mental health conditions, with 'witches' described as having the diseases of old age, of being simple-minded, silly, melancholic, lacking judgement or stupid and frivolous creatures. By the mid-seventeenth century women had to withstand another assault, but this time the language described the women on trial as delusional, miserable, continuously weeping or talking incessantly in sentences so fast others could not understand. In some instances it was also clear that the women were forced by men to behave in the way that led to a trial (see Dolan, 1994 for witchcraft trials 1584 to 1642).

The change in language and understanding did those on trial little good; if they demonstrated symptoms of mental health conditions, were infirm or had learning disabilities, their pitiful conditions were ignored and they inevitably became the victims of local abuse, ill-treatment and death. For a destitute woman enmeshed in a severe mental health condition, the end was usually conviction as a 'witch' followed by a severe beating before execution in the fire. Poor or mentally unwell men would usually fare little better, being whipped, having ears and the nose chopped off and, if convicted of spreading unrest, then having both cheeks branded with a double S for 'sower of sedition', before imprisonment and slow death through abandonment.

The authority of the witch-finders finally declined amid calls for increased state involvement as questions were asked about how witches could be in league with the devil yet not escape the might of local investigators which hardly presented a picture of satanic power. Reports began to circulate of coercion and of the accused readily pleading guilty to wildly unrealistic suggestions put by their accusers, which raised questions about the individual's abilities to even try and avoid the judgement. Even more obvious was that a scrutiny of cases in the past two hundred years consistently indicated that the vulnerable, the elderly, the poor, the sick or those with severe mental health conditions were more likely to be tried and punished. People began to ask if local communities were using such trials to dispose of their least resisting members and were being supported by the law to do so, as there was usually scant evidence to show that those who had been tried and killed were any real threat to public safety. Societal attitudes changed as individual communities began to perceive witch trials as an attack on the vulnerable, and by 1736 the witchcraft laws were finally repealed.

The voices of the people had earlier been heard in other areas of social care and had forced the state to intervene. The number of homeless children and vulnerable adults wandering the roads led to the government under Elizabeth I to order 'poor-houses' to be established in local parishes under the Poor Law (the Poor Relief Act) 1601. These were to be funded by wealthy local benefactors and so had the added bonus of ensuring that state intervention was at arm's length. Elizabeth's government was well aware of the social norms of the day regarding independence and working one's way through life, and the Poor Law should be seen as a reaction to the economic recession of that period rather than any government attempts to instigate state supported health and social care; if anything it was the opposite as the instruction for local solutions removed the monarch's responsibility for paying for care. Inevitably, the social and cultural attitudes of the early seventeenth century which viewed work as a method of improving one's character and social status (a political philosophy still adhered to by some policy makers today) was slowly brought in to the poor-houses and residents were expected to work irrespective of age. Those that were ill were housed in infirmaries, separate dwellings from the workhouses, and before long those that demonstrated mental health problems were housed in separate dwellings from the infirmaries.

The development of state intervention

By 1675 the first true workhouse institution opened in Exeter administered by the Alderman and forty elected persons (the right to vote being given only to ratepayers) and another opened in Yorkshire in 1727. Individuals with mental health conditions who could not work continued to be housed in separate areas and as their numbers continued to grow the 1774 Regulation of Private Madhouses Act was passed (Fowler, 2009). By the end of the eighteenth century almost all English counties and parishes had a locally managed workhouse and many had built their own 'asylums' to house the 'insane and lunatic'. By now state government was involved. In 1800 the Criminal Lunatics Act was passed and thereafter the numbers grew so rapidly that the County Asylum Act of 1811 made it mandatory for counties to erect and maintain their own asylums to be paid for by local ratepayers. In 1819 the Pauper Lunatic Act also allowed local aldermen to forcibly incarcerate the poor and destitute and the Criminal Lunatics Act was further amended in 1832 to ensure residents could be compulsorily detained for long periods. Life was not much better if those admitted had any goods or property; in 1828 the Chancery Lunatic Property Act allowed the county and the state to compulsorily take the goods of those admitted as part payment for their stay.

The dangerous mixture of growing population density, unemployment, new technology and industrialisation together with genuine public unease about the impact on local rates agitated the government into a legislative rush to control the growing social pressures, which only further embedded abusive, institutionalised care. People were now forcibly detained if deemed to be a public nuisance and word soon spread of the awful fate waiting for those who entered the workhouse. As Charles Dickens commented, those with a mental health condition in particular would choose to die of starvation in the streets rather than die of ill-treatment within the workhouses (Ackroyd, 2000), yet their plight was increasingly unpopular in the larger cities and in 1829 Robert Peel's

Metropolitan Police force was approved. The Poor Law Amendment Act (1834), known as the New Poor Law, was initially overseen by the Poor Law Commission then by the Poor Law Board (1847–1871), which was replaced by the Local Government Board (1871–1919), but each subsequent board could not stem the rise of abuse and neglect.

As the legislative arm of the state developed other changes were implemented. In 1820 the public decapitation of traitors was stopped and hangings were prevented from being public spectacles from 1868. Yet the law saw justice with one eye blind and one ear deaf to those with mental health conditions, who stood little chance of understanding or mercy. Gatrell (1996) recounts how an old man was hanged for bestiality with a pig in 1822 despite many parishioners including senior officials from the church and local ratepayers signing a petition stating he was mentally disturbed after suffering a trepanning (drilling a hole in the skull to release pressure, in those days without anaesthesia) following a head wound during the battle of Trafalgar. Mercy petitions had little impact; in the same year a young man shot and killed a tax collector in Caernarfon, North Wales, after he himself had suffered a blow to the head which the petitioners claimed had caused temporary insanity; he was hanged.

In 1845 the County Asylum Act was amended to allow further local growth and also for residents to work within the asylums rather than be sent to workhouses. The increased industrialisation of farming caused centuries of seasonal work availability and patterns of rural employment to disappear, forcing many workers to lose their homes and seek employment in large towns and cities which subsequently increased in population but not in jobs and income. This instigated more state interventions to manage a recession economy. In 1845 the Lunacy Act gave local ratepayers the right to remove itinerant job seekers and children who worked in the streets and chimney trades to either the workhouses, via workhouse laws, or the asylums, and in 1870 the Idiots Act permitted localities to have houses for 'imbeciles'. Still the numbers increased and the Lunacy Act was amended in 1890 to permit counties to build more asylums outside the towns and cities. However, the number of people in England and Wales diagnosed with mental health conditions, often in combination with destitution, poverty, old age and ill health, increased each time new asylums were built. In 1850 there were 7,140 'patients' in county asylums which increased tenfold in the next fifty years and by nearly another fifty thousand by 1930, and it was more than just the result of an increase in population as the rate of patients per 10,000 was only 4.03 in 1850 but was 30.14 by 1930 (Table 1.1).

As the population of the infirmaries, workhouses and asylums increased, the impact on families grew and resentment was not far from the surface; from aldermen and ratepayers who had to form boards to administer the institutions; from patients and families who were the most affected by each new piece of legislation and increasing state interference; and by local employers who chaffed at increasing breadline wages when they could pay the poor and ill much less without worrying about their welfare. There is little doubt that many of the paid officials and carers believed that the care regime they were applying was 'good' for the 'patients' but, as today, good news is not newsworthy and the media were much more interested in cases of abuse, of which there were many and increasing, and the newspapers helped feed the growing public resentment towards the Poor Laws, the Lunatic Acts and Paupers legislation which appeared to exonerate the government from responsibilities.

As early as 1844 a local teacher forced into the workhouse in Ipswich told of the matron being drunk and people dying of neglect in the infirmary. Another case reported how one poor soul was

**Table 1.1 Patients in public asylums in England and Wales
1850–1930 per 10,000 people**

Year	Patients	Rate/10,000
1850	7,140	4.03
1860	15,845	7.96
1870	27,109	12.05
1880	40,088	15.73
1890	52,937	18.34
1900	74,004	23.05
1910	97,580	27.49
1920	93,648	24.84
1930	119,659	30.14

Source: Gilbert and Scragg 1992.

held in the same bed for eleven years and in 1845, the same year as the County Asylum and the Lunacy Acts were passed, residents in the Andover workhouse in Hampshire were reported to be discovered eating marrow from old bones they were breaking as work. The marrow was their only dietary supply because the master took their food for his own use, including selling it on to others. This created such uproar that the master was sacked (though not the Board of Guardians or the medical officer who argued that the residents were well nourished), and it led to the abolition of the Poor Law Commission only for it to be immediately replaced by the Poor Law Board. Even across the years it is hard not to feel the utmost sympathy for the Andover residents, for the next master was sacked when it came to light that he had run an overcrowded and abusive workhouse at Oxford and the subsequent master was dismissed after he was found to be taking sexual advantages of female patients in the infirmary (Fowler, 2009).

Five years after the Andover case the Stepney workhouse 'inmates' were discovered to be bullied and neglected by a drunken master whilst in 1865 the matron of the Tadcaster workhouse was accused of beating inmates with weapons. Both master and matron were initially supported by their boards and only lost their posts because the number of witnesses threatened to overcome any legal proceedings. Women were frequently at risk. In 1856 the Marylebone master and his team of porters physically assaulted two young women inmates yet the guardians did not sack him and he only resigned due to public pressure. In 1866 the Poor Law Inspector for the Paddington workhouse discovered that pillows were taken from the beds of the dying to 'make them go quicker' (Fowler, 2009: 100). Legislation appeared to provide an institutionalised platform for abuse; in 1874 shortly after the implementation of the Idiocy Act it was reported that forty-seven residents of Rochdale's Infirmary were permanently secured in their beds covered in lice, scabies and bodily sores due to lying in their own faeces and urine, whilst in Norfolk several residents of the workhouse died due to medical neglect.

It was a depressingly common occurrence: finding new employees was difficult and it was easier for the guardians to employ anyone with experience and turn a blind eye to their previous employment record. As pay and social status was low for masters, matrons and asylum medical officers the temptation to steal from inmates and patients was strong. In the mid 1800s a medical superintendent earned on average up to £80 pounds per year in the workhouse infirmaries and asylums and had to purchase his own medical consumables such as dressings, ointments and tonics from his own salary. A Dr George Catch worked for a number of workhouses across London despite having a well-known reputation for poor care which included not seeing women after they had given birth and leaving women to sleep outside the workhouse gates overnight in all weathers. Perhaps it was because this practice appeared to be a widespread form of institutionalised policy. For instance, when Master George Cannon refused admittance to a mother and her child who huddled in the doorway on a bitterly painful December night in 1872, causing the child to die, the guardians supported him and his actions as he argued that he refused admission because she was drunk. In 1892 the board of Gressenhall workhouse supported the master after he refused admission to a young man who was rescued from a suicide attempt, when the master was eventually dismissed it came to light that the guardians had raised and paid for his comfortable pension. Institutionalised neglect may have been perceived as the norm and there was no medical advocacy for residents. A 1902 Parliamentary Inquiry found that workhouse and asylum doctors spent less than two hours a day with patients (only ten minutes a day in rural institutions), with the majority of care done by unqualified staff (Fowler, 2009).

During the nineteenth century the state passed eleven Acts of Parliament and Amendments (Figure 1.1) in attempts to balance the autonomy of localism with the least exchequer expenditure, but by the turn of the twentieth century it was widely accepted that localism was failing and causing deep resentment. The state had not much choice; it had to take on responsibility because legislatively they had changed mental health care too much to return to locality services. The 1834 Poor Law Amendment Act had merely sped up the process of separating the 'mentally ill' from poor workers which had started with the 1811 County Asylums Act. Originally, patients were placed apart as they were unable to work to the level of productivity required in the workhouses, but being taken from the infirmary to the asylum had the benefit of both allowing local parishes to hide their presence and also ensuring they could still work. As the twentieth century commenced workhouses were abolished and infirmaries organised into local district hospitals, whilst many faith-based and charitable organisations provided care for the wealthy, but the asylums continued to grow.

The rise of the professions

The social institutionalisation of the infirmaries, workhouses and asylums allowed opportunities for the medical fraternity to gain status if not a great deal of income. The Murders Act of 1752 had given judges authority to order the bodies of condemned murderers to be used for dissection. This helped develop the fields of anatomy, physiology and surgery (Gatrell, 1996) and by the beginning of the nineteenth century the doctor was given the responsibility for separating those individuals who were mentally disturbed, malingerers or fit enough to work (Fowler, 2009). As more infirmaries were established the doctor gained practice-based experience which, alongside the growth of Colleges and Societies, began to replace the previous apprenticeship training and more doctors gained a university education. Old titles were dropped and the surgeon-apothecary nomenclature disappeared. In 1745 the Company of Barber-Surgeons, established since 1540, renamed itself the Company of Surgeons and in 1800 gained Royal College status to stand alongside the Royal College of Physicians which kept its title (it had existed since the fifteenth century), and both were joined by the Royal College of Medicine in the eighteenth century. Meanwhile the Association of Medical

Restraining of Vagabonds Act	1572
Poor Law Act (old Poor Law)	1601
Infanticide Act	1624
Act of Coverture	1632
Act of Settlement	1662
Regulation of Private Madhouses Act	1774
Criminal Lunatics Act	1800 (Amended 1832)
County Asylums Act	1808 (Amended 1845)
Pauper Lunatic Act	1819
Chancery Lunatic Property Act	1828
Lunatics Act	1845 (Amended 1890)
Poor Law Amendment Act	1834
Education Act	1870 (Amended 1876, 1880)
Idiots Act	1886
Mental Deficiency Act	1913 (Amended 1927)
Mental Treatment Act	1930
Disabled Persons (Employment) Act	1944
Education Act	1945
Family Allowance Act	1946
National Insurance Act	1946
National Health Service Act	1948
British Nationality Act	1948
Housing Act	1949
Mental Health Act	1959
Race Relations Act	1965
Health Service and Public Service Act	1968
Chronically Sick and Disabled Persons Act	1970
Local Authority and Social Services Act	1970
Equal Pay Act	1970 (Amended 2003)
Children Act	1975
Employment Protection Act	1975
Sex Discrimination Act	1975
Education Act	1976
Race Relations Act	1976 (Amended 2000)
Education Act	1983
Mental Health Act	1983
Children Act	1989
NHS and Community Care Act	1990
Disability Discrimination Act	1995 (Amended 2004)
Employment Relations Act	1999
Disability Discrimination Act	2005
Mental Capacity Act	2005
Mental Health Act	2007
NHS Act	2010

Figure 1.1 Legislation 1572 to 2010

Officers of Asylums and Hospitals for the Insane was formed in 1841, renamed the Royal Medico-Psychological Association in 1926 and renamed again in 1971 as the Royal College of Psychiatry. The legislative arm of the state approved of such developments as can be seen by the rise of expert medical witnesses in court cases, which in turn provided status for the doctor, whilst politicians recognised that they gained more public trust if the care of the poor and the ill was supervised by learned, scientifically minded men (for the vast majority were men). This collusion and partnerships between the state and the medical profession were strengthened during the nineteenth century as the ancient acceptance of personal responsibility for oneself, family and community finally fell apart under capitalism, industrialisation and government tax regimes. The new arrangement allowed the medical professional, seeking social status, to act for both the individual and local community yet be managed by the state and policed through the law courts: an arrangement that seemed to be accepted by the growing middle classes. The voices of those with mental health conditions were little more than a whisper and were not heard as the partnership was strengthened; for example, although medical officers started to be fully employed in workhouse infirmaries from 1880 they were often inexperienced, underpaid and certainly not thought fit for management, and so they had little, if any, influence as advocates for the residents.

Meanwhile, other professions were either following or keeping up with medicine. In 1836 William Battie published his Treatise on *Insanity* (Nolan, 1993), which promulgated the view that nurses should be specifically trained to care for those with mental health conditions. Nurses were the employees of choice as the eighteenth century advanced although the title 'nurse' did not really exist as we know it today, with nurses generally viewed as 'Attendants' and many were poorly pre-pared, had little if any education and were often ex-inmates or alcoholics (Fowler, 2009). In 1703 Philippe Pinel developed his 'moral' approach to treatment for mental illness in France, stipulating compassion and kindness as interventions which were similar to the UK Quaker William Tuke's York retreat founded in 1796 which also required nurses to play an important part in interventions and care. By 1853 the Theodor Fliedner Hospital in Germany began to train and hire nurses who specialised in the field of mental health, while in the UK Florence Nightingale (1870), influenced by the Theodor Fliedner Hospital, formed the British Institute of Nursing Sisters and Mary Seacole and other contemporaries started to produce better trained nurses from 1864 onwards. In the USA a school for nurse training started at the New England Hospital for Women and Children and the first USA training school for mental health nurses commenced in 1882 at the McLean Asylum, Massachusetts. Medicine and medical supervision dominated the curriculum and it took several years for nurse tutors to be hired in New York at the Connecticut Training School in New Haven which followed Nightingale's approach (Frisch and Frisch, 2006). Initially only medical staff were appointed to directors' positions and they held superiority. The first European Nursing Association was formed in 1884 but led by a Viennese surgeon. Yet nursing as a profession was getting organ-ised: within ten years of each other the inaugural USA Nursing Conference was held at the Chicago World Fair in 1893, the Swiss Charitable Women's Organisation initiated a Nursing Commission in 1896 and in London the International Council of Nursing (ICN) was founded in 1899 with Ethel Bedford-Fenwick, Matron at St. Bartholomew's, as its first President.

History can be seen from many perspectives and it may be easy to conclude from one angle that the state effortlessly formed partnerships with the emerging professions, but that would not be the whole picture and governments did not always have it their way. Nightingale had a horror of state interference and fought actively against statutory instruments for nursing, and it was only after her death in 1910 that her views lost ground, and eventually the battle, to the equally dominant Ethel Bedford-Fenwick. She not only won statutory registration for general physical care nurses (now called adult nurses) in 1919 but also established a legally protected General Nursing Council for each of the four constituent countries making up the UK. She crowned her victory by being the first UK nurse to have her name on the new register. In the same year mental health carers gained their own trade union, the Asylum Workers', Union, which developed into today's mental health nurses. This emerging, and now statutory, group of nurses engaged in aggressive attempts to dominate each other and gain control of training and registration. The Asylum Workers' Union was needed because Bedford-Fenwick was a fierce opponent of any proposals that those caring for patients with mental health conditions should hold the title 'nurse' or be on a state register. whilst the city-dominated Nightingale Schools demanded that other, doctor-led, training schools around the UK should not be recognised by the General Nursing Councils or have their students register. Although adult nursing originally gained statutory professional recognition in 1921 it was not until 1946 that the General Nursing Councils allowed mental health 'nursing' to be formally accepted (Lester and Glasby, 2010), and even today it receives less prominence than other branches of nursing whilst the impact of chronic serious mental health conditions on physical health is only recently gaining attention.

In social care the early version of today's social worker, the Relieving Officer, was responsible for assessing Poor Law applicants within a parish and recommending to the guardians what relief, if any, should be given. Training was provided by the end of the nineteenth century, whilst across Europe the restorative practices of the health masseur became established and developed into the physiotherapy profession. In the same period the Midwives Act 1902 prescribed statutory title and status for midwives; the wise women descended from the fifteenth century had finally achieved due recognition for their part in lowering mother and child mortality.

In therapeutic interventions the rise of Freudian and Jungian psychoanalysis, with its emphasis on unconscious stimuli for emotional presentation, paralleled advances in behavioural interventions, evolutionary theory and new developments in psychology as the new century commenced. Darwin (1872) had already published his views on the links between physiological experiences and emotions whilst William James (1884) followed with similar work on emotional stimuli for physical presentations. Both were combined by the psychoanalytically trained Joseph Wolpe (1990), who developed the behavioural approach of systematic desensitisation commonly used in anxiety and phobia interventions in combination with relaxation techniques. Pavlov (1927) had also published his work on classical conditioning which demonstrated physiological predisposition to be 'trained' in response to specific stimuli.

As the nineteenth century started the state had continued to rely on the ancient practices of personal responsibility and accountability. There was no tax revenue for care, taxing the public was hugely unpopular anyway, and there was no capacity for a trained body of people to provide care. As the social status of the professions rose the governments formed alliances to gain an improved workforce in its infirmaries, workhouses and asylums and subsequent scandals dragged them further towards central control. By the twentieth century state control was in the ascendancy: the workhouses were brought under the newly formed Ministry of Health in 1919 until they were abolished fully in 1929 and replaced by infirmaries and hospitals. A new mental health act was passed in 1930 and by 1945 most health and social care professions were fully professionalised with their own colleges, royal charters and registration bodies.

The rise of managerialism

Over three centuries the organisation of care for individuals requiring mental health support had vacillated between the individual and family, state and legislators, local communities and parishes and, since 1945, the state, legislators and the professions. The deprivations caused by the Second World War had followed the unemployment and poor living standards of the 1930s and society wanted a new type of state intervention. Despite Churchill's reputation as a war leader, in 1945 his Conservative government, with its manifesto for continuing political intervention based on class and wealth and the historical emphasis on personal responsibility and less state intervention, was swept away and was replaced by his coalition deputy, Clement Atlee and the Labour government. Things should have been clearer for Churchill; in 1944 a poll had indicated that 55 per cent of people wanted a state funded health service, and throughout the war William Beveridge had been working on his review of state interventions in the fields of economics, trade, employment, health and social care which was published in 1944 to widespread public acceptance. In 1946, within a year of entering government Atlee introduced the Family Allowance Act and the National Insurance Act which gave relief to the poor, sick and the unemployed and on 5 July 1948 the Health Secretary Aneurin Bevan enacted the National Health Service Act which provided equal care and treatment, free at point of access for all citizens. Bevan was opposed by the Conservative party, the insurance industry, the British Medical Association and many charities. The medical profession had spent three hundred years gaining high social status and income; many doctors came from the middle classes and above, and they were not about to surrender all they had gained just for the sick and the needy to receive free state care. Bevan eventually offered doctors the average salary of a private consultant and sessional employment contracts so they were not full employees of the government but contracted specialists. Bevan described this in a controversial and blistering 1948 speech in the Commons as having to 'stuff their throats with gold' in order to get free healthcare for the population. Nearly seventy years later the NHS continues to be under pressure from those who wish to introduce 'market' commercialisation; many doctors still hold independent, private practices, the insurance companies provide access to financed care routes and charities are encouraged to replace state responsibilities with local interventions. The method chosen to hold the balance between the demands of the health market and state responsibilities was through a growth in general management of the professions and state resources.

In the mid-1950s the state encouraged immigration after the introduction of the British Nationality Act (1948) but there emerged a core social attitude and outlook involving racial prejudice which stubbornly remains. A 1951 census indicated that 46 per cent of the respondents saw immigration as a good way of dealing with the economy but 69 per cent would not ask a 'coloured person' into their home (Kynaston, 2008). Since then, on-going racial prejudice has, for very complex reasons, contributed towards a much higher than average incidence of mental illness in white/black mixed or black groups. This is reflected in mental health interventions, as to the present day a white/black mixed or black person has three times the chance of mental hospital admission than a white person and often they are diagnosed with the most severe type of mental conditions (Care Quality Commission, 2009).

Psychiatry continued to search for 'cures' and interventions for mental health conditions; electro-convulsive therapy was widely used from 1938 and the use of sedatives such as camphor was replaced by antipsychotic drugs in the early 1950s. Antidepressants and drugs for 'mania' came on the market from 1948 and in the 1960s the new anti-anxiolytics were used to treat anxiety. Leucotomies (lobotomies in the USA) which involved scraping away sections of brain tissue were fashionable amongst the medical fraternity whilst new advances in psychotherapeutic interventions began to overshadow psychoanalysis as new drugs and surgical interventions began to impact on individuals. The work of Albert Ellis (1962) who espoused rational emotive therapy and explored the part emotion played in negative thinking and consequent distress became better known alongside B. F. Skinner's (1972) theories of behavioural motivation, Carl Rogers's person-centred therapy (1983) and Erich Fromm's (1994) combination of psychoanalysis and existential focus. In the next decade cognitive-behavioural interventions become popular. Originally conceived by Aaron Beck in 1961 and further developed by him in 1975, cognitive behaviour therapy has continued to this day and dominates most therapeutic care in the UK and USA. In more contemporary times new interventions are slowly breaking through in areas such as multi-modal therapy (a mix of person-centred, cognitive-behavioural and other therapies), mindfulness, creative arts, physical activities and group interventions. New advances in neuro-psychology provide insights into areas of brain functioning, and there is a growing awareness not only that physical illness often co-exists alongside mental health conditions but also that more sophisticated drug regimes may be causative factors in some physical illnesses.

As the professional bodies accepted new government controls within the state and legislature partnership for the delivery of health and social care questions started to be asked about the role of the large county and city asylums. The so-called 'anti-psychiatry' movement (so-called because the movement's supporters never accepted the title), started by R. D. Laing (1960), began to question the role of psychiatric treatments in large UK asylums and the Conservative politician Enoch Powell advocated for their abolition. It took twenty-five years before they closed and as the years turned it came to light that surgical interventions did not 'cure' psychosis and had life-changing side-effects such as epilepsy, while the new drugs had their own problems, many were addictive, most caused terrible side-effects which required new drugs to control: some were lethal and even when prescribed en masse they did not seem to solve mental health care. For example scandals in care came to light in the 1960s which demonstrated neglect and cruelty in Cardiff, London and Essex.

There were also problems with nurse training which had never been resolved since Bedford-Fenwick had fought against the inclusion of mental health nurses on the state register and the on-going battles concerning the Nightingale School's attempts to introduce a national curriculum. To address these and to gain further state control, the Briggs Report (DHSS, 1972) advocated strongly against nurse training using different curriculums and led in 1979 to the new Nurses, Midwives and Health Visitors Act which helped to usher in the Conservative Margaret Thatcher's new government managerialism agenda. In 1983 the General Nursing Councils were abolished and replaced by the UK Central Council for Nursing, Midwifery and Health Visiting (UKCC) supported by four National Boards for each of the UK countries. Within three years the Boards used their new powers to approve nurse curriculums to implement a national programme in all but name whilst declaring that four 'branches' of nursing (mental health, children, general and learning disability) had their own separate and protected three-year training programmes. Later, under the national 'Project 2000' implementation programme, the UKCC and the Boards supervised the loss of the four branches as a mandatory Common Foundation Programme (CFP) took the first eighteen months of three years leaving only eighteen months left for the specialist fields. Nurse training schools were either abolished or merged first into colleges and eventually into universities which provided widening access to nursing degrees. Continuing nursing's historical predilection for in-fighting, the CFP was not universally welcomed and was criticised for diluting the specialities. By 2001 the Central Council and the four National Boards were dissolved and replaced by a single Nursing and Midwifery Council and the CFP was downgraded to one year of training to allow more time for branch specialism. Not giving up without a struggle, in the last few years supporters of state control of nurse education have brought about changes which have again diluted the specialist branches with a move to 'fields' of mental health, learning disability, health visiting, adult nursing and child nursing within a mandatory curriculum requiring integration between specialisms in a three-year undergraduate programme. But each central intervention has blurred mental health nursing which has lost its own focus, with no influential advocates from practitioners or service users for a specialist mental health nursing course. The consequent skills gap is being filled with non-nursing mental health workers now entering the care environment.

Europe was slower to develop centralised nursing or grant university education to match other healthcare specialities such as medicine. In Spain the Minister of Education and Science would not sanction recognition of a nursing degree despite the fact that courses could be undertaken in the country (Gasull, 2004); Germany only had four universities offering nursing degrees by 2004 and, like its neighbours Austria and Switzerland, had no central nursing council. Switzerland, headquarters of the International Council of Nursing since 1966, developed its own definitions of 'branches' and abolished both the mental and child health nursing programmes in 1991 and, whilst degree programmes were developed by the Red Cross, most training is at diploma level with an integrated post-graduate programme offered in three specialisms of teacher training, management and policy. In Austria nurse training continued to run at local level via hospital schools and Catholic convents, with a few universities offering programmes (Arndt, 2003) and in Russia nurse education continues to be hospital-led and medically dominated.

In social policy the 1959 Mental Health Act, which had updated previous legislation and brought together community orders, giving police holding powers and statutory guidelines on hospital detention without consent for 'patients', was amended in 1983, but by then the partnership established for nearly forty years between the state and the professions had started to fragment. Successive health ministers increasingly began to take centralised control of locally reactive care systems on the basis that what was good for London would be equally good for sparsely populated rural areas, and politicians and policy makers began to lead on what had previously been practice-led management by introducing non-clinical managers of services and provision. The tools of compliance included financial incentives, 'targets' and 'league tables' with propaganda from both leading political parties that marketisation and commercially based healthcare increased patient 'choice' and 'freedom'. Clinicians who followed the party lines were rewarded whilst those who argued for clinical-based healthcare lost influence and sometimes position. The rise of healthcare chief executives and general management provided the state with new partners; from now on the partnership between the state, profession and legislature would decay and the new, modernised partnership would be between the state, the managerial class and the market.

This was enforced by Thatcher's Conservative government and the 1990 NHS and Community Care Act, which ignored the professions as it renamed hospitals 'Trusts' and statutorily encouraged them to compete with neighbouring hospitals, to raise their own income and demonstrate they met their locality needs through centrally set targets. The old argument was back to the fore of healthcare; whether the state, the local parish or the individual should be responsible for healthcare. But now localism was devastated in the drive to the market: in four years (1990–1994), 254 hospitals closed in England and Wales whilst in fifteen years (1990–2005) only 50 new hospitals were built and 42 of these were trapped in the Private Initiative contracts where the contractor received repayment plus income from support contracts (Talbot-Smith and Pollock, 2006). This had the unexpected effect of preventing the government from pushing care responsibility to a more local level (whilst still maintaining central control) and, in an attempt to redress this issue, the Primary Care Trusts were formed in the late 1990s to take responsibility for primary and community care relationships with the local authorities. By 2010 the environment was right for new legislation to 'liberate' the NHS through the introduction of local commissioning and a partnership between the state and general practice (Department of Health, 2010). Once again those who followed the party line were rewarded whilst those who opposed the creeping privatisation of a care system held with deep affection by the population were pushed to one side. As Thomas, Burt and Parkes (2010) had already observed, when compared to the huge resistance to the closure of the UK's industrial base the privatisation agenda for healthcare was greeted with hardly any co-ordinated resistance and mostly accepted with weary acquiescence by the professions whilst the voices of the users were buried in the commercialisation of values and practices.

The state/managerial/market partnership, alongside target-driven policies, caused an expansion in auditing culture and staff found their work scrutinised to ensure both national standardisation and to encourage compliance with profit-driven organisations which increasingly took on provision previously guaranteed by the state. Care was still free at the point of 'access' but after that the 'client' or 'customer' could pay for different and quicker treatments. Professional bodies, accepting the mantra of client choice, introduced standardisation as a professional duty and practice was policed or applied by new authorities in the form of the Care Quality Commission (CQC), and the National Institute for Health and Clinical Excellence (NICE) (Thomas, 2008). Now started the period when the political parties appeared to react to media and public attitudes rather than provide political vision or leadership; populism, reassurance and re-election seemed, for all main UK political parties, to have precedence over integrity, political beliefs and the rights of people experiencing mental health conditions. For example in response to public anxieties about individuals with severe mental health conditions who had killed in their community the government reacted with the introduction of the Mental Capacity Act (2005) and the Mental Health Act (2007) whilst the CQC had to give an embarrassing public apology in 2011 after it had not responded to a series of complaints regarding poor care made by a nurse. It only intervened when the BBC broadcasted the dreadful practices in the same home using an undercover investigative method (Bower, 2011; Brindle and Curtiss, 2011).

The UK state was once again attempting to tackle the issues of local versus central control, personal versus political accountability and market freedom versus state funding. The Conservatives' 'Big Society' drive in 2010 saw more emphasis on charities and voluntary groups to adopt services previously run by local authorities so that state funding reduced and community responsibility increased. In a similar vein to the separation found in eighteenth-century workhouses, the work-worthiness assessments of those experiencing mental illness continued but ignored the market's hunger for employees who would increase production, efficiency and output on low wages. Similarly, Layard's (2005) influential but unchallenged opinions that work necessarily makes the individual happier did not take into account the interventions required by profit-driven organisations to provide people with meaningful occupations and authentic livelihoods. Layard and colleagues' superficial viewpoints suggested that mental health intervention (through talking therapies dominated by cognitive behavioural therapy (CBT)) would enhance the person's life, but the real objective appeared to be economic, with reduced state funding (Layard and Clark, 2014). Rarely did Layard and colleagues' modern twist of an ancient issue take into account the views of capitalist and commercial leaders who would seek market advantages in privately funded care and previously required legislation to protect employees from discrimination, for example the Equal Pay Act (1970, amended 2003), Employment Protection Act (1975), Sex Discrimination Act (1975), Race Relations Act (1976, amended 2000), Disability Discrimination Act (1995, amended 2004), Employment Relations Act (1999) and the Disability Discrimination Act (2005). Nevertheless, except for a few who questioned such simplicity of approach, many mental health professionals conformed, and complied with the introduction of structural interventions such as Improving Access to Psychological Therapies (IAPT) with its simplified CBT approaches and the old workhouse agenda of separating those with mental health conditions into those who could, or could not, work, and who should, or should not, receive more state support.

Despite, or perhaps because of, the rise of managerialist targets, an auditing culture and a compliant workforce, the number of abuse cases continued. As the new century started, examples came to light which mirrored the unacceptable practices that were uncovered a hundred years earlier and turned up the volume of those service users calling for their views to be taken into account; their voices were becoming louder. In 1987 Miles suggested that 40 per cent of children experiencing mental health problems were not receiving adequate care, and in 1997 BBC Bristol stated that over 400 women in mental health services were sexually, physically or emotionally abused. Nearly a decade later, Mind (2007), reported that 75 per cent of those diagnosed with a severe mental health condition were abused in their local communities yet *The Times* newspaper reported that only 68 cases of disability-aggravated crime were accepted by the Crown Prosecution Service. The abuses also entailed misuse of power, trust, personal security and income; for example in 2011 a large UK commercial care group announced they were closing homes leaving anxious residents with nowhere to live (Brindle, Goodley and Weardon, 2011). A return to the old Poor Law system of working for benefits that was first prescribed in the workhouses and not too dissimilar to the original Relieving Officer assessing applicant in the 1900s also returned in the UK's welfare system. A new system of work capability assessment introduced by the Conservative-dominated government in 2011 forced individuals with mental health conditions to undergo scrutiny to see if they 'qualified' for a lowering of their existing state benefits, lowering rather than increasing support and putting beneficiaries in a no-win situation. Within a few months Mind reported that 75 per cent of people in one survey indicated that the assessment regime was causing deteriorating mental health conditions (Taylor and Domokos, 2011) whilst suicide attempts increased (Farmer, et al. 2011).

The drive to reduce state aid and calls for a nationwide austerity drive in the UK following the 2008 financial crisis has led to a raised awareness by those experiencing mental health conditions on the front line that services have declined and user group organisations have started to resist further cuts. Representative organisations such as Mind, Making Space and Age UK increasingly provide evidence-based information demonstrating lapses in care whilst media coverage of deficiencies in care standards such as were found in Staffordshire or the commercial temptation to leave vulnerable older people to their fate when market profits slump has led to increased calls for state interventions. Perhaps the most dominant of all the pressures for improvements is in the field of negligence with increasing financial penalties and sanctions against individuals, organisations and the state having an impact on mental health care. The recently elected UK Conservative government's intention to withdraw state legal aid will potentially damage the rights of many individuals seeking court redress. Still, the current trend suggests that the voices of service users and their families are finally being heard, as can be demonstrated by the growing calls for the 'expert user' to be trained and engaged in care policies as well as governance. Service users are also getting more active inside the care system and statutory auditing groups such as the Care Quality Commission now have service users on their visit teams. In care education there is a trend to have service user representatives on interview panels when selecting university students for social work, nursing or medicine. History may indicate that the next evolution in mental health care may, therefore, include a partnership between the service users, families and carers, the state and the law with the potential for those actually using mental health services to be trained to provide care; it's been several centuries coming.

Reflective exercise

- Think about the major issues of mental health care provision today and their similarities to the past; what lessons has history given you regarding care services and how can you improve your care?
- Identify where in your professional practice the service users, families and carers have input into practice and policies; what can you do to enhance this further?
- Discuss with colleagues the development of historical state intervention; what is the ethical basis for supporting state support for individuals with a mental health condition?
- Reflect on the role of professional bodies, state auditors and inspectors; what has history taught you about their developments and what would you do to improve care scrutiny in your workplace?

References

Ackroyd, P. (2002) *Dickens*. Vintage, London.

Arndt, M. (2003) Political activity and the nurse – a professional duty? In W. Tadd (ed.), *Ethical and Professional Issues in Nursing – Perspectives from Europe*, Chapter 5, pp. 72–96. Palgrave Macmillan, Basingstoke.

Beck, A. T. (1961) An inventory of measuring depression. *Archives of General Psychiatry* 4: 561–71.

Beck, A. T. (1975) *Cognitive therapy and the emotional disorders*. Meridian, New York.

Bower, C. (2011) Care home checks. Letter in the *Guardian*, Wednesday 01/06/11.

Briggs Report (1972) *Committee on Nursing: Report of the Committee on Nursing* (Cmnd 5115). HMSO, London.

Brindle, D. and Curtiss, P. (2011) Care home abuse: ministers move to restore confidence. *The Guardian*, 1 June. https://www.google.co.uk/?gws_rd=ssl#q=Brindle%2C+D+%26+Curtiss%2C+P.+(2011)+Care+Home+abuse%3B+ministers+move+to+restore+confidence, viewed 18/11/14.

Brindle, D. Goodley, S. and Weardon, G. (2011) Fears for elderly as biggest care homes firm faces breakup. *The Guardian*, 2 June. www.theguardian.com/society/2011/jun/01/fears-elderly-care-homes-firm-breakup, viewed 18/11/14.

Burke, P. (2009) *Popular Culture in Early Modern Europe* (3rd Ed.). Ashgate Publishing Ltd, Surrey.

Care Quality Commission (2009) *Count Me In: Results of the 2009 National Census of In-Patients on Supervised Community Treatment in Mental Health and Learning Disability Services in England and Wales*. CQC, London.

Darwin, C. (1872) *The Expression of the Emotions in Man and Animals*. Murray, London.

Department of Health (1990) NHS and Community Care Act. HMSO, London.

Department of Health (2010) *Equity and Excellence: Liberating the NHS* (Cm 7881). DH, London.

Dolan, F. E. (1994) *Dangerous Familiars – Representation of Domestic Crime in England, 1550–1700*. Cornell University Press, London.

Ellis, A. (1962) *Reason and Emotion in Psychotherapy*. Stuart, New York.

Farmer, P., Jenkins. P., Grove, B., Boardman, J., Walden-Jones, B. and Watson, B. (2011) Fatal consequences of benefit changes. Letter in the *Guardian*, Wednesday 01/06/11.

Fowler, S. (2009) *The Workhouse: The People, the Places, the Life behind Doors*. The National Archives, Surrey.

Frisch, N. C. and Frisch, L. E. (2006) *Psychiatric Mental Health Nursing* (3rd Ed.). Thomson Delmar Learning, Clifton Park, New York.

Fromm, E. (1994) *The Art of Listening*. Constable, London.

Gasull, M. (2004) Interprofessional Relationships: Collaboration or Confrontation. In W. Tadd (ed.), *Ethical and Professional Issues in Nursing – Perspectives from Europe*. Chapter 6, pp. 97–112, Palgrave Macmillan, Basingstoke.

Gatrell, V. A. C. (1996) *The Hanging Tree – Execution and the English People 1770–1868*. Oxford University Press, London.

Gilbert, P. and Scragg, T. (1992) *Managing to Care – The Management of Services for People with Learning Difficulties*. Reed Business Publishing Group, Surrey.

James, W. (1884) What is an emotion? *Mind* 9, 34: 188–205.

Kynaston, D. (2008) *Austerity Britain 1945–1951*. Bloomsbury Publishing, London.

Laing, R. D. (1960) *The Divided Self*. Penguin, London.

Layard, R. (2005) *Happiness: Lessons from a New Science*. Allen Lane, London.

Layard, R. and Clark, D. M. (2014) *Thrive: The Power of Evidence-Based Psychological Therapies*. Allen Lane, London.

Lester, H. and Glasby, J. (2010) *Mental Health Policy and Practice* (2nd Ed.). Palgrave Macmillan, Basingstoke.

Miles, A. (1987) *The Mentally Ill in Contemporary Society* (2nd Ed.). Basil Blackwell, Oxford.

Nightingale, F. (1870) *Notes on Nursing: What It Is, and What It Is Not*. Appleton, New York.

Nolan, P. (1993) *A History of Mental Health Nursing in the UK*. Stanley Thornes, London.

Nurses, Midwives and Health Visitors Act (1979) HMSO, London.

Pavlov, I. (1927) *Conditioned Reflexes*. Oxford University Press, London.

Rogers, C. (1983) *Freedom to Learn*. Merrill, Columbus.

Skinner, B. F. (1972) *Beyond Freedom and Dignity*. Jonathan Cape, London.

Talbot-Smith, A. and Pollock, A. M. (2006) *The New NHS – A Guide*. Routledge, London.

Taylor, M. and Domokos, J. (2011) Experts; cuts create mental health crisis – tests for incapacity benefit harming most vulnerable people, say charities. *The Guardian*, Wednesday 01/06/11.

Thomas, M. (2008) Cognitive behavioural dimensions of a therapeutic relationship. In S. Haugh and S. Paul (eds), *The Therapeutic Relationship – Perspectives and Themes*, pp. 92–103. PCCS Books, Herefordshire.

Thomas, M., Burt, M. and Parkes, J. (2010) The emergence of evidence-based practice. In J. McCarthy and P. Rose (eds), *Values-Based Health and Social Care – Beyond Evidence-Based Practice*. Sage, London.

Wolpe, J. (1990) *The Practice of Behavioral Therapy* (4th rev. Ed.). Allyn & Bacon, New York.

2 Mental health within society and societies

Nicholas Procter, Amy Baker,
Monika Ferguson and Kirsty Baker

An introduction to mental health within society

Globally, the experience of mental illness is common. Estimates suggest that depression affects 400 million people, bipolar condition affects 60 million, and 21 million people experience schizophrenia (WHO 2014b). Mental illnesses and substance use conditions have been found to account for 7.4 per cent of the disease burden worldwide (Whiteford et al. 2013). However, the experiences and understandings of, and responses to, mental health and mental illness are not the same within all societies. To explore these differences, this chapter will begin with a focus on some of the key considerations when reviewing mental health and mental illness within various societies. It will then introduce and describe the range of common mental illnesses experienced on a global scale, while also highlighting some similarities and differences in prevalence rates between certain countries. This will be followed by a discussion of some of the major social determinants of mental illness, such as poverty, gender and isolation. The impacts of living with a mental illness, from the perspective of the individual, significant others and the broader community, will then be described. This chapter will conclude with an overview of the role that societies can play in promoting mentally healthy nations.

This chapter will consider:

- How society can influence a person's experiences and understandings of mental health and mental illness;
- The symptoms and prevalence of common mental health conditions;
- The influence of social determinants on mental health across the lifespan;
- The impact of mental illness across various life domains;
- The responsibility of societies to promote mental health through widespread initiatives.

Considerations for understanding mental health and mental illness across and within different societies

The term 'society' can be interpreted in a number of ways. In the context of this chapter, it can be thought of as a group of people connected by: proximity (or geographical space), politics, the economy, their social status, their social networks, or some other shared interest or factor (Griswold 2008). Societal differences can be considered across societies (e.g. developed versus developing countries) and within societies (e.g. rural versus metropolitan regions of a particular country). This presents complexities, as an individual can be considered to exist within one of many societies. Furthermore, individuals within a particular society can have multiple backgrounds (e.g. cultural or religious). Given increasing globalisation, it is important for health professionals to understand some of the factors that contribute to these differences with reference to mental health – this may allow for more sensitivity toward, and recognition of, an individual's perspective.

Differences within and across societies can influence how a particular society and its individuals view mental health and mental illness. For example, differences can be seen in explanatory models – that is, the beliefs and understandings about the causes, symptoms, impacts and treatments of mental illness. The dominant, Western biomedical model of illness views the causes of mental illness as predominantly biological and therefore a health professional provides a diagnosis and treatment for the illness. Under such a model, there is the use of disease- or pathology-focused language, and the individual is the focus of treatment. Other societies view mental health and illness differently, with many attributing superstitious or religious causes to mental illness. These different explanatory models can strongly influence a decision to seek help and who help is sought from. For example, those attributing biomedical causes to their mental illness may seek help from a medical professional, whereas those attributing religious causes may seek help from a religious leader. Moreover, in societies where stigma surrounding mental illness is high and there is the potential for shame to be brought to one's family upon disclosure, people may be reluctant to seek help altogether. These differences can also influence perceptions of the impact of mental illness. For example, for those in collectivist societies, an individual's experience of mental illness can be seen to influence the whole community. In Australia, Aboriginal and Torres Strait Islander communities take a whole-of-life view towards health, whereby health is seen as a balance of the body, mind, emotions, spirit and culture; it is believed that when this balance is upset for one person, the entire community can suffer (Hocking 2014).

These beliefs and understandings can also influence the way whole societies approach the care of those experiencing a mental illness. While many developed countries have focused on deinstitutionalisation and community-based care in recent decades, a report by the WHO and the Gulbenkian Global Mental Health Platform (2014) highlights how hospital-based care is the dominant model in low- and middle-income countries, with hospitals receiving an average of 70 per cent of mental health budgets. Although community-based models of care still need to be optimised, the focus on hospital care can be problematic. This level of care is often reserved for those experiencing severe and debilitating symptoms of mental illness, which can mean that many individuals experiencing less severe mental health challenges have limited access to services. There are also concerns regarding human rights violations and living conditions for those in hospital care, and this might exacerbate the experience of poor mental health.

Towards a global mental health perspective

'Global health aims to include the needs of all populations, rich and poor, across the globe, irrespective of their location, nationality, or income' (Kirmayer and Pederson 2014, p. 762). As such, global health prioritises justice and fairness in the distribution of health care globally and recognises that all countries can learn from one another to develop strategies to improve the health of all (Patel 2014). Patel (2014) argues that global mental health lies at the heart of global health given the significant reduced life expectancy of those who experience mental health conditions worldwide. But can we accurately compare higher income nations' mental health with those from lower income nations given the differences in culture, politics and wealth? Social inequality, poverty, violence and war influence mental health severely – challenges which cannot be compared to those faced in more developed countries (Lund et al. 2011). Wealth disparity between nations influences access to health care and health equality. Reporting of mental illness, humane treatment and care promoted in wealthier nations may not be realised in some less developed countries which continue to seclude people with a mental illness and can often treat those suffering neglectfully and violently (Kleinman 2009).

A global perspective of mental health assumes a Western biomedical model of understanding which does not specifically take into account the indigenous ideas of mental health and healing (Bemme and D'souza 2014). The adoption of classification systems such as the Diagnostic and Statistical Manual of Mental Disorders (DSM) and International Classification of Diseases (ICD) could negatively impact certain minority groups as cross cultural validity is questioned (Bemme and D'souza 2014). These manuals are used as a practical guide by clinicians to diagnose people with a mental health condition after thorough clinical assessment. Common symptoms are listed and linked with a label/diagnosis that enables clinicians to understand and communicate using a common language. Mental health conditions must be assessed holistically, taking into account the person's mental, psychosocial, environmental, cultural, spiritual and biological experience. Each factor is interdependent and influential in a person's lived experience, which changes over time. Accurate interpretation of the meaning behind the person's narrative is essential to gain an understanding of their true symptoms. Culture and context influence the way in which a person expresses their needs, which must be understood by the clinician in order to respond effectively. Kleinman and Seeman (2000) encourage clinicians to be open to the way in which individuals and family members communicate, understand or interpret their own or someone else's mental illness or mental well-being. Cultural context must be at the forefront of the clinician's mind when carrying out an assessment, as particular symptoms may be attributable to common cultural experiences. For example, symptoms of schizophrenia may be attributable to a mind-body imbalance, or a spiritual possession as the mind, body and spirit are viewed as one whole. Cultural explanatory models attempt to understand the deeper meaning of what something is called, how it affects the person and how it might be treated (Procter et al. 2014). Cultural competence ensures sensitivity toward a person's identified race, religion, language, social class, customs and rituals which enrich the individual's identity and assists them in making sense of the world. The clinician who is able to adapt their own values and perceptions of the world and put themselves in another person's shoes will be more likely to gain therapeutic trust and commence the important therapeutic relationship.

Worldwide prevalence of mental health conditions

The World Mental Health Survey conducted by WHO between 2001 and 2003 surveyed ten developed countries (United States, New Zealand, Japan, Belgium, France, Germany, Italy, the Netherlands, Spain and Israel) and seven less developed countries (Nigeria, South Africa, Colombia, Mexico, Ukraine, Lebanon and People's Republic of China). A summary of the rates of mental health conditions in each country is shown in Figure 2.1. Overall, it was found that more than one third of those people from the United States, New Zealand, France, Colombia and Ukraine experienced a lifetime mental health condition. More than a quarter of respondents from Belgium, Germany, Lebanon, Mexico, Netherlands and South Africa experienced a lifetime mental health condition and more than one sixth of respondents in Israel, Italy, Japan and Spain experienced a lifetime mental health condition (Kessler et al. 2009). The People's Republic of China and Nigeria reported a significantly lower prevalence of lifetime mental health conditions, however this may not be a true reflection of actual prevalence and may be due to under reporting (Kessler et al. 2007). The ABS found that approximately one in five Australians experience a mental health condition each year, with anxiety and depression the most commonly reported (ABS 2007).

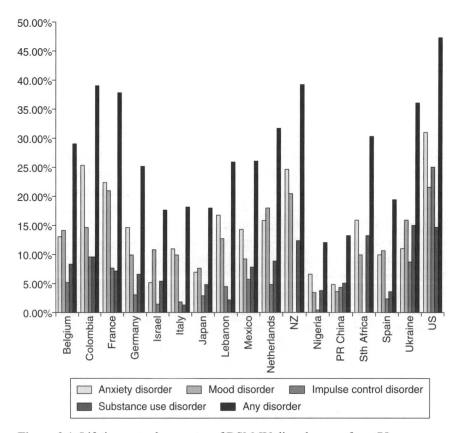

Figure 2.1 Lifetime prevalence rates of DSM-IV disorders as of age 75

Source: Adapted from Kessler et al. 2007, p. 172.

Such data must be considered objectively, taking into account the underestimated prevalence of mental health conditions due to stigma and a reluctance of people to disclose their illness. This bias is even stronger in less developed countries that would not otherwise conduct research in this area of health or use common diagnostic manuals as a way to understand and treat mental health conditions (Kessler et al. 2009).

The following sections will outline some of the most commonly experienced mental health conditions across societies, with a focus on conditions typically experienced in adulthood. More specific information about mental health conditions at the different life stages will be detailed in later chapters.

Anxiety conditions

Worldwide, the most frequently experienced mental health conditions are anxiety disorders which are reported to be higher in Western developed countries. For example, the United States report a 31.0 per cent prevalence of anxiety disorders compared with Mexico which reports a 14.3 per cent prevalence of anxiety disorders (Kessler et al. 2007). Anxiety is a normal part of life and mild anxiety is considered productive, such as the anxiety experienced prior to an interview or when faced with a threat. Anxiety is best understood by the 'fight or flight' response, which is the activation of the autonomic nervous system which stimulates adrenaline and noradrenaline, resulting in an increase in heart rate, blood pressure and breathing rate (Puri and Treasaden 2010). When anxiety becomes irrational or unmanageable over a prolonged time period, it may be assessed and classified as an anxiety disorder. Anxiety disorders are classified as a mental illness, and consist of consistent fear and worry which affects most aspects of a person's functioning and impacts on their ability to perform required daily tasks (Thomasson 2014).

Anxiety conditions feature feelings of fear, tension and worry, causing surges of autonomic arousal of the peripheral nervous system. This is associated with thoughts of immediate threat, hypervigilance in preparation for perceived danger and escape behaviours. This experience can be so overwhelming that it interferes with a person's day-to-day functioning as the person avoids anxiety provoking situations. A diagnosis may be given following thorough assessment of a person's experience, including their thoughts and behaviours. These diagnoses include generalised anxiety, panic disorder, social phobia, agoraphobia, obsessive compulsive disorder and post-traumatic stress disorder (APA 2013). Four of the most commonly experienced anxiety conditions include generalised anxiety disorder, agoraphobia, social anxiety disorder and panic attacks.

Generalised anxiety disorder

Generalised anxiety disorder is characterised by excessive worry about a variety of events or activities and is considered out of proportion to the actual likelihood or impact of the anticipated event (APA 2013). Adults with generalised anxiety disorder often worry about routine life circumstances such as their own and others' health, finances and minor matters such as impending appointments and household chores. This worry is excessive and can occur without precipitants. Physical symptoms are likely to accompany this worry such as feelings of restlessness, poor-quality or broken sleep, being easily fatigued and feeling on edge.

Agoraphobia

Agoraphobia is characterised by intense fear or anxiety triggered by the idea of an inability to escape a situation. This generally occurs on public transport, in open spaces such as the park, enclosed spaces such as the supermarket, standing in a crowd, or alone outside of the home (APA 2013).

Social anxiety disorder

Social anxiety disorder, or social phobia, is marked by intense fear or anxiety triggered in social situations in which the person feels scrutinised by others and negatively judged. The person fears they will show signs of anxiety such as sweating, tripping over their words or trembling, resulting in the individual avoiding feared social situations by subtly avoiding eye contact with others or refusing to attend gatherings at all.

Panic attacks

Panic attacks can occur as a result of the previously described anxiety disorders. This involves a sudden surge of intense fear which peaks within minutes and can trigger biological symptoms of palpitations, sweating, nausea, dizziness and paraesthesia. Expected panic attacks can occur when the person is faced with anxiety provoking situations that have historically induced anxiety or a panic attack. For others, there may be no obvious precipitant to a panic attack and can occur when the person is at rest. Worry given to panic attacks and their consequences usually involves fear of cardiac arrest, embarrassment and a sense of losing control. Maladaptive behaviours can occur which aim to minimise the likelihood of a panic attack and include avoidance of physical exertion, leaving the home, shopping, travelling or attending social events (APA 2013).

Mood disorders

Mood disorders are the second most prevalent set of mental health conditions after anxiety, and are reported to be more common in Western developed countries (Kessler et al. 2009). Major unipolar depression is predicted to become the leading cause of disability worldwide by 2020 (Murray et al. 1996). The impact of a mood disorder on the person can be immense and can influence many aspects of a person's life including socialisation, relationships, employment and their physical health. Mood disorders most often include major depressive disorder and Bipolar 1 and 2 disorders.

Major depressive disorder

Major depressive disorder is a classic condition consisting of at least two weeks' duration of changes in affect, cognition and neuro-vegetative functions, such as a change in appetite, energy, libido, concentration or sleep. It is important to delineate between normal sadness or grief as a result of events such as the loss of a loved one or a relationship break-up, and a diagnostic mood disorder in which a persistent depressed mood is evident with an inability to anticipate happiness or pleasure (APA 2013). The disorder causes significant distress or impairment in important areas of functioning such as relationships and occupation. Symptoms include depressed mood or loss of interest or pleasure, along with five or more of the following symptoms:

1   feelings of inappropriate guilt or worthlessness,
2   significant weight loss or weight gain,
3   psychomotor agitation/retardation,

4   recurrent thoughts of death,
5   insomnia or hypersomnia,
6   impaired concentration,
7   fatigue (APA 2013).

Bipolar 1 disorder

Bipolar 1 disorder meets criteria for at least one episode of mania and frequent episodes of major depression, discussed above. A manic episode is characterised by at least one week's duration of persistent abnormally elevated or irritable mood with goal directed activity or increased energy and is not caused by a medical condition or substance use. The severe mood disturbance negatively impacts on the person's social or occupational functioning and may require emergency treatment to prevent harm to themselves or others. Psychotic symptoms may be present and, in almost all instances, will require treatment. The person will also experience at least three of the following symptoms to a significant degree and which denote a noticeable change from their normal behaviour:

- engaging in risk-taking activities such as unprotected sex, excessive spending or unwise business arrangements,
- psychomotor agitation or increased goal directed activity,
- inflated self-esteem or grandiosity,
- flight of ideas or racing thoughts,
- distractibility or inattentiveness,
- reduced need for sleep,
- pressured speech (APA 2013).

Bipolar 2 disorder

Bipolar 2 disorder meets criteria for a current or past episode of major depression, as discussed above. The person will also experience an episode of hypomania which is characterised by at least four days of persistent abnormally elevated or irritable mood with goal directed activity or increased energy and is not caused by a medical condition or substance use. During this time three or more of the symptoms of mania, discussed above, are evident. The episode is not severe enough to cause marked impairment to the person's social or occupational functioning and does not require hospitalisation. If psychotic features are evident, the diagnosis is defined as manic (APA 2013).

Personality disorder

Personality disorder refers to an enduring pattern of inner experience and behaviour that is in stark contrast to the expectations of the person's culture. The person's emotional behaviours are intense and are a response to the way in which they interpret self-experience and the perception of others around them. The personality traits are persistent and maladaptive, causing significant functional impairment or distress in the person's functioning.

Personality disorders are classified by their specific symptoms and are listed as: paranoid personality disorder, schizoid personality disorder, schizotypal personality disorder, antisocial personality disorder, borderline personality disorder, histrionic personality disorder, narcissistic personality disorder, avoidant personality disorder, dependent personality disorder, obsessive-compulsive personality disorder (APA 2013).

Post-traumatic stress disorder

Post-traumatic stress disorder (PTSD) is the development of symptoms following exposure to one or more traumatic events which include, but are not limited to: war, threatened or actual assault, threatened or actual sexual violence, domestic violence, kidnapping, torture, incarceration, natural or human-made disasters and severe motor vehicle accidents (APA 2013). The traumatic event is re-experienced with recurrent, involuntary and intrusive recollections of the incident, in particular in the form of distressing dreams. Flashbacks can occur briefly following exposure to a trigger of the event but leave the person in a state of hyper-arousal and intense psychological distress. Common symptoms of PTSD include recurrent distressing memories and dreams of the event, intense psychological distress from exposure to triggers, avoidance of stimuli associated with the event, and negative changes in cognitions and mood associated with the event (APA 2013).

Schizophrenia

Schizophrenia is a psychotic disorder characterised by changes in one or more of the following domains:

- Delusions: fixed beliefs that are not amenable to change in light of contradictory evidence. Themes may be persecutory, referential, somatic, religious or grandiose in nature and are deemed bizarre and not reflective of the cultural norms with which that person identifies.
- Hallucinations: uncontrollable perceptual experiences that occur without an external stimulus, most commonly in the form of an auditory experience. This symptom may be described as a voice or voices that are perceived as distinct from the person's own thoughts. It is important to note that hallucinations may be a normal experience in certain cultural contexts, such as the phenomenon of mediums who receive information from spirits of the deceased in the form of auditory or visual perceptions that are not available to others (Roxburgh and Roe 2014).
- Disorganised thinking: this is reflected in the person's speech, which can be confusing as the person switches between topics or gives unrelated answers to questions asked. The symptom must be severe enough so as to substantially impair effective communication.
- Grossly disorganised or abnormal motor behaviour: this may be evident in persons with unpredictable agitation or playful, childlike behaviours that lead to difficulties in functioning or completing activities of daily living. In contrast to this, catatonic behaviour is characterised by a marked decrease in reactivity to the environment which may result in bizarre posturing, mutism, staring or grimacing.

- Negative symptoms: these are characterised by diminished emotional expression in the face and behaviours that would usually occur when interacting with others. Avolition can be observed in people who have difficulty in motivated self-initiated activities, resulting in the person sitting for extended periods of time, or having difficulty interacting with their environment (APA 2013).

Feeding and eating disorders

Feeding and eating disorders are commonly seen in adolescence and can persist into adulthood. Two of the more common feeding and eating disorders are anorexia nervosa and bulimia nervosa. Anorexia nervosa is characterised by restriction of energy intake relative to output, resulting in significant low body weight that is less than minimally expected. The person suffers from intense fear of gaining weight with persistent lack of recognition of the seriousness of the low body weight (APA 2013). High-income countries report higher incidence of anorexia nervosa though the true incidence of rates in lower-income countries is uncertain, with hidden rates of the condition being culturally sanctioned (APA 2013). Suicide risk is heightened in eating disorders and reported to occur in 12 per 100,000 individuals experiencing anorexia nervosa per year (APA 2013).

In contrast to anorexia, people diagnosed with bulimia nervosa engage in binge eating of large amounts of food without control and then purposefully vomit, use laxatives, fast or exercise in order to avoid weight gain. This pattern occurs at least once a week for three months or longer. Self-evaluation is excessively influenced by body shape and dissatisfaction with their natural weight (APA 2013).

Social determinants of mental health and mental illness

As outlined above (pp. 23–25), different individuals, cultures and societies attribute unique causes to mental health and mental illness. Taking a Western perspective, there are a number of suggested determinants associated with mental health and mental illness. Often, these are categorised as risk and protective factors, some of which are distinct and others which exist at opposite ends of a spectrum. Risk factors refer to those which may reduce mental health and may increase an individual's vulnerability to, and severity of, mental illness, whereas protective factors refer to those which contribute to reduced exposure to risk and/or act as a buffer against the experience of mental illness. Risk and protective factors can be categorised into some key domains: individual factors (attributes and behaviours, such as an individual's innate and/or learned ability to manage their thoughts and feelings); genetic and biological factors (such as chromosomal abnormalities); and social factors (e.g. cultural, economic, political and environmental influences). Some of these can be modifiable (e.g. income) whereas others are not (e.g. genetics). Collectively, these factors help to explain an individual's current state of mental health and/or illness.

Here, we focus on some of the more general social determinants – that is, those factors which are determined and influenced by the society or societies with which an individual identifies. Exposure to social determinants often begins before birth and accumulates across the lifespan (WHO and

Calouste Gulbenkian Foundation 2014b). How such factors have more of an influence in some societies and cultures than others will be discussed. It is important to remember that these socially determined risk factors are just one set of influences, and will interact in various ways with factors in other domains (e.g. individual and biological factors). This will be explored in later chapters. While it is not possible to discuss all of the social determinants here, some of the widely regarded influences include: poverty, economic environment, trauma, gender, isolation and social attitudes/norms.

Poverty

Taking a global perspective, one of the most widely acknowledged social factors influencing mental health and illness is poverty. Currently, global estimates suggest that 1.2 billion people are living in extreme poverty, that is, existing on less than $1.25 per day (World Bank 2014) and that 11.3 per cent of people in 34 developed countries are living in relative poverty, that is, those who have less access and resources considered sufficient to live within their particular county (OECD 2014). The association between poverty and poor mental health is well established. One large review found associations between poverty and common mental disorders in low- and middle-income countries in over 70 per cent of the 115 studies included (Lund et al. 2011). These trends are also seen in developed countries. Evidence from the United Kingdom indicates that the prevalence of a common mental disorder increases as household income decreases (Ceverill and King 2009). This trend is more pronounced for men than for women, with men in the lowest income bracket being three times more at risk than those in the highest. A similar relationship was found for suicidal thoughts and behaviours, with these being most prevalent among individuals in the lower income bracket (Nicholson, Jenkins and Meltzer 2009).

Poverty has a number of associated consequences which can contribute to poor mental health. These consequences can be material, such as lack of choice about where to live, poor housing conditions, nutrition and clothing, and lack of access to health care and transport (Patel et al. 2007, Stansfeld et al. 2008). Such consequences may contribute to feelings of hopelessness (Patel and Kleinman 2003) and being unable to access basic resources may contribute to low self-esteem (Stansfeld et al. 2008). Other factors can influence mental health more indirectly – for example, the lack of access to adequate nutrition may influence mood and concentration (Stansfeld et al. 2008). There are also many social implications. For example, poor housing conditions may mean that individuals in poverty are often living in over-crowded environments, with a lack of space for positive social interactions within and external to the family (Stansfeld et al. 2008). There are also associations between poverty and risk of violence (Patel and Kleinman 2003). Finally, the association between poverty and mental health is considered to be bi-directional, whereby poverty increases the risk of mental illness, and those with a mental illness are at risk of drifting into, or remaining in, poverty (WHO 2012).

Economic environment

Although many people will never experience poverty, changes to the economic environment can also influence mental health. This was seen recently during the global financial crisis which resulted in widespread unemployment and underemployment (ABS 2013) and consequently, loss of housing and other resources for numerous individuals. A number of studies have found associations between the crisis and mental health outcomes worldwide. For example, a study of over 10,000 people in Spain showed an increase in the number of mental health presentations in primary care from 2006 to 2010, which were particularly related to mortgage repayments and unemployment (Gili et al. 2013). Similarly, a longitudinal study of 1973 older Australians two to four years before the crisis, and then again during the crisis, showed an increase in symptoms of depression and anxiety (Sargent-Cox, Butterworth and Anstey 2011).The crisis also had similar effects on unemployed migrant workers in eastern China (Chen et al. 2012). In Greece, the prevalence of suicidal ideation and reported suicide attempts increased during this time; those who were particularly vulnerable were people with depression, men, married individuals, those experiencing financial strain, those with low interpersonal trust, and those with a history of suicide attempts (Economou et al. 2013). The crisis had other flow-on effects, such as reductions in health care funding to support mental health, which further compounded the impact of the crisis on those who required mental health services (Procter, Papadopoulos and McEvoy 2010).

Trauma

While there is evidence to suggest that early adversity – such as the experience of trauma – can have benefits for mental health (e.g. psychological growth and resilience), it is also widely established that it can contribute to mental deterioration and mental illness later in life (Green et al. 2010). While later chapters will further explore the links between trauma and poor mental health at certain life stages, the links between trauma and mental illness are particularly prominent among certain social groups, and can be influenced by the political and government context of a particular society. A pertinent example is war-related trauma and violence. A detailed review of 161 articles related to adult refugees and other conflict-affected persons from 40 different countries concluded that certain traumatic experiences (e.g. torture) are strongly related to PTSD and depression (Steel et al. 2009). Further, there is growing recognition of risk factors which may develop upon arrival in a new country as a result of fleeing from trauma. Evidence indicates high levels of anxiety, depression, PTSD, self-harm and suicidal ideation among asylum seekers and refugees in held detention in Western countries, and that the severity of mental health concerns increase with time in detention (Robjant, Hassan and Katona 2009).

Within some countries, the trauma associated with colonisation (a process which is largely driven by a society's dominant government) has had a recognisable influence on the mental health and well-being of indigenous societies. For example, recent data suggest that Indigenous Australians are twice as likely as non-Indigenous Australians to report either high or very high levels of psychological distress (AIHW 2011). Government policies – such as assimilation and child removal – have been identified as causes of such trauma and long-term social disadvantage, contributing to mental illness (Hocking 2014). Other contributors associated with government policies and increased risk of diminished well-being include widespread grief and loss, cultural dislocation and identity issues, economic and social disadvantage, physical health problems, incarceration, violence, and substance use (Zubrick et al. 2010). Similarly, in New Zealand, the prevalence of experiencing a mental health condition in the past twelve months is almost 10 per cent higher for Māori and almost 5 per cent higher for Pacific Island people than for the total New Zealand population (Foliaki et al. 2006). It is suggested that one of the key factors contributing to this is the relative socio-demographic disadvantage of these groups (Foliaki et al. 2006).

Gender

The WHO (2014b) stresses that gender is another predictor of mental illness, with global figures indicating a higher prevalence among women than men (largely accounted for by higher rates of depression among the former). The WHO (2014a) states that: 'Gender determines the differential power and control men and women have over the socioeconomic determinants of their mental health and lives, their social position, status and treatment in society and their susceptibility and exposure to specific mental health risks.' For women, this has been attributed to the disadvantage that stems from gender inequality (a socially determined concept), the lower status attributed to women in many countries and their socially defined roles, meaning that they are often subject to violence. Globally, it is estimated that 35 per cent of women have experienced physical and/or sexual violence, usually by an intimate partner (WHO 2013). Reported rates of intimate partner violence vary between countries: as low as 16 per cent in East Asia to as high as 66 per cent in sub-Saharan Africa. Intimate partner violence can lead to stress, fear and social isolation, suggesting why women who have been exposed to such violence are almost twice as likely to experience depression as those who have not (WHO 2013). Moreover, gender inequality means that many women are unable to gain an education or earn an income, and consequently are more at risk of experiencing poorer mental health, such as stress and anxiety (WHO 2014a).

There are various examples of the influence of gender differing within Western societies, and across different mental health experiences. One UK study showed a higher prevalence of alcohol use and dependence among men than women, for any age group and regardless of ethnicity (white, black, south Asian), whereas eating disorders were more common among women (Thompson, Brugha and Palmer 2009). In a similar example, reported rates of suicide in Australia are higher among men than women (ABS 2012). While there are many suggested reasons for this difference, it may be attributed to the social attributes or expectations of men and women, whereby there has traditionally been greater acceptance of women discussing their emotions than men. See Chapters 7 and 8 for further exploration of gender differences.

Isolation, marginalisation and social exclusion

Exclusion from society and one's community can be experienced by a range of people for a variety of reasons, and can contribute to the experience of poor mental health. Examples include refugees separated from their families and country of origin, and the elderly who typically live alone in many individualistic societies. The WHO (2014d) explains that social exclusion prevents individuals from fully engaging in their community/social life which:

> consists of dynamic, multi-dimensional processes driven by unequal power relationships interacting across four main dimensions – economic, political, social and cultural – and at different levels including individual, household, group, community, country and global levels. It results in a continuum of inclusion/exclusion characterised by unequal access to resources, capabilities and rights which leads to health inequalities.

Isolation may be experienced by those who work away from their family, friends and community. Changing economic situations have seen increases in the number of people undertaking Fly-in-Fly-Out (FIFO) work, largely for the mining and natural resources industry. By nature, FIFO work involves working away from one's usual place of residence for a period of time (e.g. up to four weeks at a time), working longer than usual shifts (e.g. 12 hours compared to the typical 8 hours), and often staying in shared housing/camps. A recent report Australian FIFO workers found that the predominant stress experienced by these individuals was separation from their family and/or home (Lifeline WA 2013). Other stresses were associated with lengthy shifts and lack of adequate sleep, leading to fatigue. Although the majority of the sample (over 900 FIFO workers) showed low levels of psychological distress, there was a greater likelihood of experiencing distress and having a psychological disorder than in the average Australian population. There is also evidence to suggest that rates of suicide are higher among those in the mining industry, and that this is accounted for by relationship problems experienced as a result of the work (McPhedran and De Leo 2013).

Social isolation is not solely experienced by those who are physically isolated, but also by those who experience stigma and consequent isolation from their community on a daily basis. One such example is people who identify as lesbian, gay, bi, transgender and intersex. In Australia, it is estimated that these individuals are twice as likely to experience anxiety and three times as likely to experience depression than the rest of the population (beyondblue 2014). A recent review of the literature (Johnson and Amella 2014) explored this notion of isolation in adolescents who identify as lesbian, gay, bi or transgender (LGBT), finding that multiple common forms of isolation are experienced: social isolation from family, friends and school in terms of a lack of social support, lack of contact with the LGBT community, social withdrawal and victimisation; emotional disconnect from others; and cognitive isolation resulting from a lack of access to information about homosexuality.

Social beliefs, attitudes and norms

Commonly held social beliefs, attitudes and norms can also contribute to risk factors for mental illness. A prime example is alcohol abuse and misuse, which has a well-established link as a risk factor for the development of poor mental health. In many societies, substance use conditions are more common among men, and this has been partially attributed to societal attitudes surrounding substance use behaviour (WHO 2012). Contrasts in attitudes towards substance consumption in Western metropolitan and rural environments can also account for this. For example, one study explored differences in alcohol, tobacco and illicit substance use in students (aged 12–15 years) in the US and Australia, finding higher lifetime and current use in rural compared to urban areas (Coomber et al. 2011). Interviews with Australian adults living in rural locations highlighted the 'normalisation' of alcohol consumption in these regions and the potential for exclusion from social activities for individuals who do not consume alcohol. The link between these social attitudes and norms and poor mental health may be compounded in societies or communities with other risk factors (e.g. lack of access to mental health service and stigma in rural communities). Another example is eating disorders, which have commonly been more prevalent in developed countries and fuelled, in part, by social attitudes valuing thinness, as emphasised in the media (e.g. print, television, popular figures). Until recently, these were not seen in other societies; however, expansion and globalisation of the media has been associated with an increase in indicators of eating conditions in non-Western countries (Becker et al. 2002).

Another notable risk factor linked to social attitudes and norms is help-seeking behaviour. It is widely accepted that early intervention and treatment can reduce the long-term impact of mental illness: however, many individuals do not seek help. There are a number of potential reasons for this across different societies and communities. For example, in rural communities, notions of stoicism and self-reliance (Fuller et al. 2000) may account for lower help-seeking compared to those living in metropolitan communities. Refugee and asylum seeker communities may be reluctant to seek help due to cultural beliefs stipulating that the individual should be able to 'control' their own thoughts and emotions (Prasad-Ildes and Ramirez 2006), and attitudes/beliefs regarding service confidentiality (Blignault et al. 2008) and trustability (Minas, Klimidis and Kokanovic 2007). These may contribute to lower access to mental health services (Australian Government Department of Health 2014).

The impact of living with a mental illness

The lives of people with a mental illness can be impacted by many factors, including the effects of an illness itself, treatment or medication side-effects, stigma, social exclusion, as well as limited access to services, support and resources. People with a mental illness may also experience a profound degree of loss (Baker, Procter and Gibbons 2009). This section discusses a range of issues directly and indirectly related to mental illness which impact not only on people living with a mental illness, but also their supports and society more generally.

Impact on identity and aspects of the self

The onset and presence of mental illness may bring about a range of changes to a person's identity and selfhood. Some changes to the self may occur due to symptoms of mental illness, whereas others can stem from treatments such as medication or electroconvulsive therapy (ECT). In addition, changes to a person's sense of self-concept may also arise from social influences, such as stigma, which will be explored further on page 39. Some effects on a person's identity – such as a loss of hope or sense of purpose in life – may have profound consequences for a person's well-being and recovery, as well as the well-being of those around them.

The often unpredictable nature of many mental illnesses can impact profoundly on a person's sense of self, including how they think, feel and behave. For example, depression may make it difficult for a person to initiate or engage in certain activities, including self-care tasks such as getting dressed or eating (Baker and Procter 2014). Mental illness may deeply affect a person's routine, including their sleeping pattern. A person may sleep excessively or experience a severe lack of sleep, both of which can have a major impact on other aspects of the person's life and the lives of those around them. A loss of energy or motivation, stemming from the symptoms and consequences of mental illnesses, such as depression, may also cause difficulties in everyday life (Baker and Procter 2014). An excess of energy, experienced during mania, can also hold grave consequences for a person's ability to function and process the world around them. For a person experiencing psychosis, a loss of reality, insight, judgement and other severe changes to the self may take place.

Delusions may be present, causing a person to have false beliefs, such as the presence of special powers or that they are under constant surveillance by police. Hallucinations may cause a person to see, hear, smell or taste things which are not actually present. Such experiences can severely impact on the way a person interacts with the world and can be confusing and distressing for the person experiencing psychosis, as well as for those around them.

Compared with the general population, people with a serious mental illness (SMI) – such as psychotic disorders and major mood disorders – die earlier and experience more medical illnesses (Viron and Stern 2010). In those with SMI, the prevalence of obesity, metabolic syndrome, diabetes mellitus, symptoms of cardiovascular disease and respiratory disease exceed that of the general population by at least two times (Scott and Happell 2011). A host of factors are thought to contribute to the increased prevalence of chronic diseases in people with SMI, including poor diet, sedentary behaviour, smoking, drug and alcohol misuse and risky sexual behaviours (Scott and Happell 2011). In addition, many medications and other treatments for mental illness carry side-effects, some of which can severely impact on a person's sense of self. Negative side-effects stemming from medications for mental illness may include extreme lethargy, negative body image, difficulties in sexual functioning, reduced fitness levels and a loss of motivation, judgement or memory. Involuntary treatment in hospital can also impact on people with a mental illness. The loss of freedom (Jeffs 2009) and control over one's life experienced during hospitalisation has been perceived to lead to a loss of dignity (Nilsson, Nåden and Lindström 2008). Other losses which may arise from being hospitalised include: time, support from others, memory (from ECT), and the ability to relate to others, with many of these having profound or long-lasting effects on people with a mental illness.

The way mental illness is understood and described can also have powerful implications. For example, when people define a person with a mental illness as a 'schizophrenic' or 'manic depressive', these labels totalise that person as a mental illness. Non-totalising descriptions, such as 'a person with schizophrenia', are preferred, as the identities of those who experience mental illness are far more than simply a label or an illness. On a much deeper level, mental illness can impact on a person's sense of purpose in life or their hope for the future. Loss of hope is commonly described within the literature on mental illness (Beeble and Salem 2009, Bradshaw, Armour and Roseborough 2007). As a factor in the prediction of suicide (Schrank, Stanghellini and Slade 2008), it is imperative that loss of hope is addressed. It is important to consider the range of ways in which mental illness may impact on identity and other aspects of the self, as a person's attitudes and beliefs play a crucial part in their own recovery journey. Furthermore, it should be noted that not all impacts of mental illness are necessarily negative. Some people with a mental illness report positive aspects or opportunities arising from this experience. For example, Young and Ensing (1999) note that through the process of recovery, people often revive parts of themselves which they assumed were lost because of mental illness. Mental illness may also be associated with positive traits or abilities, such as creativity and openness to different experiences that may occur for people with bipolar disorder (Galvez, Thommi and Ghaemi 2011).

Impact on relationships and social participation

Mental illness can have a profound impact on a person's relationships with others and broader social roles and activities in the community. People with a mental illness commonly report loneliness or that their social needs are not addressed adequately (Borba et al. 2011; Nilsson, Nåden and Lindström 2008), with the loss of relationships or contacts being a major contributor (Mauritz and van Meijel 2009). Loss of relationships for people with a mental illness can range from friends and family members to colleagues or community contacts. For people with a mental illness, relationship losses have been described in terms of 'not belonging', the loss of place in a social milieu (Mauritz and van Meijel 2009) and a lack of fellowship and relief (Nilsson, Nåden and Lindström 2008). Roles or other aspects of relationships may be lost, such as the loss of social status or credibility, parenthood in losing relationships with children (Fernandez, Breen and Simpson 2014) or a sexual self (Quinn and Browne 2009).

Factors thought to lead to the loss of relationships or social opportunities for people with a mental illness include: stigma (Proudfoot et al. 2009), frequent changes in living arrangements, lost employment or educational opportunities (Chernomas, Clarke and Marchinko 2008), as well as their mental health condition itself (Borba et al. 2011). Furthermore, losses that may emerge due to mental illness, such as the loss of reality, self-respect or ability to communicate, may lead people to inadvertently sever ties with their loved ones. Karp (1996: 28) describes this as the paradox of greatly desiring connection whilst being: 'simultaneously deprived of the ability to realize it'. Even in times of great distress and need, such as an acute hospitalisation, this dilemma may create challenges both for people who have a mental illness trying to reach out to others, and for others trying to reach out to them.

Studies have consistently demonstrated that a large proportion of people with a mental illness feel stigmatised and that stigma has major implications for well-being. Stigma is manifested by stereotyping, fear, embarrassment, anger, rejection and avoidance (WHO 2005). Consequences of being stigmatised, either directly or indirectly, are extensive and include shame, humiliation and despair (Carr and Halpin 2002), along with the potential loss of opportunities (Corrigan 2002), for example, in being hired or approved for a rental property (Bradshaw, Armour and Roseborough 2007). Stigma and discrimination influence various aspects of community living, including education, personal safety, employment and social activity and has been cited by mental health consumers as a reason for not seeking help. As a result of stigma, social exclusion and a fragile sense of self-worth, people with a mental illness may find it difficult to connect with others and engage in social activities (Young and Ensing 1999).

The citizenship of people with a mental illness can also be impacted. Citizenship refers to the rights and privileges of members in a democratic society as well as the responsibilities these rights engender, which, historically, have been restricted for people with a mental illness (Ware et al. 2007). Thus, citizenship involves having choices such as participating in clubs, voting, going to school, having intimate relationships or even choosing to do none of these (Mezzina et al. 2006). Importantly, social integration and exercising one's citizenship involve growth and development for people with a mental illness, rather than simply an alleviation of symptoms. In addition, public perceptions about the causes of mental illness may hold implications for its 'social acceptance', including levels of tolerance in the community (Schnittker 2008). For people with mental health conditions which are more highly stigmatised, such as schizophrenia, a loss of moral status can occur, having major implications for a person (Yang and Kleinman 2008) and their family.

Impact from – and on – broader societal issues

Given that the impact of mental illness can extend beyond the individual to their wider society, this section briefly considers several critical societal issues which mental illness may impact on, and conversely, which can impact upon the outcomes for people affected by mental illness.

Factors facing some people with a mental illness, which can profoundly impact on their ability to engage in society adequately include a dire financial situation or poverty (Davidson et al. 2005), dependence on public transport or restricted housing opportunities (Bradshaw, Armour and Roseborough 2007). Issues of adequate housing and homelessness can be significant for people affected by mental illness. For example, people with a SMI are over-represented in the homeless population (Kirkpatrick and Byrne 2009). A range of factors, including stigma, reduced incomes, difficulties in everyday functioning and fluctuations in symptoms, often mean that people with a SMI are unable to compete for market rental housing or have difficulty gaining entry to social and supporting housing units (Kyle and Dunn 2008). Furthermore, existing living arrangements may be lost at the point of hospitalisation for people with a mental illness (Forchuk et al. 2006). For people with a mental illness, provision of adequate housing is an important factor for achieving and maintaining health (Kyle and Dunn 2008) and being in recovery, including reconnecting with family, gaining employment and planning for the future (Kirkpatrick and Byrne 2009).

Challenges and losses in the area of education and employment are commonly reported due to mental illness. For example, people with bipolar disorder reported that the inability to create consistency in life resulted in disruption and discontinuation in education, employment and career development (Inder et al. 2008). Other reasons why people with a mental illness may lose work include the symptoms of mental illness, a loss of abilities or skills, as well as attitudes or beliefs, such as a loss of self-esteem (Baker and Procter 2014). Productivity loss from mental illness covers a range of situations, including absenteeism, presenteeism and work-cutback (Stang et al. 2007), as well as lower rates of workforce participation (Lindström et al. 2007) and premature mortality (Insel 2008). Unlike many other medical disorders, losses to society in the form of costs for mental illness are more often derived from indirect than direct costs, such as public income support payments and the effect of reduced educational attainment (Insel 2008). For example, across the entire US population in 2002, SMI was estimated to result in a loss of $193.2 billion in personal earnings (Kessler et al. 2008).

Another area which mental illness can impact on and which can influence mental health outcomes is healthcare. Compared with the general population, many people with a mental illness receive inferior healthcare (Mitchell, Malone and Doebbeling 2009; Viron and Stern 2010). Inequalities in healthcare for people with mental illness can occur due to a range of reasons, including attitudes of care providers, poorly integrated care and reduced access to care (Viron and Stern 2010). The issue of reduced access can be pronounced for people from culturally and linguistically diverse (CALD) backgrounds, who may experience further difficulties due to language barriers, unfamiliar health systems and differing beliefs of the causes and treatments for mental illness.

Promoting mental health within a whole-of-health framework

This chapter has highlighted the role that societies and social factors can play in contributing to mental illness, and the profound influence that mental illness can have on individuals and societies. In turn, this raises questions about the role that societies can play in promoting mentally healthier nations and addressing mental illness. In a recent report, the WHO recognised that mental health conditions share many common features with physical health conditions (e.g. similar underlying causes and consequences), and that these conditions often co-occur (WHO and Calouste Gulbenkian Foundation 2014a). As such, the WHO has called for actions to promote mental health within a whole-of-health approach, implemented across multiple sectors, i.e., not just the health sector, but also education, environment, housing, welfare, etc. The WHO (2014c) also stresses that promoting mental health 'involves actions to create living conditions and environments that support mental health and allow people to adopt and maintain healthy lifestyles', along with 'a climate that respects and protects basic civil, political, socio-economic and cultural rights'. The WHO (2014c) further argues for the importance of early intervention initiatives, which seek to provide early access to services to prevent and/or reduce the long-term impacts of poor mental health.

Collins et al. (2013) discuss some of the challenges associated with such change, given that integration of mental health care will require local, national, and global-level shifts. It also involves integrating change at the level of the community and challenging traditional approaches to service delivery, such as the one-to-one service delivery by a highly trained mental health professional (Kazdin and Rabbitt 2013). In addition to these changes, societies (at various levels) can play a role in promoting mental health by encouraging social supports and social connectedness, as well as reducing stigma and improving mental health literacy. These are just several elements which may contribute to mentally healthier nations, and which can be achieved through both widespread campaigning as well as initiatives targeted at particular at-risk groups. Some examples of these will be briefly discussed in this section.

Promoting social support and social connectedness

It should now be evident that isolation and disconnection from family, friends and one's community can contribute to an increased risk for poor mental health. At the other end of the spectrum, social support and social connectedness can play an important role in an individual's mental health. Kawachi and Berkman (2001) highlight how social ties can be useful, whether or not individuals are under stress. Social supports can provide emotional sustenance (e.g. love and care), as well as coping assistance (e.g. empathy and validation of feelings), which can be offered by significant others, including those who have also experienced poor mental health (Thoits 2011). Social support can also mitigate other risk factors for mental illness across the lifespan, providing protection at times of distress and/or trauma such as loss of employment and family breakdown (Commonwealth of Australia 2009). For example, a study of 1152 women exposed to intimate partner violence found that those with higher social support had significantly reduced risk of poor mental health (Coker et al. 2002). Similarly, a study of 63 resettled Sudanese refugees in Australia found that the perceived level of social support from one's ethnic community after relocation predicted symptoms of PTSD, anxiety and somatization. (Schweitzer et al. 2006). Perceived social support can also be a factor in encouraging help-seeking behaviours (Gulliver, Griffiths and Christensen 2010).

The need for improved social support and opportunities for social connection is becoming increasingly addressed. On example is the Men's Sheds initiative, which has been established in numerous developed nations, such as Australia, New Zealand, Ireland and the UK. Men's Sheds aim to address social isolation by connecting men with other members of their communities in a physical space, and offer opportunities to engage men about their health and well-being in a non-traditional health setting (Australian Men's Sheds Association 2011). This initiative seeks to reduce disparities in mental health which may be associated with factors such as social constructions of the roles of males, reduced tendency for men to talk due to cultural perceptions or suggestions that men should refrain from talking about feelings and emotions, less interest in their own health and well-being, and a reluctance to seek help. While empirical evidence for these initiatives is in the early stages, there is some evidence to suggest that Men's Sheds promote learning (Wilson and Cordier 2013), and encourage social connectedness, camaraderie and an inclusive environment (Hansji, Wilson and Cordier 2014). In a study of Men's Sheds users in Australia, one participant explained: 'The main reason I think I came down to the Shed here was . . . not so much [to] get involved in all the making things . . . it was more to do with . . . getting out of the house and meeting some new friends' (Hansji, Wilson and Cordier 2014, p. 5).

In addition to these targeted programs, widespread initiatives can also promote social support. For example, in Australia, 'R U OK' day encourages people to ask each other if they are okay, on the grounds that encouraging people to talk about their concerns and showing support might reduce the risk of suicide (RU OK? 2014). Such initiatives clearly have an important potential to improve mental health, yet they often require funding and government support in order to be sustainable. This highlights the need for national and international policies to prioritise mental health.

Reducing stigma and enhancing mental health literacy

Again referring to developed countries, there are increasingly widespread initiatives aimed at raising awareness and educating the general public about mental health in order to reduce stigma and enhance mental health literacy. Examples include: Like Minds, Like Mine in New Zealand; See Me in Scotland; and beyondblue in Australia. Often, these campaigns are run in national media (e.g. television and online) and can be both general and specific to certain at-risk groups. Such initiatives can reduce the stigma associated with mental illness by raising awareness that these are common and treatable experiences. Many of these campaigns are co-designed and incorporate narratives of people with lived experience of mental illness, which helps to demystify and destigmatise mental health conditions and encourage help-seeking. Improved mental health literacy – that is, knowledge of mental illness prevention, symptom recognition, help-seeking and treatment options, and mental health first aid to support others (Jorm 2012) – is another aim of these campaigns. Jorm (2012) argues that there is a discrepancy between mental and physical health literacy, with the general public being less knowledgeable about the former. With global levels of help-seeking for mental health concerns being relatively low, particularly for those individuals in low- and middle-income countries (WHO 2014b), such campaigns have the potential to encourage greater service use. Again, these would not be available without support from national and international policy, demonstrating the responsibility that society has to promote mental health and approaches to maintaining mental health.

Conclusions

This chapter has introduced the notion that although mental illness is common worldwide, there are many differences in the experience of mental health and illness across and within societies. In particular, it has highlighted the importance of considering the differences in the way that societies experience, understand and respond to mental health and mental illness. A range of common types of mental illness, such as anxiety conditions and mood disorders, were outlined, with the observation that some of these are more prevalent in certain societies than others. The presence of social determinants (such as poverty and gender) and how these interact with other risk and protective factors to explain an individual's current state of mental health was also explored. Further, this chapter explored the profound impact that mental illness can have not only on the individual, but also their support networks, significant others, and wider community. The important role that societies can play in promoting mental health and well-being, particularly through initiatives to improve social connectedness, reduce stigma and enhance mental health literacy, was also highlighted. The considerations raised in this chapter should be kept in mind as readers progress through the subsequent chapters of this book. Having an understanding of these concepts will encourage a comprehensive view of mental health and mental illness.

Reflective exercises

- Ask your friends to talk about how the society and culture with which an individual identifies might influence their personal views of mental health and mental illness. Is there a common view?
- Think about common global mental health difficulties and how they differ between wealthy and poor countries; what would you do to improve mental health in different cultures?
- Imagine you fall ill while in a foreign country and must communicate your needs to people who do not understand your language. Describe the range of emotions you might be feeling. How would you expect the health clinician to care for you?
- Describe some ways in which mental illness can impact on a person's relationships with others. How can people experiencing mental illness be supported by those around them and the wider community?

References

ABS (Australian Bureau of Statistics) 2007, *National survey of health and wellbeing: Summary of results*, cat. no. 4326.0, ABS, Canberra.

ABS 2012, *Gender indicators, Australia, Jan 2012*, cat. no. 4125.0, viewed 1 December 2014, <www.abs. gov.au/ausstats/abs@.nsf/Lookup/by+Subject/4125.0~Jan+2012~Main+Features~Suicides~3240>.

ABS 2013, *Underemployed workers, Australia, Sep 2011*, cat. no. 6265.0, viewed 3 December 2014, <www.abs.gov.au/ausstats/abs@.nsf/Lookup/6265.0Main+Features3Sep+2011>.

American Psychiatric Association (APA) 2013, *Diagnostic and statistical manual of mental disorders: DSM-5*, 5th edn, APA, Arlington, Va.

Australian Government Department of Health 2014, *Fact sheet: Mental health services for people of culturally and linguistically diverse (CALD) backgrounds*, viewed 1 April 2014, <www.health.gov. au/internet/main/publishing.nsf/Content/mental-multi-fact>.

AIHW (Australian Institute of Health and Welfare) 2011, *The health and welfare of Australia's Aboriginal and Torres Strait Islander people, an overview 2011*, cat. no. IHW 42, AIHW, Canberra.

Australian Men's Shed Association 2011, *What is a Men's Shed?*, viewed 1 December 2014, <www.mensshed.org/what-is-a-men%27s-shed/.aspx>.

Baker, AEZ and Procter, NG 2014, 'Losses related to everyday occupations for adults affected by mental illness', *Scandinavian Journal of Occupational Therapy*, vol. 21, no. 4, pp. 287–294.

Baker, AEZ, Procter, NG and Gibbons, T 2009, 'Dimensions of loss from mental illness', *Journal of Sociology and Social Welfare*, vol. 36, no. 4, pp. 25–52.

Becker, AE, Burwell, RA, Gilman, SE, Herzog, DB and Hamburg, P 2002, 'Eating behaviours and attitudes following prolonged exposure to television among ethnic Fijian adolescent girls', *British Journal of Psychiatry*, vol. 180, pp. 509–514.

Beeble, ML and Salem, DA 2009, 'Understanding the phases of recovery from serious mental illness: The roles of referent and expert power in a mutual-help setting', *Journal of Community Psychology*, vol. 37, no. 2, pp. 249–267.

Bemme, D and D'souza, NA 2014, 'Global mental health and its discontents: An inquiry into the making of global and local scale', *Transcultural Psychiatry*, vol. 51, no. 6, pp. 850–874.

beyondblue 2014, *Lesbian, gay, bi, trans and intersex (LGBTI) people*, viewed 3 December 2014, <www.beyondblue.org.au/resources/for-me/lesbian-gay-bi-trans-and-intersex-lgbti-people>.

Blignault, I, Ponzio, V, Rong, Y and Eisenbruch, M 2008, 'A qualitative study of barriers to mental health service utilisation among migrants from mainland China in south-east Sydney', *International Journal of Social Psychiatry*, vol. 54, no. 2, pp. 180–190.

Borba, CPC, DePadilla, L, Druss, BG, McCarty, FA, von Esenwein, SA and Sterk, CE 2011, 'A day in the life of women with a serious mental illness: A qualitative investigation', *Women's Health Issues*, vol. 21, no. 4, pp. 286–292.

Bradshaw, W, Armour, MP and Roseborough, D 2007, 'Finding a place in the world: The experience of recovery from severe mental illness', *Qualitative Social Work*, vol. 6, no. 1, pp. 27–47.

Carr, V and Halpin, S 2002, *Stigma and discrimination,* Commonwealth of Australia, Canberra.

Ceverill, C and King, M 2009, 'Common mental disorders', in S McManus, H Meltzer, T Brugha, P Bebbington and R Jenkins (eds), *Adult psychiatric morbidity in England, 2007: Results of a household survey*, The Health and Social Care Information Centre, Social Care Statistics, UK, pp. 25–52.

Chen, L, Li, W, He, J, Wu, L, Yan, Z and Tang, W 2012, 'Mental health, duration of unemployment, and coping strategy: A cross-sectional study of unemployed migrant workers in eastern China during the economic crisis', *BMC Public Health*, vol. 12, no. 1, doi:10.1186/1471-2458-12-597. URL: www.biomedcentral.com/1471-2458/12/597.

Chernomas, WM, Clarke, DE and Marchinko S 2008, 'Relationship-based support for women living with serious mental illness', *Issues in Mental Health Nursing*, vol. 29, pp. 437–453.

Coker, AL, Davis, KE, Arias, I, Desai, S, Sanderson, M, Brandt, HM and Smith, PH 2002, 'Physical and mental health effects of intimate partner violence for men and women', *American Journal of Preventive Medicine*, vol. 23, no. 4, pp. 260–268.

Collins, PY, Insel, TR, Chockalingam, A, Daar, A and Maddox, YT 2013, 'Grand challenges in global mental health: Integration in research, policy, and practice', *PLoS Medicine*, vol. 10, no. 4, e1001434.

Commonwealth of Australia 2009, *Fourth National Mental Health Plan – An agenda for collaborative government action in mental health 2009–2014*, Commonwealth of Australia, Canberra.

Coomber, K, Toumbourou, JW, Miller, P, Staiger, PK, Hemphill, SA and Catalona, RF 2011, 'Rural adolescent alcohol, tobacco, and illicit drug use: A comparison of students in Victoria, Australia, and Washington State, United States, *Journal of Rural Health*, vol. 27, no. 4, pp. 409–415.

Corrigan, PW 2002, 'Empowerment and serious mental illness: Treatment partnerships and community opportunities', *Psychiatric Quarterly*, vol. 73, no. 3, pp. 217–228.

Davidson, L, Borg, M, Marin, I, Topor, A, Mezzina, R and Sells, D 2005, 'Processes of recovery in serious mental illness: Findings from a multinational study', *American Journal of Psychiatric Rehabilitation*, vol. 8, no. 3, pp. 177–201.

Economou, M, Madianos, M, Peppou, LE, Theleritis, C, Patelakis, A and Stefanis, C 2013, 'Suicidal ideation and reported suicide attempts in Greece during the economic crisis', *World Psychiatry*, vol. 12, no. 1, pp. 53–59.

Fernandez, ME, Breen, LJ and Simpson, TA 2014, 'Renegotiating identities: Experiences of loss and recovery for women with bipolar disorder', *Qualitative Health Research*, vol. 24, no. 7, 890–900.

Foliaki, SA, Kokaua, J, Schaaf, D and Tukuitonga, C 2006, 'Twelve-month and lifetime prevalences of mental disorders and treatment contact among Pacific people in Te Rau Hinengaro: The New Zealand Mental Health Survey', *Australian and New Zealand Journal of Psychiatry*, vol. 40, no. 10, pp. 924–934.

Forchuk, C, Ward-Griffin, C, Csiernik, R and Turner, K 2006, 'Surviving the tornado of mental illness: Psychiatric survivors' experiences of getting, losing, and keeping housing', *Psychiatric Services*, vol. 57, no. 4, pp. 558–562.

Fuller, J, Edwards, J, Procter, N and Moss, J 2000, 'How definition of mental health problems can influence help seeking in rural and remote communities', *Australian Journal of Rural Health*, vol. 8, pp. 148–153.

Galvez, JF, Thommi, S and Ghaemi, N 2011, 'Positive aspects of mental illness: A review in bipolar disorder', *Journal of Affective Disorders*, vol. 128, pp. 185–190.

Gili, M, Roca, M, Basu, S, McKee, M and Stuckler, D 2013, 'The mental health risks of economic crisis in Spain: Evidence from primary care centres, 2006 and 2010', *The European Journal of Public Health*, vol. 23, no. 1, pp. 103–108.

Green, JG, McLaughlin, KA, Berglund, PA, Gruber, MJ, Sampson, NA, Zaslavsky, AM and Kessler, RC 2010, 'Childhood adversities and adult psychiatric disorders in the national comorbidity survey replication I: Associations with first onset of DSM-IV disorders', *Archives of General Psychiatry*, vol. 67, no. 2, pp. 113–123.

Griswold, W 2008, *Cultures and societies in a changing world*, 3rd edn, Pine Forge Press, California.

Gulliver, A, Griffiths, KM and Christensen, H 2010, 'Perceived barriers and facilitators to mental health help-seeking in young people: A systematic review', *BMC Psychiatry*, vol. 10, no. 113, viewed 1 December 2014, <www.biomedcentral.com/1471-244X/10/113>.

Hansji, NL, Wilson, NJ and Cordier, R 2014, 'Men's Sheds: Enabling environments for Australian men living with and without long-term disabilities', *Health and Social Care in the Community*, in early view, doi: 10.111/hsc.12140.

Hocking, D 2014, 'The social and emotional well-being of Aboriginal Australians and the collaborative consumer narrative', in N Procter, HP Hamer, D McGarry, RL Wilson and T Froggatt (eds.), *Mental health: A person-centred approach*, Cambridge University Press, Victoria, Australia, pp. 51–71.

Inder, ML, Crowe, MT, Moor, S, Luty, SE, Carter, JD and Joyce, PR 2008, '"I actually don't know who I am": The impact of bipolar disorder on the development of self', *Psychiatry*, vol. 71, no. 2, pp. 123–133.

Insel, TR 2008, 'Assessing the economic costs of serious mental illness', *American Journal of Psychiatry*, vol. 165, no. 6, pp. 663–665.

Jeffs, S 2009, *Flying with paper wings: Reflections on living with madness*, The Vulgar Press, Carlton North, Australia.

Johnson, MJ and Amella, EJ 2014, 'Isolation of lesbian, gay, bisexual and transgender youth: A dimensional concept analysis', *Journal of Advanced Nursing*, vol. 70, no. 3, pp. 523–532.

Jorm, AF 2012, 'Mental health literacy: Empowering the community to take action for better mental health', *American Psychologist*, vol. 67, pp. 231–243.

Karp, DA 1996, *Speaking of sadness: Depression, disconnection and the meanings of illness*, Oxford University Press, New York.

Kawachi, I and Berkman, LF 2001, 'Social ties and mental health', *Journal of Urban Health*, vol. 78, no. 3, pp. 458–467.

Kazdin, AE and Rabbitt, SM 2013, 'Novel models for delivering mental health services and reducing the burdens of mental illness', *Clinical Psychological Science*, doi: 10.1177/2167702612463566.

Kessler, RC, Angermeyer, M, Anthony, JC, de Graaf, R, Demyttenaere, K, Gasquet, I, De Girolamo, G, Gluzman, S, Gureje, O, Haro, JM, Kawakami, N, Karam, A, Levinson, D, Mora, MEM, Oakley

Browne, MA, Posada-Villa, J, Stein, DJ, Tsang, CHA, Aguilar-Gaxiola, S, Alonso, J, Lee, S, Heeringa, S, Pennell, B-E, Berglund, P, Gruber, MJ, Petukhova, M, Chatterji, S and Üstün, TB 2007, 'Lifetime prevalence and age-of-onset distributions of mental disorders in the World Health Organization's World Mental Health Survey Initiative', *World Psychiatry*, vol. 6, no. 3, pp. 168–176.

Kessler, RC, Heeringa, S, Lakoma, MD, Petukhova, M, Rupp, AE, Schoenbaum, M, Wang, PS and Zaslavasky, AM 2008, 'Individual and societal effects of mental disorders on earnings in the United States: Results from the National Comorbidity Survey Replication', *The American Journal of Psychiatry*, vol. 165, no. 6, pp. 703–711.

Kessler, RC, Aguilar-Gaxiola, S, Alonso, J, Chatterji, S, Lee, S, Ormel, J, Üstün, TB and Wang, PS 2009, 'The global burden of mental disorders: An update from the WHO World Mental Health (WMH) Surveys', *Epidemiologia e Psichiatria Sociale*, vol. 18, no. 1, pp. 23–33.

Kirkpatrick, H and Byrne, C 2009, 'A narrative inquiry: Moving on from homelessness for individuals with a major mental illness', *Journal of Psychiatric and Mental Health Nursing*, vol. 16, pp. 68–75.

Kirmayer, LJ and Pederson, D 2014, 'Toward a new architecture for global mental health', *Transcultural Psychiatry*, vol. 51, no. 6, pp. 759–776.

Kleinman, A 2009, 'The art of medicine, global mental health: A failure of humanity', *The Lancet*, vol. 374, pp. 603–604.

Kleinman, A and Seeman, D 2000, 'Personal experience of illness', in GL Albrecht, R Fitzpatrick and SC Scrimshaw (eds), *Handbook of social studies in health and medicine*, Sage, London, pp. 230–243.

Kyle, T and Dunn, JR 2008, 'Effects of housing circumstances on health, quality of life and healthcare use for people with severe mental illness: A review', *Health and Social Care in the Community*, vol. 16, no. 1, pp. 1–15.

Lifeline WA 2013, *FIFO/DIDO mental health research report 2013*, viewed 3 December 2014, <www.rawhire.com.au/sites/default/files/fifo_dido_mental_health_research_report_2013.pdf>.

Lindström, E, Eberhard, J, Neovius, M and Levander, S 2007, 'Costs of schizophrenia during 5 years', *Acta Psychiatrica Scandinavica*, vol. 116, no. 435, pp. 33–40.

Lund, C, De Silva, M, Plagerson, S, Cooper, S, Chisholm, D, Das, J, Knapp, M and Patel, V 2011, 'Poverty and mental disorders: Breaking the cycle in low-income and middle-income countries', *The Lancet*, vol. 378, no. 9801, pp. 1502–1514.

Mauritz, M and van Meijel, B 2009, 'Loss and grief in patients with schizophrenia: On living in another world', *Archives of Psychiatric Nursing*, vol. 23, pp. 251–260.

McPhedran, S and De Leo, D 2013, 'Suicide among miners in Queensland, Australia: A comparative analysis of demographics, psychiatric history, and stressful life events', *SAGE Open*, doi: 10.1177/2158244013511262.

Mezzina, R, Borg, M, Marin, I, Sells, D, Topor, A and Davidson, L 2006, 'From participation to citizenship: How to regain a role, a status, and a life in the process of recovery', *American Journal of Psychiatric Rehabilitation*, vol. 9, no. 1, pp. 39–61.

Minas, H, Klimidis, S and Kokanovic, R 2007, 'Depression in multicultural Australia: Policies, research and services', *Australian and New Zealand Health Policy*, vol. 4, no. 16, viewed 1 April 2014, <www.anzhealthpolicy.com/content/4/1/16>.

Mitchell, AJ, Malone, D and Doebbeling, CC 2009, 'Quality of medical care for people with and without comorbid mental illness and substance misuse: Systematic review of comparative studies', *The British Journal of Psychiatry*, vol. 194, pp. 491–499.

Murray, JL, Lopez, AD, World Health Organisation, World Bank, Harvard School of Public Health 1996, *Global health statistics: A compendium of incidence, prevalence, and mortality estimates for over 200 conditions*, World Health Organisation, Geneva.

Nicholson, S, Jenkins, R and Meltzer, H 2009, 'Suicidal thoughts, suicide attempts and self-harm', in S McManus, H Meltzer, T Brugha, P Bebbington and R Jenkins (eds), *Adult psychiatric morbidity in England, 2007: Results of a household survey*, The Health and Social Care Information Centre, Social Care Statistics, UK, pp. 71–88.

Nilsson, B, Nåden, D and Lindström, UÅ 2008, 'The tune of want in the loneliness melody – loneliness experienced by people with serious mental suffering', *Scandinavian Journal of Caring Sciences*, vol. 22, pp. 161–169.

OECD 2014, *Society at a glance 2014: OECD social indicators*, OECD Publishing, viewed 3 December 2014, <dx.doi.org/10.1787/soc_glance-2014-en>.

Patel, V 2014, 'Why mental health matters to the globe', *Transcultural Psychiatry*, vol. 51, no. 6, pp. 777–789.

Patel, V and Kleinman, A 2003, 'Poverty and common mental disorders in developing countries', *Bulletin of the World Health Organization*, vol. 81, no. 8, pp. 609–615.

Patel, V, Flisher, AJ, Hetrick, S and McGorry, P 2007, 'Mental health of young people: A global public-health challenge', *The Lancet*, vol. 369, no. 9569, pp. 1302–1313.

Prasad-Ildes, R and Ramirez, E 2006, 'What CALD consumers say about mental illness prevention', *Australian e-Journal for the Advancement of Mental Health*, vol. 5, no. 2, viewed 1 April 2014, <amh.e-contentmanagement.com/archives/vol/5/issue/2/article/3332/what-cald-consumers-say-about-mental-illness>.

Procter, NG, Babakarkhil, A, Baker, A and Ferguson, M 2014, 'Mental health of people of migrant and refugee background', in N Procter, HP Hamer, D McGarry, RL Wilson and T Froggatt (eds.), *Mental health: A person-centred approach*, Cambridge University Press, Victoria, Australia, pp. 917–216.

Procter, N, Papadopoulos, I and McEvoy, M 2010, 'Editorial: Global economic crises and mental health', *Advances in Mental Health*, vol. 9, pp. 210–214.

Proudfoot, JG, Parker, GB, Benoit, M, Manicavasagar, V, Smith, M and Gayed, A 2009, 'What happens after diagnosis? Understanding the experiences of patients with newly-diagnosed bipolar disorder', *Health Expectations*, vol. 12, pp. 120–129.

Puri, BK and Treasaden, IH 2010, *Psychiatry: An evidence-based text*, Hodder Arnold, London.

Quinn, C and Browne, G 2009, 'Sexuality of people living with a mental illness: A collaborative challenge for mental health nurses', *International Journal of Mental Health Nursing*, vol. 18, no. 3, pp. 195–203.

Robjant, K, Hassan, R and Katona, C 2009, 'Mental health implications of detaining asylum seekers: Systematic review', *The British Journal of Psychiatry*, vol. 194, no. 4, pp. 306–312.

Roxburgh, EC and Roe, CA 2014, 'Reframing voices and visions using a spiritual model. An interpretative phenomenological analysis of anomalous experiences in mediumship', *Mental Health, Religion and Culture*, vol. 17, no. 6, pp. 641–653.

RU OK? 2014, 'RU OK? A conversation could change a life', viewed 1 December 2014, <www.ruok.org.au/>.

Sargent-Cox, K, Butterworth, P and Anstey, KJ 2011, 'The global financial crisis and psychological health in a sample of Australian older adults: A longitudinal study', *Social Science and Medicine*, vol. 73, no. 7, pp. 1105–1112.

Schnittker, J 2008, 'An uncertain revolution: Why the rise of a genetic model of mental illness has not increased tolerance', *Social Science and Medicine*, vol. 67, no. 9, pp. 1370–1381.

Schrank, B, Stanghellini, G and Slade, M 2008, 'Hope in psychiatry: A review of the literature', *Acta Psychiatrica Scandinavica*, vol. 118, no. 6, pp. 1–13.

Schweitzer, R, Melville, F, Steel, Z and Lacherez, P 2006, 'Trauma, post-migration living difficulties, and social support as predictors of psychological adjustment in resettled Sudanese refugees', *Australian and New Zealand Journal of Psychiatry*, vol. 40, no. 2, pp. 179–187.

Scott, D and Happell, B 2011, 'The high prevalence of poor physical health and unhealthy lifestyle behaviours in individuals with severe mental illness', *Issues in Mental Health Nursing*, vol. 32, pp. 589–597.

Stang, P, Frank, C, Yood, MU, Wells, K and Burch, S 2007, 'Impact of bipolar disorder: Results from a screening study', *Primary Care Companion Journal of Clinical Psychiatry*, vol. 9, no. 1, pp. 42–47.

Stansfeld, S, Weich, S, Clark, C, Boydell, J and Freeman, H 2008, 'Urban-rural differences, socio-economic status and psychiatric disorder', in H. Freeman and S. Stansfeld (eds), *The impact of the environment on psychiatric disorder*, Routledge, New York, pp. 80–126.

Steel, Z, Chey, T, Silove, D, Marnane, C, Bryant, RA and Van Ommeren, M 2009, 'Association of torture and other potentially traumatic events with mental health outcomes among populations exposed to mass conflict and displacement: A systematic review and meta-analysis', *The Journal of the American Medical Association*, vol. 302, no. 5, pp. 537–549.

Thoits, PA 2011, 'Mechanisms linking social ties and support to physical and mental health', *Journal of Health and Social Behavior*, vol. 52, pp. 145–161.

Thomasson, J 2014, 'Anxiety disorders', *Australian Nursing and Midwifery Journal*, vol. 21, no. 6, pp. 26–27.

Thompson, J, Brugha, T and Palmer, B 2009, 'Eating disorders', in S McManus, H Meltzer, T Brugha, P Bebbington and R Jenkins (eds), *Adult psychiatric morbidity in England, 2007: Results of a household survey*, The Health and Social Care Information Centre, Social Care Statistics, UK, pp. 135–149.

Viron, MJ and Stern, TA 2010, 'The impact of serious mental illness on health and healthcare', *Psychosomatics*, vol. 51, no. 6, pp. 458–465.

Ware, NC, Hopper, K, Tugenberg, T, Dickey, B and Fisher, D 2007, 'Connectedness and citizenship: Redefining social integration', *Psychiatric Services*, vol. 58, no. 4, pp. 469–474.

Whiteford, HA, Degenhardt, L, Rehm, J, Baxter, AJ, Alize, JF, Erskine, HE, Charlson, FJ, Norman, RE, Flaxman, AD, Johns, N, Burstein, R, Murray, CJL and Vos, T 2013, 'Global burden of disease attributable to mental and substance use disorders: Findings from the Global Burden of Disease Study 2010', *The Lancet*, vol. 382, no. 9904, pp. 1575–1586.

WHO (World Health Organization) 2005, *WHO resource book on mental health, human rights and legislation: Stop exclusion, dare to care*, WHO, Geneva.

WHO 2012, *Risks to mental health: An overview of vulnerabilities and risk factors*, WHO, Geneva.

WHO 2013, *Global and regional estimates of violence against women: Prevalence and health effects of intimate partner violence and non-partner sexual violence*, WHO, Geneva.

WHO 2014a, *Gender and women's mental health*, viewed 3 December 2014, <www.who.int/mental_health/prevention/genderwomen/en/>.

WHO 2014b, *Mental disorders. Fact sheet N°396*, viewed 3 December 2014, <www.who.int/mediacentre/factsheets/fs396/en/>.

WHO 2014c, *Mental health: strengthening our response. Fact sheet N°220*, viewed 3 December 2014, <www.who.int/mediacentre/factsheets/fs220/en/>.

WHO 2014d, *Social determinats of health – social exclusion*, viewed 3 December 2014, <www.who.int/social_determinants/themes/socialexclusion/en/>.

WHO and Calouste Gulbenkian Foundation, 2014a, *Integrating the response to mental disorders and other chronic diseases in health care systems*, WHO, Geneva.

WHO and Calouste Gulbenkian Foundation, 2014b, *Social determinants of mental health*, WHO, Geneva.

WHO and Gulbenkian Global Mental Health Platform 2014, *Innovation in deinstitutionalization: A WHO expert survey*, WHO, Geneva.

Wilson, NJ and Cordier, R 2013, 'A narrative review of Men's Sheds literature: Reducing social isolation and promoting men's health and well-being', *Health and Social Care in the Community,* vol. 21, pp. 451–463.

World Bank 2014, *Measuring poverty overview*, viewed 3 December 2014, <www.worldbank.org/en/topic/measuringpoverty/overview#1>.

Yang, LH and Kleinman, A 2008, '"Face" and the embodiment of stigma in China: The cases of schizophrenia and AIDS', *Social Science and Medicine*, vol. 67, no. 3, pp. 398–408.

Young, SL and Ensing, DS 1999, 'Exploring recovery from the perspective of people with psychiatric disabilities', *Psychiatric Rehabilitation Journal*, vol. 22, no. 3, pp. 219–232.

Zubrick, S, Dudgein, P, Gee, G, Glaskin, B, Kelly, K, Paradies, Y, Scrine, C and Walker, R 2010, 'Social determinants of Aboriginal and Torres Strait Islander social and emotional wellbeing', in N Purdie, P Dudgeon and R Walker (eds), *Working together: Aboriginal and Torres Strait Islander mental health and wellbeing principles and practice*, Commonwealth of Australia, Canberra, pp. 75–90.

3 Mental health within different ethnic groups and minorities

Richard Mottershead, Vijaya Kumardhas and Charles Masulani Mwale

Introduction

This chapter will explore barriers and cultural beliefs that interfere with seeking help and the utilisation of mental health services by different ethnic groups and minorities. Intolerance of mental health issues, the power of stigma and shame, and religious beliefs within different ethnic groups and minorities will be discussed. Research undertaken by Conner et al. (2010) shows that ethnic minorities are noted to be intolerant of mental health problems and do not talk openly about mental health problems, and are therefore reluctant and embarrassed to seek help. Intolerance and the presence of stigma is affirmed by Higgins et al. (2007) who explain that in some cultures men with mental health illness are labelled as 'freaks' and female patients described as being 'possessed' and 'witches'.

   This chapter will specifically cover four main themes: cultural barriers, language, religion and how stigma, shame and fear can influence mental health. The experiences of health professionals and people with mental health issues will be explored in order to create an understanding of the idioms of distress, cultural constructions and explanatory health beliefs within the ethnic minorities.

This chapter will consider:

- The mental health challenges that are associated with engaging with different ethnic groups and minorities;
- The current understanding of specific challenges to mental health within different ethnic groups and minorities;
- The mental health care and support needs of different ethnic groups and minorities;
- The current understanding of specific barriers to mental health utilisation within different ethnic groups and minorities;
- Culturally endorsed coping strategies within different ethnic groups and minorities;
- The increased risks associated with mental health within ethnic groups and minorities.

Background

According to Suckling (2008), the black and minority ethnic (BME) population is made up of distinct groups with their own identity recognised by themselves and others. This refers to people of African, African Caribbean, Bangladeshi, Indian, East African, Asian, Pakistani, Chinese, Vietnamese, South Asian descent and white populations from Eastern Europe, Turkey, the Middle East and Ireland. Culture refers to the ideas, customs, and social behaviour of a particular people or society (Gary, 2005). This chapter will explore connections between the culture of ethnic minorities and mental health care in order to benefit Western mental health practitioners who serve the ethnic groups within their culturally diverse communities. Corrigan et al. (2004) argue that mental health remains imbued with connotations that serve as barriers to seeking help and treatment, whilst Gary (2005) states that the reasons why many people avoid the mental health treatment that they need are not fully understood.

Although O'Connor and Vandenberg (2005) highlight that health services must satisfy the needs of culturally diverse communities, Knifton (2012) points out that inconsistencies exist in both access to and quality of mental health care for ethnic minority groups, which leads to their under-utilisation. Choi and Gonzales (2005) reveal the most significant barriers to seeking mental health treatment in the ethnic minority as shame and guilt, cultural and language barriers, fear and distrust of the system and lack of information. Goodchild (2012) argues that language barriers can prevent people with mental health problems from accessing treatment, and O'Mahony and Donnelly (2007) identify that differing values and standards set by individuals help develop thinking or behaviour which may pose a barrier between health providers and service user. Donnelly (2006) had earlier stipulated that cultural values have been found to have an influence in the ethnic minorities' reaction to health and illness. In a study by Conner et al. (2010) it was noted that African Americans were significantly less likely to seek help for mental health problems and there was some suggestion that this specific group may be utilising informal strategies, such as religion and self-reliance, to cope with their psychological symptoms. Conner et al. (2010) further suggest that denial is also articulated as a barrier to accessing mental health services as people may not disclose, even resorting to lying to others and denying depression to themselves due to not wanting their family members to worry. Whaley and Hall (2009) state that religion is a dominant force in the lives of the majority of African Americans and has a significant effect on coping and help seeking when they have mental health problems. Within Middle Eastern culture it has been noted that mental health has been viewed as an evil spirit and, therefore, sufferers visit traditional healers for help (Goodchild, 2012). However, it has been acknowledged that mental health has a long history of considering religious beliefs as pathological, for example Freud's characterisation of religion as mass delusion and immature regression as cited in (O'Connor and Vandenberg, 2010).

Conner et al. (2010) in another study found that participants expressed fear in the Black community about repercussions associated with mental illness and seeking treatment or therapy, as this was associated with life time records and jeopardising job opportunities. Conner et al. (2010) further highlight that African Americans received substandard care and treatment from mental health services when compared to their white counterparts, which instilled fear and made them afraid of the consequences that accompany admitting to having a mental health problem. Brown (2010) confirms negative attitudes towards mental health which have also been identified as a barrier to treatment and therapy engagement by some ethnic minorities. It has been highlighted that some ethnic communities are intolerant of mental health problems and have great difficulty in talking openly about these types of health problems (Conner et al., 2010). Intolerance of mental health problems is highly associated with stigma and shame attributes and how this affects their family as a whole and their status in their local communities.

Societies often have shared beliefs which can influence how mental health is viewed and dealt with: see Chapter 2 for further insights. It has been noted that the Western belief system has a common rationality whereby individuals who deviate from it may be defined as ill (O'Connor and Vandenberg, 2010). This, therefore, may result in delayed help-seeking for fear of social consequences and misdiagnosis of people from other cultures and beliefs because their behaviour may be misconstrued as bizarre when isolated from its cultural context (Sonethavilay et al., 2011). Hence, this leads to many people experiencing difficulties in accessing the health care system. Barrio, cited in Higgins et al. (2007), suggests that Western provision models of mental health may not be appropriate for people from ethnic minorities. In other countries, mental health services may even produce negative care and support outcomes for some people when their cultural values and attitudes are not understood. Lukoff et al. (1992) have reported that cultural insensitivity can have a negative impact when religious beliefs are examined out of the context of cultural frameworks which may then be considered pathological. In the 1990s, practitioners were recommended to use caution in utilising the Diagnostic and Statistical Manual of Mental Health Disorders, DSM-IV (now DSM-5, APA, 2013) without being culturally sensitive to the individual service users needs (Lukoff et al., 1992). There has, however, been a recognition of the short-fall within the DSM with considerable efforts now being placed on ensuring that the DSM-5 would become a more culturally sensitive diagnostic tool. This will be discussed further within the relevant section of this chapter.

In the UK, the government aim is to close the inequality gap within the BME populations. The growth of multiculturalism in the UK and other countries brings about cultural traits and practices in health which present complicated challenges to health provision and policies when striving to provide equitable access (POST, 2007). Research undertaken by Eichelman (2007) suggests that psychiatry and mental health professionals have started to employ a more holistic approach, which takes into account religion and spirituality. Evidence suggests that there is now some acceptance of what has been perceived as anti-religion by psychiatrists (Eichelman, 2007). In addition, in its Guiding Statement on Recovery the National Institute of Mental Health in England (2005) state in Guiding Principles III and XI for the delivery of recovery-oriented mental health services that service users' culture should be understood for them to recover more quickly. This report stresses the consideration of a holistic approach which includes psychological, emotional, spiritual, physical and social needs.

Cultural issues

Conner et al. (2010) identified cultural beliefs as one of the barriers to treatment and therapy in the ethnic minorities, stating that some black minorities do not tolerate individuals suffering from any forms of mental health. It has been debated widely that people from ethnic minorities do not talk openly about their mental health issues, this being partly due to the belief that this personal information is confidential to the sufferer (Thompson and Bazile, 2004; Conner et al., 2010). Thompson and Bazile (2004) also suggested that this could be due to the fact that some ethnic minority families believe they are able to cope with the person's mental health issues and should be able to deal with these problems themselves and without having to involve any outsiders. Shim et al. (2009) further suggest that some people are often uncomfortable when sharing personal information with people from different cultural backgrounds. Gary (2005) has reported that a mental health diagnosis in some ethnic minorities can affect family reputations, status in the community and may even compromise relationships with their neighbours. Dastjerdi et al. (2012) highlighted that people who do access mental health services are sometimes left with no option but to engage with outsiders as third party interpreters are often needed, especially when language becomes a significant barrier. Within the United States, it has been noted that such internalising mental health concerns are linked to the way 'Black folks' are raised (Conner et al, 2010). The authors give an example of a participant in their study who responded to a researcher and said 'that's the way us Black people were brought up, what goes on in your house stays within as a family secret'.

Not surprisingly, people will attempt not to disclose some of their issues, purposely misconstrue their symptoms, decline to answer some questions and deliberately give wrong responses to save face in community (Dastjerdi et al., 2012). Thompson et al (2004) suggest that mental health problems are viewed as a significant sign of weakness in the ethnic minorities and therefore a great many people are reluctant to seek help and are most likely to disengage from services.

To meet this identified short-fall within the DSM-5 a working group was established with the aim of creating a research agenda for at that time the proposed DSM-5 (Kupfer et al., 2002). The American Psychiatric Association (APA, 2013) aimed to improve the diagnosis and care for people of all backgrounds with a specific focus on incorporating a greater cultural sensitivity throughout the manual. As highlighted by Sonethavilay et al. (2011) the way that different cultures access health care systems can vary greatly and throughout the DSM-5 development process the working groups sought to utilise culturally determined criteria so that they would be more equitable across different cultures (APA, 2013). As an example, the DSM-5 addresses cultural concepts of distress, exploring methods in which different cultures explain symptoms. The American Psychiatric Association (2013) has further created a cultural formulation interview guide which aims to support health practitioners to assess cultural factors influencing a person's perspectives of their symptoms and provide treatment/therapy options.

Language

The second theme identified as a barrier is language. Effective communication is imperative when engaging with people in mental health treatment or therapy, especially during initial contact and when starting to develop some rapport (Atdjian and Vega, 2005). According to Dastjerdi et al. (2012) and Shim et al. (2009) language is the most prominent barrier that impedes access to and provision of mental health services and hinders the development of therapeutic alliances between professionals and service users. Bartlett et al. (2011) further suggest that language barriers have led to increased levels of psychopathology, misdiagnoses and an unclear understanding of symptoms when care givers do not speak the same language as the service user. Bartlett et al. (2011) go on to clarify that it is difficult for a person to explain their concerns and needs to health care providers if they have limited English proficiency, and this then hinders them from knowing how the health care system works. It was reported that in Canada, Iranian people became so frustrated with language and communication difficulties that this led to miscommunication and misunderstanding and they stopped seeking help (Dastjerdi et al., 2012). This led to a reduction in visiting doctors, not following recommended treatment and, ultimately, led to getting help from informal resources which in some cases resulted in critical situations. It has been reported that interpreters are not always used in clinical practice and this then may lead to less translation of cultural context (Atdjian and Vega, 2005). People seeking mental health services thrive on comfortable discussions with service providers, but this is clearly unachievable if professionals do not understand a person's language and cannot communicate effectively (Donnelly et al., 2011). Evidence suggests that while a little effort to speak a person's language by health professionals has some positive outcomes and makes the person feel valued, respected and relaxed during interactions, it is not a satisfactory solution (Bartlett et al., 2011). In some countries communication problems are becoming less of an issue as more of the younger generation are fluent in English and most people are registered with doctors from their own backgrounds (Panos and Panos, 2000). Dastjerdi et al. (2012) have described how some Iranian people in Canada were reluctant to learn the native language and preferred to locate an Iranian doctor in order to be able to communicate competently.

Trusted bilingual family members or trained interpreters are important as resources available to people who have language barriers and they are shown to facilitate self-disclosure if the cultural norm is to allow more disclosure of mental health issues (Bauer and Alegria, 2010; Dastjerdi et al., 2012). Cultural competency is believed to be enhanced by utilising interpreters, although they tend to be the gatekeepers of the information, selecting what information to convey by drawing their personal agendas and beliefs into interactions (Sonethavilay et al., 2011; Dastjerdi et al., 2012). This could be because the interpreters might be uncomfortable discussing issues such as sexuality or may want to minimise or exaggerate pathology (Sonethavilay et al., 2011). Some ethnic minorities feel disempowered by communication barriers and may sometimes resort to their family and friends as sources of information (Dastjerdi et al., 2012). Donnelly et al. (2011) state that using family members as interpreters can be detrimental as it fails to give out the exact message due to family involvement in their family member's situation and could potentially make things worse. Donnelly et al. (2011) also identified that some prefer not to ask their partners to be their interpreters as they believe they would use their mental health status against them to exert power over their marital relationships. This then leads to a person's preference for professional interpreters, which ensures to at least some degree that their information will remain confidential (Dastjerdi et al., 2012). Tribe and Lane (2009) argue that using interpreters is beneficial to the health services and also cost effective, as the cost of educating and training them is less than that of misdiagnosis or lack of treatment or therapy until a medical crisis happens.

Religion

Whaley and Hall (2009) suggest that religious themes can be interpreted as an indication of strong cultural beliefs. It is dominant in African Americans and has a significant impact on coping behaviours and influences help-seeking for mental health problems. Gearing et al. (2010) stress that health professionals may benefit from assessing whether their own beliefs, religion and spirituality might interfere with their judgements. Within the UK, the Nursing and Midwifery Council's Standards for Pre-Registration Nurse Education (NMC, 2010) highlighted the need for the general public to trust newly qualified graduate nurses to engage with them and their family or carers within their cultural environment in an accepting and anti-discriminatory manner free from harassment and exploitation. Graduate nurses must now demonstrate and evidence an understanding of how culture and religion can impact on illness and disability (NMC, 2010).

Conner et al. (2010) and O'Mahony and Donnelly (2007) highlight that some ethnic minorities usually turn to God for their mental health problems, emphasise their relationship with God and believe in healing through the Bible and prayer. Conner et al. (2010) reported that people believe in giving their burdens to God, trusting in the guidance of the holy spirit as they believe God is elevated above the doctor. For example, within the Hindu faith there is evidence of guidance being sought from astrology and intervention in issues relating to mental distress (O'Mahony and Donnelly, 2007). Conner et al. (2010) and Whaley and Hall (2009) also highlight that people turn to religion as a coping strategy when they lose faith in mental health services. Whitley et al. (2006) established that West Indians in Montreal were reluctant to access mental health services as they believed in the curative power of non-medical interventions, notably God, and to a lesser extent traditional folk medication. Goodchild (2012) argues that ethnic minorities are more likely to consult their ethnic group leaders and other informal support systems rather than health professionals. Donnelly et al. (2011) suggest that religious beliefs are held because these are a vital support in coping with mental health problems and that self-dialogue through prayer provides a person with a source of hope, reconciliation and strength which in turn improves their mental wellbeing. Donnelly et al. (2011) go on to argue that although spiritual beliefs can be a source of strength they can also present barriers to seeking mental health provision. Mohr and Huguelet (2004) suggest that religion can offer solutions to human insufficiencies and can be a protective factor against suicide in people with schizophrenia. O'Mahony and Donnelly (2007) have reported that faith and spirituality can have a positive impact and help in reducing anger, coping with traumas and assisting in clear and positive thinking as well as providing a source of personal peace.

Bal (1989) argues that there is no evidence that recourse is made to traditional healers instead of formal services as it appears that where help is sought from these sources it is usually in addition to Western medicine instead of it. In contrast, Huguelet and Koenig (2009) debate that being 'over spiritual' can be detrimental as it sometimes prevents people from accessing mental health services. Conner et al. (2010) further argue that psychiatrists are more likely to believe that religion and spirituality can have a negative impact on their patients.

Religious practices have been linked to and mistaken for religious delusions although religiosity is not necessary for their development (O'Connor and Vandenberg, 2005). It has been noted that religious delusions are often persecutory, by the devil or demons, or grandiose, believing to be God, Jesus or an angel (Wilson, 1998). There is some evidence of practitioner bias towards their own faith and cultures. For example, Whaley and Hall (2009) indicate that health professionals gave lower ratings of psychopathology to patients processing the religious beliefs of Catholicism and Mormonism, but religious content reflecting views of Black Muslims were judged to represent severe psychopathology. Davies et al. (2001) argue that health professionals assess the extent of distress linked with the existence of symptoms, particularly hallucinations, in order to determine whether religious beliefs in psychotic symptoms are non-pathological.

In conclusion, Whaley and Hall (2009) have reported that the Structural Clinical Interview for DSM education and training may prevent bias related to religious themes and other cultural beliefs.

According to O'Connor and Vandenberg (2010) this will enable health practitioners to assess beliefs on the basis of the relative social standing of the religions from which these are derived.

Stigma, shame and fear

It is important that more is understood about the complexities of stigma and shame when considering ethnic minorities and mental health. Stigma can generally be defined as having psychological and social attributes that can result in others experiencing fear, rejection, prejudice and evident discrimination (Shim et al., 2009). Steen and Jones (2014) have defined shame as 'a universal, adaptive and common emotional response to exposure of easily-hurt aspects of the self' (p. 1), and some people are more vulnerable to it than others (Wiklander et al., 2003). Steen and Jones (2013) in an earlier paper have described how shame within normal limits 'is a socially adaptive emotion and relates to the need to present a positive image of oneself to others by not transgressing established norms' (p. 5). Shame can give rise to self-criticism and this can lead to personal scornfulness without the necessity of the disapproval of others. To experience strong shame can be both socially isolating and emotionally tormenting (Steen and Jones, 2014). There is evidence to show that when people receive care in mental health settings this can lead to feelings of shame and stigma because of their situations (Jones and Crossley, 2008). The American Psychiatric Association (2000) suggests that when health professionals provide a psychiatric diagnosis such as schizophrenia and paranoia then stigma is a possible outcome. Thompson and Bazile (2004) further state that people who had no prior experience with mental health services believed that the stigma of mental illness together with the shame and embarrassment linked to it was a significant barrier to seeking treatment. Hines-Martin et al. (2004) suggest that the BME community may have negative attitudes towards mental health and some are reluctant in seeking professional help. However, Diala et al. (2001) and Shim et al. (2009) do not agree with this and instead state that people from the ethnic minority are less likely to feel embarrassed about mental health problems and would 'definitely' seek help from services. Gary (2005), Shim et al. (2009) and Conner et al. (2010) address the notion of the ethnic minority suffering double stigma due to their group affiliation and getting a diagnosis of mental health problems as their communities are less accepting. Conner et al. (2010), Gary (2005) and Shim et al. (2009) go on to highlight that the stigma associated with mental health deters people from most populations, but particularly from minority populations, from accessing mental health treatment and can lead to mortalities and morbidities that could have been prevented and treated. However, Corrigan et al. (2004) and Gary (2005) suggest that even if treatment is sought many are not compliant with the treatment regime and will disengage from mental health services. Knifton (2012) argues that the public continues to link danger and unpredictability with severe and enduring mental illness such as schizophrenia and psychosis, which leads to social distance and isolation. However, Conner et al. (2010) present an argument against this by identifying internalised stigma where an individual with a mental illness internalises the public's beliefs, either real or perceived, and applies them to how they feel.

In some cases, admissions and restrictive treatments under the Mental Health Act 2007 (as cited in Care Quality Commission, 2011) are enforced within ethnic minorities and this can instil fear that compulsory treatment might lead to a lifetime record and interfere with career prospects (Fernando, 2003; Conner et al., 2010). Compulsory admissions and restrictive measures can be attributed to fear amongst health practitioners and the diagnostic process which takes little account of cultural variations (Knifton, 2012). Cochrane and Sashidharan (1995) found that black people suffer similar mental disorders as their white counterparts but receive alternative forms of care or may not gain access to care as they may find it aversive.

Stigma can exist amongst families who in turn can be stigmatised in the community, leading to shame, guilt and loss of face along with secrecy about conditions to friends, family and health services (Yeung, 2004). Providers who engage with cultures from firm communities and families should consider the impact and/ importance of stigma (Knifton, 2012).

Families can also become affected as they try to defend against feelings of shame along with stigmatisation caused by their connection with a family member's mental illness. Stigma and shame might therefore impede a person's recovery and difficulties can be passed on across generations within families (Steen and Jones, 2013).

Conclusions

Inconsistencies exist in both access to and quality of mental health care for ethnic minority groups, which consequently leads to their under-utilisation. Literature suggests that there is insufficient guidance for culturally competent workers, which hinders work with people from different cultural and ethnic backgrounds. Lack of guidance often puts strains on the relationship between service users and health professionals. Western models of mental health care may not be applicable to people from ethnic minorities and other countries and may even produce negative outcomes. More research is needed to understand the cultural and social factors that influence health practitioner approaches as people with mental health problems are still frequently stigmatised. The development of a more culturally sensitive DSM-5 (2013) and the utilisation of a cultural formulation interview may help to ensure a rich data stream for future studies. As stigma, shame and fear are recognised barriers which take several forms, often relating to underlying cultural and religious beliefs, for example framing mental health problems as a punishment from God or a sin caused by spirits or jinn. Assessment of people's culture and beliefs is paramount for diagnosis and treatment or therapy planning. Religion is a dominant force in the lives of many ethnic minority groups and evidence suggests that it has a significant impact on coping when they have mental health problems.

Recommendations for future practice provision

Cultural competence should be incorporated within undergraduate and continuing professional development health and social care programmes in order to prepare future practitioners to provide integrated complex and bespoke care for diverse populations.

Clinicians should be aware that holding religious beliefs, even when having a more pronounced presentation within the service user's life, may be the result of seeking solace rather than a delusional belief as classified in the Diagnostic and Statistical Manual of Mental Health Disorders (APA, 2013).

Service users in remission should be referred to informal support networks or third sector charitable organisations so they may share experiences, remain concordant with treatment and alleviate their feelings of stigma, fear and shame.

Mental health services should have continuous access to interpreters for linguistic and sign language needs.

Case study 3.1

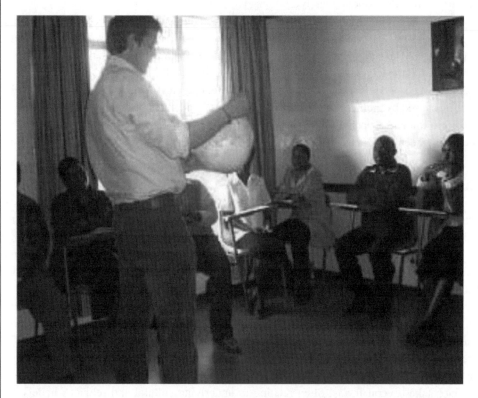

Figure 3.1 Facilitating learning and understanding about mental health and wellbeing

Mr Singh, an Indian national who has been in the country for three months working as an Engineer for an Indian contractor. Within this period he has experienced several cultural shocks and changes, which he feels to be quite strange. He is failing to cope with his present situation and wishes to return home. Coming to this country was initially a relief from the personal distress he went through in his own country due to family issues and a divorce, but he has now received news from relatives that Sheriffs in his own country are about to impound his property for maintenance to his former wife and children. His new wife has told him that as a man he has to be bold and she sees these problems as minor but he is becoming more and more depressed. His employers insist that he has to serve for at least two years, otherwise he has to pay back the funds they have invested in him. With on-going stress and continued pressure he has been having sleepless nights and losing interest in the things he used to enjoy and is becoming more and more withdrawn. Following a lot of persuasion from a workmate, he consults a Liberian psychologist who works at a nearby clinic, but this psychologist only speaks French and charges exorbitantly. He feels that he cannot trust any interpreter and is now resigned to agreeing with his wife that he should deal with his problems alone.

Case Study 3.2

Mrs Kumar is a 28-year old woman who has only received primary education and speaks only Bihari (an Indian) language. She has been married for 8 years and has no children and resides in the UK. Mrs Kumar is from a middle class family and her husband works as a manager in a cotton mill.

Ten months ago, Mrs Kumar, suddenly became overzealous in her religion and started performing pujas (prayers) throughout the night. She has stated that she is a Goddess and any women in need can come to her and they will receive help. Mrs Kumar has also started to exhibit unusual behavior such as dancing in front of the image of a deity god. People from the neighborhood have started coming to her house for the puja, and see her as a holy person. Her abnormal behavior is becoming violent and aggressive and now her family members have started calling her a crazy, mad lady. Mrs Kumar was admitted to an acute psychiatric care unit after she became violent towards her husband, running up and down the street claiming that her husband had killed her baby.

She has been diagnosed as experiencing an acute psychotic attack and was prescribed antipsychotic drugs. The mental health team could not communicate with her as she speaks only Bihari. Her husband was visiting her once a week and with family members once in a while as the hospital was far away from her home. Mrs Kumar's husband travelled by public transport and never disembarked from the bus in front of the hospital but two stops away and then walked to the hospital. He was afraid that if people knew his wife was mentally ill his family reputation and status in the community would be affected and his family would be stigmatized. So he continued doing this for the first few months, then, gradually, Mrs Kumar's husband started reducing his visits to see his wife and her family members never visited her at the hospital. Mrs Kumar kept crying saying that she wanted to go home. However, she has been disowned by her family and they refuse to take any responsibility for her and would not allow her to return home. She remains in the mental health unit and is managed by antipsychotic drugs. Plans to re-engage with her family are on-going and support from social services and local community groups is being planned. This case is not going to be easily resolved and many challenges for the mental health team are foreseen.

Case Study 3.3

Ms Hajjar, a 20-year old Arabic student is studying in the 2nd year of the Bachelor of Science (B.Sc) degree program. She lives in the UAE with her parents and nine other siblings. She is the sixth child having five older brothers and three sisters younger than her.

Past History: *A few months after Ms Hajjar enrolled at the university she started showing abnormal behavior. She become inattentive and not concentrating when attending lectures. She began to miss lectures, not hand assignments in on-time and thus getting low grades. She was*

(continued)

(continued)

also demonstrating distractive behavior, such as fidgeting and laughing without any reason when she did attend lectures. One night she was found lying in the entrance of the University premises and a Civil Defense Officer accompanied Ms Hajjar to the emergency department. Her vital signs and physical investigations were normal and she was discharged. In the meantime, Ms Hajjar has expressed to her friends that she wants to end her life because her boyfriend has decided to end their relationship. Shortly after this disclose [sic] she attempts to commit suicide by taking a caffeine drink with several Paracetamol tablets. In addition, some students have now reported that she has threatened to jump from the first floor of the university building. A friend has also prevented her from leaping in front of speeding vehicles and a security guard has found her lying under a parked car. Her parents were informed of these events and they were asked if their daughter could be taken to a mental health unit for further assessment and treatment. The Arabic translator was asked to give this information to her parents. Her parents were shocked and could not believe her behavior. However, they refused to take her to a mental health unit. Instead they chose to take her to their own physician as they believed she was weak or some family enemies had performed black magic on her. After a physical checkup by the physician she was referred to a psychiatrist who diagnosed a 'depressive psychosis with mood liability'. Despite her parents' objections Ms Hajjar was prescribed antidepressant medication. Her academic performance started to improve whilst she complied with the treatment.

After a year Ms Hajjar stopped taking her prescribed antidepressants and relapsed. She now refuses to go for any follow-up as her family fear that if their friends and neighbours know of her illness, then no one will marry her due to the stigma and shame of mental illness in Arab culture. She is once again not performing well in her studies. After several discussions with her parents she has now been referred back to the mental health unit for further management. Ms Hajjar says that mental illness means that she is insane, her family will neglect her and she would be distant from Allah as she is refusing to co-operate in her care management.

Reflective exercise

- After reading this chapter and case studies, can you describe and think about some of the barriers and cultural beliefs that would stop a person from an ethnic group seeking help from mental health services?
- Can you identify the increased risks associated with mental health within ethnic groups and minorities?
- Can you think about how you would communicate with a person who speaks very little English and what resources would you be able to use to enable you to communicate?
- Consider how your own personal biases and beliefs may affect your decision making when assessing a person with a mental health problem from an ethnic minority group and how you will recognise these and provide holistic care to meet their needs.

References

American Psychiatric Association (1994) *Diagnostic and statistical manual of mental health disorders.* 4th ed. Washington, DC: American Psychiatric Association.

American Psychiatric Association (2000) *Diagnostic and statistical manual of mental disorders.* 4th ed. text rev. Washington, DC: American Psychiatric Association.

American Psychiatric Association (2013) *Diagnostic and statistical manual of mental health disorders.* 5th ed. Washington, DC: American Psychiatric Association.

Atdjian, S. Vega, W.A. (2005) Disparities in mental health treatment in US racial and ethnic minority groups: implications for psychiatrists. *Psychiatric Services.* 56 (12), 1600–1602.

Bal, S. S. (1989) *The cross cultural symptomatology of psychological distress.* Unpublished doctoral dissertation. University of Birmingham.

Bartlett, R. Williams, A. Lucas, R. (2011) A common language is so basic. *Mental Health Nursing.* 32, 608–609.

Bauer, A.M. Alegria, M. (2010) Impact of patient language proficiency and interpreter services use on the quality of psychiatric care: a systematic review. *Psychiatric Services.* 61 (8), 765–773.

Brown, C. (2010) Depression, race and treatment seeking behaviour and attitudes. *Journal of Community Psychology.* 38, 350–368.

Care Quality Commission (2011) *Monitoring the Mental Health Act in 2010/11*: Annual report on the exercise of its functions in keeping under review the operation of the Mental Health Act 1983. Care Quality Commission, Newscastle upon Tyne, NE1 4PA.

Choi, N.G. Gonzales, J.M. (2005) Geriatric mental health clinicians' perceptions of barriers and contributors to retention of older minorities in treatment: an exploratory study. *Clinical Gerontologist.* 28, 3–25.

Cochrane, R. Sashidharan, S. P. (1995) *Mental health and ethnic minorities: a review of the literature and implications for services.* Birmingham: University of Birmingham and Northern Birmingham Mental Health Trust.

Conner, K. Copeland, V. Grote, K. Rosen, D. Albert, S. McMurray, M. L. Reynolds, C.F. Brown, C. Koeske, G. (2010) Barriers to treatment and culturally endorsed coping strategies among depressed African-American older adults. *Aging and Mental Health.* 14 (8), 971–983.

Corrigan, P.W. Markowitz, F.E Watson, A.C. (2004) Structural levels of mental illness stigma and discrimination. *Schizophrenia Bulletin.* 30, 481–491.

Dastjerdi, M. Olson, K. Ogilvie, K. (2012) A study of Iranian immigrants' experiences of accessing Canadian health care services: a grounded theory. *International Journal of Equity in Health.* 11, 55.

Davies, M.F. Griffin, M. Vice, S. (2001) Affective reactions to auditory hallucinations in psychotic, evangelical, and control groups. *British Journal of Clinical Psychology.* 40.

Diala, C.C. Muntaner, C. Walrath, K. Nickerson, K. LaVeist, T. Leaf, P. (2001) Racial/ethnic differences in attitudes toward seeking professional mental health services. *American Journal of Public Health.* 91, 805–807.

Donnelly, T. (2006) The health-care practices of Vietnamese-Canadian women: cultural influences on breast and cervical cancer screening. *Canadian Journal of Nursing Research.* 38, 82–101.

Donnelly, T. Hwang, J.J. Este, D. Ewashen, C. Adair, C. Clinton, M. (2011) If I was going to kill myself, I wouldn't be calling you. I am asking for help: challenges influencing immigrant and refugee women's mental health. *Mental Health Nursing.* 32, 279–290.

Eichelman, B. (2007) Religion, spirituality and medicine. *American Journal of Psychiatry* 164 (12), 1774–1775.

Fernando, S. (2003) *Cultural diversity, mental health and psychiatry. The struggle against racism.* Hove, UK: Brunner-Routledge.

Gary, F.A. (2005) Stigma: barrier to mental health care among ethnic minorities. *Mental Health Nursing.* 26, 979–999.

Gearing, R.E. Alonzo, D. Smolak, A. McHugh, K. Harmon, S. Baldwin, S. (2010) Association of religion with delusions and hallucinations in the context of schizophrenia: limitations for engagement and enhancement. *Schizophrenia Research.* 1–14.

Goodchild, S. (2012) Lifting the clouds. *Mental Health Today.* 8–9.

Higgins, L. Dey-Ghatak, P. Davey, G. (2007) Mental health nurses' experiences of schizophrenia rehabilitation in China and India: a preliminary study. *International Mental Health Journal of Nursing.* 16, 22–27.

Hines-Martin, V.P. Usui, W.S. Furr, A. (2004) A comparison of influences on attitudes towards mental health services in an African-American and White community. *Journal of National Black Nurses Association.* 15, 17–22.

Huguelet, P. Koenig, H.G. (2011) Religion and spirituality in psychiatry. *Mental Health, Religion and Culture.* 14 (1), 79–81.

Jones, A. Crossley, D. (2008) In the mind of another: shame and acute psychiatric inpatient care: an exploratory study in progress. *Journal of Psychiatric and Mental Health Nursing.* 15, 749–757.

Knifton, L. (2012) Understanding and addressing the stigma of mental illness with ethnic minority communities. *Health and Social Review.* 21 (3), 287–298.

Kupfer, D.J. First, M.B. Regier, D.A (2002) *A research agenda for the DSM 5.* Washington DC: American Psychiatric Association.

Lukoff, D. Lu, F. Turner, R. (1992) Toward a more culturally sensitive DSM-IV: psychoreligious and psychospiritual problems. *Journal of Nervous and Mental Disease.* 180 (11), 673–682.

Mohr, S. Huguelet, P. (2004) The relationship between schizophrenia and religion and its implications for care. *Swiss Med Weekly.* 134, 369–376.

NIMHE (2005) *Guiding statement on recovery.* http://studymore.org.uk/nimherec.pdf (accessed 01/09/15).

Nursing and Midwifery Council (2010) *Standards for pre-registration nursing education.* London: NMC.

O'Connor, S. Vandenberg, B. (2005) Psychosis or faith? Clinicians' assessment of religious beliefs. *Journal of Consulting and Clinical Psychology.* 73 (4), 610–616.

O'Connor, S. Vandenberg, B (2010) Differentiating psychosis and faith: the role of social norms and religious fundamentalism. *Mental Health, Religion and Culture.* 13 (2), 171–186.

O'Mahony, J.T. Donnelly, T.T (2007) The influence of culture on immigrant women's mental health care experiences from the perspectives of mental care providers. *Issues in Mental Health Nursing.* 28, 453–471.

Panos, P.T. Panos, A.J. (2000) A model for a cultural sensitive assessment of patients in health care settings. *Social Work Health Care.* 31, 49–62.

Parliamentary Office of Science and Technology (2007) Ethnicity and health. *Postnote.* 276 (Jan).

Shim, R.S. Compton, M.T. Rust, G. Druss, B.G. Kaslow, N.J. (2009) Race-ethnicity as a predictor of attitudes toward mental health treatment seeking. *Psychiatric Services.* 60 (10), 1336–1341.

Sonethavilay, H. Miyabayishi, I. Komori, A. Onimuru, M. Washio, M. (2011) Mental health needs and cultural barriers that lead to misdiagnosis of South Asia refugees: a review. *International Medical Journal.* 18 (3), 169–171.

Steen, M. Jones, A. (2013) Maternal mental health: stigma and shame. *The Practising Midwife.* 16 (6), 5.

Steen, M. Jones, A. (2014) The burden of stigma and shame. *Midwives.* 2, 5–6.

Suckling, R. (2008) *Black and minority ethnic population mental health needs in Doncaster.* Retrieved from www.rdash.nhs.uk/ . . . /Black-Minority-Ethnic-Population-Mental-Health-Needs-Assessment-in-Doncaster (accessed 01/09/15).

Thompson, K. Melia, K.M. Boyd, K.M (2005) *Nursing ethics.* 4th Ed. London: Elsevier Livingstone.

Thompson, S. Bazile, A. (2004) African Americans' perceptions of psychotherapy and psychotherapists. *Professional Psychology: Research and Practice.* 35(1), 19–26.

Tribe, R. Lane, P. (2009) Working with interpreters across language and culture in mental health. *Journal of Mental Health Nursing.* 18 (3), 233–241.

Whaley, A.L. Hall, B.N. (2009) Effects of cultural themes in psychotic symptoms on the diagnosis of schizophrenia in African Americans. *Mental Health, Religion and Culture.* 12 (5), 457–471.

Whitley, R. Kirmayer, L.J. Groleau, D. (2006) Understanding immigrants' reluctance to use mental health services: a qualitative study from Montreal. *Canadian Journal of Psychiatry.* 51 (4), 205–209.

Wiklander, M., Samuelsson, M. Åsberg, M. (2003) Shame reactions after suicide attempt. *Scandinavian Journal of Caring Sciences.* 17 (3), 293–300.

Wilson, E.O. (1998) *Consilience: the unity of knowledge.* New York: Alfred A. Knopf.

Yeung, E. (2004) *Improving accessibility to mental health services for Chinese people.* Liverpool, UK: Merseyside Health Action Zone.

4 Mental health during pregnancy and early parenthood

Mary Steen and Ben Green

Introduction

During pregnancy and the first year following childbirth, anxiety and stress are a common phenomenon and can stand alone or present as co-morbidities and predispose women to other mental health problems (Steen and Steen 2014). Pregnant women and new mothers throughout the world are susceptible to mental health problems that can have adverse affects on their physical health and also be detrimental to the health and well-being of their infant, which can lead to bonding and attachment issues (Steen et al. 2013). Women who suffer from an existing mental health illness are at an increased risk of relapse during pregnancy. Birth trauma can also be a trigger for a mental health problem and some women can develop anxiety and stress, and suffer post-traumatic stress disorder (PTSD), which may lead to maternal exhaustion and depression. In severe cases mental health problems can lead to maternal suicide and even infanticide (CMACE 2011).

This chapter will focus on highlighting the needs of pregnant women and mothers who are at risk of developing or have an existing mental health problem. The chapter will be introduced by a brief exploration of how a pregnant woman's or new mother's background, life style, environment and fear of being judged and perceived by society as a 'bad mother' can affect her general health and well-being and contribute to mental health problems. This will be followed by a discussion regarding the evidence and recognition of mild to moderate mental health problems such as anxiety and stress, phobias, panic symptoms, baby blues, antenatal depression, postnatal depression (including paternal), eating disorders, links with alcohol and substance use; and then more severe mental health conditions such as puerperal psychosis, schizophrenia and bipolar disorder will be covered. The implications of taking prescribed medication during pregnancy and when breast feeding will be considered. In addition, building resilience as a preventative measure and the benefits of social support and psychological therapies will be discussed. Disguised real life case scenarios will be included to give the reader an insight into some pregnant women's and mothers' experiences of mental health problems and the care and support given to help these women to develop coping strategies and improve their mental health and well-being.

This chapter will consider:

- The risks of mental health problems during pregnancy, childbirth and in the first year following birth;
- The evidence and recognition of mild, moderate and severe mental health problems;
- The care and support needs of women who are at risk of developing or have an existing mental health problem during the childbirth continuum;
- How mental health problems during pregnancy and the transition to motherhood can affect partners and other members of the family;
- The increased risks of mental health problems for fathers during this time period;
- The influence of social determinants and expectations during pregnancy and when becoming a mother.

Mental health and motherhood

Socio-economic and life events

There are several socio-economic and life events that can have an impact on a pregnant woman's health and well-being status. Childhood experiences, relationships with family members, friends and own peer group can affect how a woman perceives herself. Her personality and life style behaviours also play a part as do personal relationships with a partner. Family violence, sexual abuse and poverty are known risk factors that can trigger mental health issues and being a single mother and a teenager can increase the risk further (Steen et al. 2013). Young deprived mothers are more likely to misuse drugs and alcohol and have safeguarding issues to contend with (National Treatment Agency for Substance Misuse 2010). Many of these pregnant women live stressful and disorganised lives. During pregnancy they may conceal or minimise their alcohol and drug use, often fearing that their baby will be placed in care, which often is the outcome. CMACE (2011) reported a case where a young mother who was a substance user committed suicide shortly after her baby was placed in care. Guilt, shame, loss and being judged contributed to her poor mental health state.

Mental health intervention

It is noteworthy that up to 16 per cent of women may require a mental health intervention during the antenatal and postnatal period (NICE 2008). There is some evidence that women who are substance users and who attend treatment programmes are likely to have better antenatal care and better general health than those who do not (National Treatment Agency for Substance Misuse 2010). NICE (2007a) recommend that a stepped care level of treatment is adopted and this be incorporated in a mental health care pathway, which facilitates referral to appropriate services. Psychological therapies have been demonstrated to be effective in the treatment of mild to moderate mental health problems (NICE 2007a) but the Improving Access to Psychological Therapies (IAPT) strategy indicates a lower threshold for access to women in pregnancy (IAPT 2009). Many vulnerable women will not attend for antenatal care. It is, therefore, vitally important that maternity services work closely and share information with the woman's General Practitioner and addiction services to identify these at risk women and then involve the mental health team to address associated mental health problems.

Motherhood

In today's society mothers are increasingly expected to invest heavily to enhance their child's physical, social, intellectual and emotional development; balancing their time, energy, finances and own physical and emotional health can take its toll (Kingdon 2009). Fear of being judged and perceived by society as a 'bad mother' can contribute to a woman's belief in her ability to mother. Second-wave feminist research during the 1960s and 1970s highlighted and advanced understanding of the linkages between gender and mental health, with women much more likely than men to suffer from anxiety and depression (Busfield 2010). In particular, Gavron (1968) identified how the gender division of labour, where women are principally associated with the domestic sphere, impacts on women's mental health. Around the same time, Oakley (1979), in her seminal study of first time mothers, demonstrated the disjuncture between women's expectations of motherhood and their actual experiences. More recent research by Gattrell (2005) and Miller (2007) highlights the persistence of this disjunction, the realities of mothers' continued engagement in the labour force and their increasing agency in challenging how childbirth and motherhood should be, for example, medical discourse, natural childbirth discourse, the ideology of motherhood and intensive mothering discourse, in order to maintain their 'sanity'.

Some mothers from culturally and linguistically diverse (CALD) backgrounds are at increased risk of becoming socially isolated when not residing in their country of origin. Language barriers, lack of opportunities to integrate with local communities and different cultural and traditional aspects of motherhood can all play a part in predisposing these women to mental health problems. Mental health problems are often hidden and a taboo subject in many cultures around the globe. Stigma and shame is associated with mental health and this can contribute to pregnant women and new mothers not seeking help and support (Steen and Jones 2013). It is, however, noteworthy that a recent review has reported that similar patterns of mental illness are prevalent in pregnant women and mothers residing in East Asia when compared with rates reported in Western countries (Schatz et al. 2012).

Balancing family life and work commitments can take its toll and affect general health and well-being and exacerbate mental health problems. That said, many women from various backgrounds can develop good coping strategies to maintain a good level of health and well-being regardless of what life throws at them; they take on the caretaker role of the family and adjust to motherhood without too many problems. There is emerging evidence that demonstrates that when a mother has good family support this helps her remain mentally well (Gjerdingen et al. 2009;

Stapleton et al. 2012). When family support is lacking she is vulnerable and can be susceptible to mental health problems. A recent study of low-income Mexican American families examined cortisol reactivity in infants born to mothers who had experienced stress during pregnancy and found an association between higher cortisol reactivity in infants and lower partner support during the pregnancy (Luecken et al. 2013).

Pregnancy, birth and becoming a mother are major life events that require good support and care for a woman to sustain good health and well-being status. CMACE (2011) recommend pre-conceptual counselling and care for women with a history of a mental health problems so that planning for adjustments can be made for pregnancy and following birth. There is also emerging evidence that a befriending approach and social support is beneficial (Darcy et al. 2011; Robinson et al. 2014). Steen (2007) reported that pregnant women and mothers who attended a maternal health and well-being community programme highly valued the opportunity of meeting others and the social support they received. There is evidence that local community peer support, sometimes referred to as 'community mothers' can be beneficial (Johnson et al. 2000; Molloy 2007). These local mothers are able to befriend and support other mothers who are feeling alone and isolated. Trust is developed and they are seen to be non-judgemental, approachable and know the reality of living in the local community. This is confirmed by further evidence reported by Robinson et al. (2014) who have demonstrated clear benefits to show how befriending and peer support help women to stay mentally well.

Women and mental health during the childbirth continuum

Anxiety and stress during pregnancy

Even though pregnancy is associated with a happy life event which is often planned but sometimes not, women can suffer from varying degrees of anxiety and stress. Fear of the unknown, past life events, current life events, changes to personal relationships, work related stress and a dissatisfaction with changing body image can contribute to some women having what can be classified as mild, moderate or severe anxiety and stress (Bergman et al. 2007; Lavender 2007; NICE 2007a). Prevalence rates may be under-estimated and variations have been reported to be between 8 and 24 per cent (Rubertsson et al. 2003; van Bussell et al. 2006),

Pregnant women in Western societies who suffer severe anxiety and stress are usually identified and referred to the specialist mental health team. In the UK, women who suffer mild to moderate anxiety and stress are usually cared for by a community midwife and the primary care team. These women are more difficult to identify and therefore it is vitally important that woman during their pregnancy have continuity of care and carer. Furber et al. (2009) conducted an exploratory study and interviewed pregnant women and three emerging themes were identified. The three themes that emerged were the cause of, and the impact of, ways of controlling their self-reported mild to moderate distress. This study demonstrated that past life events, previous childbirth experiences and current pregnancy worries contributed to anxiety and stress. Mild to moderate anxiety and stress often took over the women's lives and they used both positive and negative coping strategies to try and manage their anxiety and stress.

Midwives and other health professionals need to be alert to women's emotional and psycho-social well-being during pregnancy and will need to watch for signs and symptoms of anxiety and stress. The link between mental health and physical symptoms needs to be recognised. Anxiety and stress are associated with several cognitive, behavioural and autonomic symptoms (Steen and Steen 2014). Palpations, headaches, dizziness, restlessness, insomnia, gastric problems, urinary frequency and muscular tension and pain are often present and may be overlooked. Distinguishing between the normal transition of physical and emotional/psychological changes that occur during pregnancy and following birth and recognising episodes of anxiety and mild to moderate levels of depression is a challenge for health professionals (Robertson et al. 2004). In addition, raised cortisol levels in pregnancy due to anxiety and stress can increase the risk of hypertension, pre-eclampsia, premature labour and intra-uterine growth restriction (Field et al. 2010; Yu et al. 2013).

Routinely enquiring about how a woman is coping with her pregnancy and her support mechanisms will assist to identify women at risk of anxiety and stress and create an opportunity to offer additional care and support to meet their individual needs.

Building resilience for better maternal mental health

Local community support groups can help pregnant women to build confidence and resilience and this local support can continue following birth. The mental health charities Mind and the Mental Health Foundation in the UK recently developed a resilience triad model to help people remain mentally well. Recently, this resilience model has been piloted with pregnant women and vulnerable mothers who are at risk of developing mental health problems (Robinson et al. 2014). The evaluation report clearly demonstrates improved maternal mental health and well-being when the resilience triad model is used to facilitate local community care and support for pregnant women and new mothers. This triad model focuses on building resilience to mental health problems by assisting people to acquire a range of coping strategies, build self-esteem and confidence in

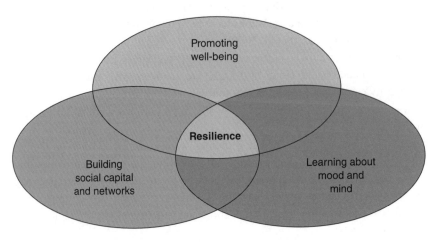

Figure 4.1 Striving for better maternal mental health

relation to a triad model which encompasses well-being, psychological therapies and social capital (Holloway 2013). Positive activities are advocated, such as exercising outdoors (for example, pram walks), building social networks (befriending) and increasing awareness of how to manage anxiety and stress based on principles of low intensity cognitive behavioural therapy (CBT) and mindfulness (Figure 4.1).

Holloway (2013) describes how 'resilience is not an inherent quality with which you are born and . . . not simply an ability to "bounce back"'. Resilience involves being able to face challenging circumstances whilst also maintaining a positive mental health status; it is an important life skill that enables a person to cope with the highs and lows of life and is closely associated to how confident a person is and their level of self-esteem. Developing skills and coping strategies to be resilient during pregnancy and when becoming a mother is essential for maintaining maternal mental health.

Agoraphobia and panic attacks

Agoraphobic behaviour is frequently associated with panic attacks (Bandelow et al 2006; Ramnero and Ost 2007) and has been linked to anxiety and stress during pregnancy (Furber et al. 2009). Panic attacks are intense episodes of anxiety associated with a variety of bodily symptoms such as palpitations, dizziness, tremor, sweating, hyperventilation and dry mouth. Sufferers may feel they are about to die and be extremely frightened. They may last 1–10 minutes until intervention, or until the person develops some form of self-control. A woman can achieve better control if she learns about the biological basis of her symptoms of panic disorder or is helped to generate her own model of how to cope with panic, maybe by teaching her how to employ easy relaxation techniques. In Figure 4.2

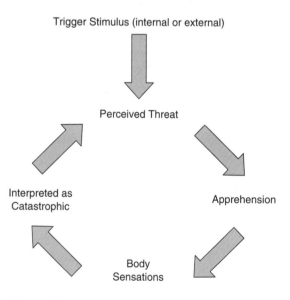

Figure 4.2 Cognitive model of panic disorder

we see how the cycle of panic develops. Interventions such as explanations of bodily symptoms lead to the person no longer interpreting them as necessarily catastrophic, and relaxation methods can inhibit the cycle too.

Women with panic attacks may become dependent on alcohol or other substances, or come to rely on anxiolytic drugs like benzodiazepines. There is sometimes an overlap with other mental health problems, such as depression or PTSD. It is, therefore, vital to exclude hormonal and physical health problems, for example hyperthyroidism, before diagnosing a panic disorder. In addition, a psychiatric label can sometimes cause a physical problem to be overlooked and this can lead to a fatal outcome, for example, a pulmonary embolism.

Antenatal depression

Pregnancy was always generally thought to have an uplifting effect on mood and women were seen as more or less protected against depression. Even amongst midwives knowledge about the condition is limited. Nevertheless, for some women depressed mood is a problem during pregnancy. Antenatal depression has become more recognised in recent years and has been linked with poor partner and family support (Schatz et al. 2012).

There is some suggestion that it is linked to adult depression and life circumstances and then linked to postnatal depression following birth (Robertson et al. 2004). There is also growing evidence that antenatal depression is associated with several risk factors, such as increased levels of anxiety and stress suffered when a woman has a complicated pregnancy and is at increased risk of a difficult birth (Andersson et al. 2004). This can result in a premature or intra-uterine growth restricted baby (Field et al. 2010), which is then linked to post-partum depression (van Bussell et al. 2006). In addition, impaired maternal–fetal attachment is also linked to antenatal depression (Lindgren 2001) and developmental problems in the infant (Deave et al. 2008).

Researchers exploring women's experiences of antenatal depression have reported emotional loneliness (Bennett et al. 2007; Raymond 2009). It is worth noting that antenatal domestic violence is highly associated with antenatal depression in women (Flach et al. 2011) and is correlated with later childhood behavioural problems (probably mediated through maternal depression). Practitioners need to be mindful to seek out and eliminate underlying causes of depression. Research suggests that intervention antenatally to treat symptoms of depression may prevent more severe postnatal depression later (Clatworthy 2012). Levels of distress, antenatal depression and stress about the parenting role are reduced by help-seeking behaviour in women and antenatal interventions to treat depression improve engagement and well-being (Milgrom et al. 2011).

Where there is a history of depression in fathers (Areias et al. 1996), this is linked to an increased risk of a father also susceptible to anxiety and stress during pregnancy and antenatal depression (Ramchandani et al. 2008).

Eating disorders

Eating disorders (ED) can affect the health and well-being of some pregnant women and new mothers. An eating disorder is a complex compulsion to eat in a way which disturbs physical,

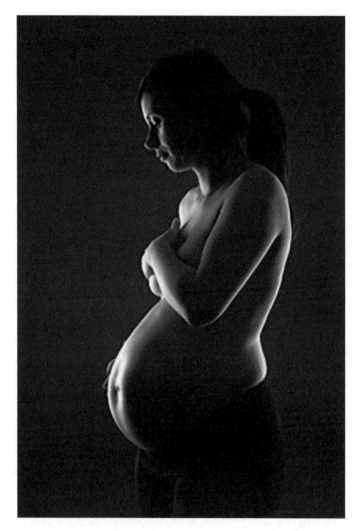

Figure 4.3 Maternal-fetal attachment

social, emotional and psychological health (NICE 2004). See the Glossary of mental health terms for a description of common types of eating disorders. Eating disorders appear to be more common in young women, and dysfunctional eating behaviours if not recognised and treated can develop into an addiction (Wolfe 2005). There is often a history of psycho-social problems and some form of abuse within the young woman's life (Little and Lowkes 2000). Mitchell and Bulik (2006) have highlighted that women living with an eating disorder are at risk of their dysfunctional eating behaviour exacerbating during pregnancy and after giving birth. In addition, those women who have previously experienced such disorders may be at risk of a recurrence during pregnancy because of significant issues around change in body image, weight gain and major life transition.

Gieleghum et al. (2002) raised concerns that even though women with an eating disorder are at increased risk of poor maternal and fetal outcomes, disclosure by them seldom occurs. Therefore, health professionals need to be alert to possible physical, emotional, psychological and behavioural indicators to detect an eating disorder and offer supportive care. Body Mass Index (BMI) may be an indicator to a possible eating disorder. For instance, a BMI <18.5 is associated with Anorexia Nervosa and a BMI >40 is associated with Bulimia Nervosa (Hudson et al. 2007). Specifically relating to pregnancy, there may be a history of difficulties in conceiving and poor pregnancy outcomes such as miscarriage, stillbirth, intra-uterine growth restriction (IUGR), premature birth and congenital abnormalities. Other physical indicators such as tooth decay, a persistent sore throat, digestive problems such as heartburn, difficulty swallowing and constipation are possible indicators of an eating disorder.

Complaints of general malaise, persistent backache and leg cramps (they are more at risk of mineral loss from their bones and osteoporosis), signs of dehydration and frequent complaints about urinary and bowel problems may also be indicators. A pregnant woman with previous or current eating disorders may demonstrate signs of anxiety and stress, low self-esteem, feelings of guilt and being ashamed, poor body image and a history of mental health problems where she has self-harmed or even attempted suicide. In general she appears to be struggling to cope with life and the pregnancy. She has poor family support and there may be a history of taking prescribed drugs such as antidepressants and slimming pills. During pregnancy she may be reluctant to discuss dietary intake and may deny having any eating problems. She may also be very anxious about weight increase during pregnancy and can appear obsessive about losing weight in the immediate postnatal period. If she has children, they may have eating problems such as overeating or food refusal (Little and Lowkes 2000).

Asking questions about eating habits and patterns needs be undertaken very sensitively. Initially, general questions about how she is feeling, how she is coping with her pregnancy, her family life and what social support she has may give an opportunity to then ask more direct questions about her eating habits, patterns, likes and dislikes of food types (Steen 2009). Documenting concerns is paramount, as is also discussing with the woman a referral to the local mental health team who can offer additional care and support from an eating disorder specialist. There is evidence that women with an eating disorder can positively modify their eating behaviours whilst pregnant as they want to provide a good nutritional intake for their developing baby, but they may go back to their dysfunctional eating behaviour following birth and are at increased risk of postnatal depression (Mitchell and Bulik 2006; NICE 2004, 2007a).

Long term follow up with an eating disorder specialist is often necessary to prevent the woman from relapsing. The most common treatments for eating disorders are cognitive and other behavioural therapies and these have been reported to help many women but this take time and women may need several years of therapy (NICE 2004, 2007a). An eating disorder specialist will aim to focus the woman on her negative thoughts towards food and weight, then support the woman to enable her to recognise 'triggers' and then replace the negative thoughts with more positive ones that are rational and healthy. Often other mental health problems will also need to be worked through (Steen 2009).

Eating Disorder: a case scenario

Helen booked late for antenatal care. She arrived unexpectedly at the clinic when she was approximately 28 weeks gestation. The midwife knew her from a previous pregnancy and was aware that she had several social issues and little family support. The clinic was busy and the midwife was running late with the appointments as there had been some other social problems to sort out with a few of the women attending. Therefore, she could not book Helen at the clinic but arranged to go visit her at home later in the day. The midwife's first impression of Helen was that she looked tired and very pale. She reflected and remembered that she had a history of miscarriage and intra-uterine growth restriction (IUGR). The midwife arrived at Helen's home around 4 pm and Helen's little girl was present.

Whilst taking her booking history, the midwife noticed that Helen was coughing a lot and complained of a sore throat. Helen put it down to being 'run down and not looking after herself'. When the midwife asked her about her diet, Helen disclosed that she had little appetite and was suffering from constipation. The midwife was aware that there had been some concern in her last pregnancy about domestic violence and she had a history of self-harming as a teenager, although Helen never disclosed this. She appeared generally unwell and possibly dehydrated as she was constipated and also complained of general aches and pains in particular, affecting her lower back and legs. The midwife was concerned about Helen's mental health state as she was not happy about being pregnant and when gently asked how she was coping she showed signs of being upset. Her partner had left her and she was struggling to cope with life in general. The midwife referred her to the mental health team and arranged to visit her weekly. During the weeks that followed there was a concern that Helen's baby was not growing and developing as well as expected and a growth scan confirmed this. Helen's pregnancy was monitored closely and she attended the consultant-led unit.

Helen's sister agreed to care for her little girl when she went into labour at term. She gave birth to a baby boy who weighed 2300 g and showed physical signs of IUGR. He fed well in the postnatal period which pleased Helen. During this time she disclosed to her midwife how she felt guilty for not eating properly during her pregnancy. When sensitively questioned about this she discussed how she had struggled to eat properly for a few years and it was particularly a problem when she was stressed and had relationship problems. In addition, her little girl's eating habits were a concern to her health visitor and she was underweight. This alerted the midwife to the possibility of an eating disorder and this was discussed with her general practitioner and the mental health team.

Long term follow up with an eating disorder specialist was arranged to help her to focus on her negative thoughts towards food and then support her to recognise 'triggers' and then replace these negative thoughts with positive thoughts to eat healthier. The mental health team continued to support her and she was coping fairly well with her new baby and she had her sister and some friends to support her.

Existing mental health conditions

Women with existing mental illness such as schizophrenia and bipolar disorder may develop relapses of their condition during pregnancy, especially if compliance with maintenance medication is lost (NICE 2007a). Close working relationships between health professionals is essential and regular meetings for advance care planning for various contingencies is vital. In these cases specialist midwives with mental health expertise are extremely valuable in formulating birth plans and supporting women. The situation can become difficult to manage if women are adamant they will not take medication 'for the baby's sake'. In Western societies admission to an all-female Psychiatric Intensive Care Unit (PICU) during pregnancy may be justified in such cases, with liaison with the local Mother and Baby Unit to see if attempting to keep mother and baby together following birth is at all feasible. A pregnant women with schizophrenia may also need to be admitted to a PICU. There is some evidence that a pregnant women with schizophrenia is at an increased risk of poor pregnancy and neonatal outcomes (Nilsson et al. 2002). There may be a denial of the pregnancy even though physical changes are occurring and this can lead to not receiving the care and support she desperately needs. Following birth, specialist care and support is essential as the new mother is also at increased risk of failing to bond with her baby and this leads to a poor mother–infant attachment.

During episodes of bipolar disorder, the risk of suicide increases. Judgement may be impaired during mania and, due to elation and dis-inhibition, a woman may make unwise decisions such as overspending or being promiscuous, increasing her risk of acquiring a sexually transmitted disease (STD) or becoming pregnant. The various mood stabilisers (such as valproate and lithium) are associated with cardiovascular and neural tube birth defects. Pregnancies in bipolar women need to be carefully planned with adjustments to medication. Misuse of alcohol during hypomania may increase the risk of fetal alcohol syndrome and a family history of bipolar disorder has been shown to increase the risk of a woman developing puerperal psychosis following childbirth (NICE 2007a). In the UK, a recent landmark case which was referred to the courts highlighted how ethically challenging the area of severe mental illness can be in the context of pregnancy. A woman referred to as Miss B (to safeguard her anonymity) was given the right to an abortion, despite an NHS hospital trust ruling that claimed she was not of sound mind and therefore incapable of making a decision. Suffering from bipolar disorder, the pregnant woman claimed that having the baby would likely result in her suicide and killing the baby. The judge ruled in favour of Miss B on the grounds that denying her an abortion would be a 'total affront to her autonomy' and he didn't accept the claim that she was lacking in capacity (Ensor 2013). It is, therefore, imperative that pregnant women with severe mental health problems are listened to and their wishes respected.

There is some evidence to suggest that an increase of obsessive compulsive behaviours may occur perinatally (Chaudron and Nirodi 2010), such as intrusive ideation in the mothers about the baby's health or safety, coupled with, say, washing compulsions or cleaning rituals. Difficulties in pregnancy such as oedema and prolonged labour have been proposed as potential risk factors for further study (Vasconcelos et al. 2007). In patients who attended a mental health obsessive compulsive disorder (OCD) clinic, out of the 78 women in the ever being pregnant group (ever pregnant group), 32.1 per cent (n = 24) had OCD onset in the perinatal period (perinatal-related group), 15.4 per cent in pregnancy, 14.1 per cent at postpartum, and 1.3 per cent after miscarriage (Forray et al. 2010). This indicates that for females suffering from OCD, the perinatal period is a time when symptoms are highly likely to reveal themselves. Some specific scales such as the perinatal obsessive compulsive scale (POCS) have been developed to measure perinatal OCD (Lord et al. 2011).

The possibility of a woman remaining in her own home, supported by a health care team, will be considered if the woman's mental health state is assessed as being not severe enough to warrant admission as an in-patient. If she is deemed at risk of harming herself or her baby then admission to the nearest Mother and Baby Unit may be necessary. Women with existing mental health illness are at risk of relapses and psychotic episodes following birth and every case needs to be assessed on its own merits.

Drug use and pregnancy

Mothers using substances are statistically more likely to have infections such as Hepatitis B Virus (HBV) and Human Immunodeficiency Virus (HIV), have an increased incidence mental illness and be prone to poor social support and thus require a deal of proactive planning and care (APA 2012). Mothers using cocaine are at increased risk of hypertension and pneumothorax. Underlying mental health conditions are associated with illicit drug misuse – conditions such as PTSD, personality disorder, psychosis and alcoholism. Increased risks to the fetus include fetal alcohol syndrome, infection, malnutrition, and neonatal withdrawal from drugs such as opiates. Neonates may have low birth weight, increased developmental abnormalities and be born prematurely.

Grandey et al. (2002) found that 1 per cent of mothers using maternity services were substance users and a third of their babies were in withdrawal and required special care units. Various studies have found that these mothers were more likely to be victims of violence, to present late in pregnancy, have less antenatal care, increased mental health morbidity and neglect social roles (Thompson and Kingree 1998; Hans 1999).

Medication and the fetus

Approximately 7 per cent of mothers in their childbearing years suffer from a mental illness (NICE 2007a). This, combined with the fact that many pregnancies are generally 'unplanned', means that there is a significant risk that the developing fetus might be exposed to psychotropic drugs. First trimester exposure is associated with abnormal organ formation and third trimester exposure is linked to withdrawal effects in the neonate. For instance, neonatal withdrawal symptoms can be seen with some antidepressant and antipsychotic drugs. As no drug can be deemed wholly safe, the policy of avoiding drugs during pregnancy (especially in the first trimester) is the wisest course. This is only counterbalanced if the risk, for example, of suicide or severe relapse of psychosis, is a serious concern.

Of all the many drugs that the developing fetus might be exposed to the so-called tricyclic antidepressants are relatively safe in terms of any risk of malformations, but if used in the third trimester can lead to withdrawal symptoms in the neonate. There is less certainty about the serotonin re-uptake inhibitors (SSRIs) and malformations. Of the antipsychotics the older style phenothiazines, like chlorpromazine, are associated with a small risk of malformations. Haloperidol is thought to be relatively safe as is olanzapine, a newer antipsychotic drug. The outlook for women, say with a bipolar disorder, taking mood stabilisers is of more concern and careful advice about contraception and planning pregnancies needs to be given on initial prescription and repeated thereafter. Of the various mood stabilisers lithium is definitely associated with fetal cardiac abnormalities, for example Fallot's tetralogy, while sodium valproate and carbamazepine are associated with neural tube defects and phenytoin is associated with facial cleft defects.

Care and support

Problems with motivation may make pregnant women and newly delivered mothers with severe mental health conditions less likely to engage proactively with health professionals and this may impair compliance with health advice. This in turn may affect a pregnant woman or mother's ability to cope with everyday life activities, therefore necessitating careful planning with mental health services, their family, social services and community support.

It is vitally important to involve the woman's family to support her. Living with a mental health condition has its challenges and living with someone who has a mental health condition can also be very difficult. Fear of not being able to cope will be a strong emotion for some women and their family members. There is still an element of stigma and shame attached to mental illness and a woman and her family will be fearful of how other people in society will react to her and to some extent to her family as a whole (Steen and Jones 2014). A woman-focused and family-included approach to care and support is required as this will benefit all concerned.

Childbirth and mental health

The medicalisation of childbirth

Traditionally throughout history, birth has been a social event that takes place within the nurturing setting of the home and a communal celebration. During the 1970s and 1980s a technocratic approach to birth gained momentum with the growing use of biomedicine and the power of obstetrics within the health service (Harris 2012). The assumption that being in a hospital was a safer environment to give birth rather than the home led to the majority of women giving birth in hospital with the use of machinery and being treated as a patient. Birth became a medical event rather than a social event and this has had a major impact on how birth is viewed by society as a whole. There is evidence emerging that this technocratic approach to birth is having detrimental effects on some women's health and well-being (Emerson 1998; Murphy 2003; Newnham 2014). This approach has had an effect on women's confidence and ability to give birth normally. A growing phenomenon of the 'fear of birth' continues to affect many women's views of childbirth: some become very anxious, even depressed and fretful during pregnancy (Melender 2002; Steen and Jones 2012). Sudden unexpected interventions and events during labour and birth can lead to tokophobia (morbid fear of childbirth). In severe cases mental health problems may lead to maternal suicide (CMACE 2011).

Fear of childbirth

Fear can be acquired by suggestion or association and can manifest itself in dread and dismay, even terror, depending on the nature of the stimulus and a person's personality (Tucker 2003). The bible teachings have instilled a generic fear of childbirth and the 'Curse of Eve' has given women a reason to fear birth. Genesis 3:16 quotes *'Unto the woman he said, I will greatly multiply thy sorrow and thy conception; in sorrow thou shalt bring forth children . . . '*

For many women over the centuries this has been the case until the great advances of science and living conditions played their role in improving the health and well-being of women (Steen and Jones 2012). There is no doubt that great advances in the care of expectant mothers and their babies have contributed to better maternal and fetal outcomes, but *medicalisation* and more recently the *media's* portrayal of birth have contributed to this generic fear of childbirth. Fear of childbirth has had an effect on women's confidence and ability to give birth normally. This fear continues to affect many women's views of childbirth, and may lead to maternal request for caesarean section.

Tokophobia is a complex but rare condition where women need to be supported by a range of healthcare professionals, including midwives, obstetricians and occasionally perinatal mental health specialists. This collaborative approach can help a woman to be less anxious and understand the normal physiological process of birth and prepare for birth feeling supported. The most appropriate choice of birth environment and how to give birth to meet her individual needs is vitally important in her care and being actively listened too and counselling can also help (NICE 2007b; RCOG 2011).

Post-traumatic stress disorder (PTSD)

For most mothers birth is a happy, rewarding and life-affirming milestone in their lives. However, in Western countries it is estimated that around 1.5 per cent to 6 per cent of mothers experience PTSD following childbirth complications which, whether due to inherent pathology or clinical negligence, mean that the mother's life or the child's life can be threatened or serious injury may result (Andersen et al. 2012). However, social and cultural differences between countries and different assessment scales used to identify women with PTSD following birth may influence the reporting of prevalence rates. For example, a higher rate of prevalence (17 per cent) for PTSD following birth in a study undertaken in Iran has recently reported by Shaban et al. (2013).

The researchers reported a strong relationship between anxiety and depression and the mother's occupation. In addition, it is now acknowledged that women can develop PTSD following birth involving unexpected obstetric procedures and complications and in some women symptoms can last for several months (Ayers and Pickering 2001; Beck 2004; Leeds and Hargreaves 2008). PSTD is associated with high trait anxiety, pre-existing fear of childbirth, other physical and/or mental health problems during pregnancy and a previous traumatic birth experience and history of child sexual abuse (Ayers and Pickering 2001; Bailham and Joseph 2003; Soet et al. 2003).

During birth trauma heightened states of arousal and fear can engender PTSD, a moderately severe psychiatric disorder encompassing nightmares, anxiety and panic, flashbacks (intrusive thoughts) and avoidance behaviour. Depending on the outcome of such traumatic injuries chronic ill health may lead to adjustment disorder (or secondary depression) which can be treated by antidepressants or cognitive behavioural therapy (CBT). Loss of the baby and loss of future reproductive ability are both bereavements and are sometimes complicated by depression, again treatable by antidepressants or CBT with the addition of elements of grief therapy.

Just as with couple depression (this is where one partner in a couple is depressed and there is a heightened risk of depression in the other), there is often a sharing of PTSD symptoms across the mother-father dyad – where trauma symptoms are experienced by one these are correlated with trauma symptoms in the other (Iles et al. 2011). Staff attitudes can contribute to the development of PTSD, with disinterested or nervous midwives adding to fear levels during emergency caesarean procedures (Tham et al. 2010).

Post-traumatic stress disorder: a case scenario

A 30 year old primigravida who had opted for active management of the third stage of labour had difficulties delivering the placenta. It became apparent that the placenta was abnormally attached. Following IM injection with syntometrine and cord-controlled traction (CCT) by a newly quali-fied midwife the placenta was not delivered. This was uncomfortable to the point of pain for the woman. A senior midwife was summoned who again repeated CCT, but with greater force, leading to more severe pain, anxiety and stress and tending to panic for the woman. Finally a junior doctor was called who removed the placenta manually by dividing the placenta from the uterine wall with her fingers bit by bit until eventually the placenta came away. No anaesthetic was involved and subsequently the woman developed a heavy blood loss and infection as complications of the pro-cedure. The woman said that she had been screaming and in great pain throughout the procedure.

Thereafter, she had nightmares from which she awoke in a panicky, sweaty state. Her sleep was poor, and she felt low in mood. She chose to avoid hospitals, doctors and midwives because of the reminder of feelings of panic and fear experienced in their presence. She could not be driven past the hospital where her baby was delivered. Her libido was absent even six months after the delivery. She felt constantly on edge, was irritable and easily startled. She suffered intrusive memories of the doctor's angry face shouting at her not to 'be stupid' and the feeling of the doctor's hand inside her uterus. A diagnosis of post-traumatic stress disorder (PTSD) was made and there was some response to antidepressants and CBT, but the woman was very clear with her therapist that she would 'never' contemplate having another baby.

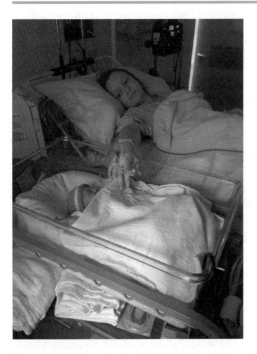

Figure 4.4 First touch, following emergency C-S, susceptible for PTSD

Care and support

It is important in promoting the normality of birth and even when complications occur that the woman and her partner are fully informed and consent is given to the interventions and care necessary. The woman and her partner must be supported in a caring and compassionate way to reduce fear and anxiety.

Mental health following birth

Transient psychological disorder (baby blues)

A transient psychological disorder commonly referred to as the baby blues is relatively common, being experienced by about 1 in 3 mothers (Steen 2011). Baby blues refer to transient feelings of weepiness or pessimism occurring within days of birth and lasting just hours or days, and certainly no more than a week postnatally. The lowered mood is typically relatively mild in nature and may be accompanied by tiredness and insomnia. The causes may include a psychological reaction to apprehension or anxiety about the birth, physiological reaction and the genuine physical exhaustion felt, or a sociological reaction and the realisation that a life event has finally occurred. Other causes may include a biological switch in hormone levels with withdrawal from previously high levels of progesterone and oestrogen. Whatever the cause the symptoms of baby blues usually disappear with support and some reassurance and without the need for specialist intervention.

Baby blues: a case scenario

A first time mother on her 3rd postnatal day: felt weepy, didn't know why, just started to cry, very emotional, query anti-climax following the pregnancy and birth, over tired, not had much sleep, feels hormonal, breasts engorged and aching, baby not fixing on properly, perineum hurting from stitches, house a mess. Midwife arrived to undertake a postnatal visit and recognised baby blues, she sat and listened to the woman's concerns and reassured her that she appeared to have the baby blues which many women have after giving birth but it would subside with help and support. It was decided that the woman's partner would take their newborn out for a stroll in the pram and the woman would take herself off to bed and get some very needed sleep. The woman had the midwife's contact details if she needed a chat later in the day and another visit was arranged for the next day. The next day was much better, the woman had had some sleep and felt able to cope, her breasts were not as engorged and her baby was able to fix on and feed well, stitches were still causing some pain but bathing, cool packs and analgesia were helping to alleviate this, her own mother had come around and tidied up. She was going to take another nap in the afternoon and was gaining confidence in her ability to be a 'mother'.

4.5.2 *Postnatal depression*

This is also sometimes called postpartum depression; postnatal depression (PND) is defined as a depressive illness within a year of birth. Symptoms include excessive low mood, poor sleep, poor concentration, altered appetite, increased tiredness, low self-esteem, social withdrawal, lack of interest or pleasure, increased irritability and reduced sex drive. In more severe forms suicidal ideation and plans can form and be accompanied by psychotic features such as delusions of guilt or worthlessness and auditory hallucinations. In different studies PND can affect between 5 and 25 per cent of mothers (Gaynes et al. 2005). A recent study in Spain found depression in 9.3 per cent and 4.4 per cent of mothers at 3 and 12 months postpartum respectively (Escriba-Aguir and Artazcoz 2011). However, there is some evidence that PND prevalence may be higher in some developing countries (Fisher et al. 2012). A cross-section study undertaken in Karnataka, South India screened a sample of 123 women who attended a rural maternity hospital and reported rates of PND to be around 45 per cent in the immediate post birth period and then at 6–8 weeks following birth (Johnson et al. 2015). PND was associated with mood swings during pregnancy, being stressed, having a low-esteem, staying with maternal family and being away from their husbands. In Indian societies, risk factors such as low income, lack of education, multiparity, congenital malformations, disappointment that infant is female, husband's use of alcohol, difficult relationship with mother-in-law and history of depression within the family have been found to be associated with PND (Hegde et al. 2012).

There is debate as to whether PND is a separate illness confined to the postnatal period or to be seen as a depressive episode that is likely to be part of a recurrent affective disorder and also linked to antenatal depression. The prevalence of depression in parents postnatally is not that different from the prevalence of depression in adults. Risk factors include a past psychiatric history of depression, poor relationship with partner, adverse temperament in the infant, lack of support, being a single parent, being a smoker, amongst others (Beck 2001). Recent studies have additional factors: being a younger mother, being less educated and being impoverished (Darcy et al. 2011) and intimate partner violence (IPV) (Valentine et al. 2011 and Garabedian et al. 2011), and having suffered previous miscarriages/stillbirths (Blackmore et al. 2011). Causes of PND are not well understood –hypothetical causes may include sleep deprivation and exhaustion (perhaps due to infant temperament problems or colic), hormonal shifts (Soares and Zitek 2008), iron deficiency (Beard et al. 2005) and socioeconomic factors.

Midwives and doctors are advised to enquire early in the pregnancy about any family and personal history of serious mental illness so referrals and specialised expertise can be arranged (NICE 2008). However, screening for mental health problems during pregnancy is much debated. There are a number of validated screening tools for depression (Sanders 2006) and the Edinburgh Postnatal Depression Scale (EPDS) is a well recognised ten-question scale used to screen for postnatal depression (Cox et al. 1987). NICE (2008) do not recommend using the scale antenatally.

PND is associated with poorer quality of life for mother and child at follow up over a year later (Darcy et al. 2011). Social support is a necessary adjunct, with deployment of the full resources of the multi-disciplinary team being helpful. At times admission to an inpatient unit may be necessary particularly where there are issues of suicide risk and third party risks to the baby whether through neglect or depression-driven delusional action. Effective treatments include antidepressants, interpersonal therapy and CBT (Sockol et al. 2011). In the UK, recent work has focused on training health visitors with additional cognitive behavioural and person-centred therapy skills to deploy in helping women with PND (Morrell et al. 2011). In the UK, Australia and New Zealand, specialist midwife posts have been created to specifically focus on women with mental health issues and to promote a care pathway that encourages a joint up teamwork approach.

PND: a case scenario

Mary was a 24 year old single mother who lived with her mother. She had been tearful and withdrawn before the birth of her daughter Ann. This was observed and documented by her midwife and a GP referral was made. Mary's mood improved transiently following the baby's arrival. On transfer of care to the health visitor, the community midwife discussed Mary's health and well-being during her pregnancy and then following the birth of her baby. At six weeks, the health visitor made a home visit and found Mary to be very withdrawn and almost silent. On questioning she became tearful and said that Ann was waking her every hour or so at night and that she felt exhausted. Mary said that although her Mum had been looking after Ann in her bedroom at night for the past week to give Mary some sleep, Mary said she thought she had no future and that the world would be better off without her, and Ann. Mary was referred to the mental health team. In-patient admission was deemed not necessary and community care was given. PND is treatable and Mary's mental health improved with, initially, antidepressants, then cognitive therapy and by attending local support groups and home visits from a volunteer befriender.

Paternal mental health

The issue of paternal mental health around the time of childbirth is only now being taken relatively seriously. For many years the mental health of fathers has either been neglected or been the target of sexist humour. The twentieth century's popular view of the subject can be encapsulated in the ribald humour of the film *Carry On Doctor* (1967) where Charles Hawtrey played a husband who shared his wife's pregnancy and symptoms. Hawtrey's fictional case was probably a depiction of *Couvade syndrome* (or sympathetic pregnancy, long recognised in the medical literature since antiquity as a rare male psychological reaction to pregnancy). The focus on adult mental health around pregnancy has always been firmly placed on maternal mental health until recently.

Paternal postnatal depression

In the last decade or so, there have been various papers describing serious researches into paternal postnatal depression. Firstly, there have been researches into the scope of the problem. Skari et al. (2002) 'clinically important psychological distress' a few days after childbirth in some 13 per cent of fathers with 2 per cent of fathers having 'severe intrusive stress symptoms'. However, after six weeks they found that these levels of distress fell to a level found in the general population. However, this return to normal cannot always be guaranteed. Paulson et al. (2009) found that 10 per cent of fathers were depressed at 9 months. Sherr et al. (2006) identified depression in 12 per cent and anxiety in 30 per cent of the fathers of children aged 6 years and under in North London. Infant crying and sleep problems seem to particularly correlate with depression – where these problems are present up to 30 per cent of fathers have abnormal depression scores (as measured on the Edinburgh Postnatal Depression Scale) (Smart and Hiscock 2007). A Spanish study found depression in 9.3 per cent and 4.4 per cent of mothers and 3.4 per cent and 4.0 per cent of fathers at 3 and 12 months post-partum respectively, (Escriba-Aguir and Artazcoz, 2011).

Paternal depression also has effects on child development. Ramchandani et al. (2008) looked at the development of child psychopathology in association with male postnatal depression. They followed 10,975 fathers and their children for seven years and found that postnatal paternal depression (measured by the Edinburgh Postnatal Depression Scale) was associated with psychiatric disorder in the children seven years later – these mainly being oppositional defiant/conduct disorders. This association appears to be independent of maternal postnatal depression. (Ramchandani et al. 2008). An earlier study of Ramchandani's on a similarly large cohort of 12,884 fathers found an association between male postnatal depression and adverse emotional and behavioural outcomes in their children at 3.5 years old, with conduct disorders in boys (Ramchandani et al. 2005). Postnatal male depression may be a major predictor for impaired parental competence during the first months after birth (Ferketich and Mercer, 1995). Paternal depression at 9 months post childbirth has also been linked to a reduced tendency to read to the child and impaired development of the child's vocabulary (Paulson et al. 2009).

There are various risk factors that might predict which fathers might develop male postnatal depression. These risk factors include a past psychiatric history of depression in fathers (Areias et al. 1996), higher prenatal depression and anxiety scores (Ramchandani et al. 2008), being the father of twins (Vilska et al. 2009), early infant crying and sleeping problems (Smart and Hiscock 2007), excessive crying in the infant (van den Berg et al. 2009) and maternal postnatal depression (Edhborg et al. 2005). Amongst father of twins conceived through assisted reproduction treatment (ART) they show no difference in terms of depression rates compared to fathers of singletons during pregnancy. However, at two months and one year after delivery fathers of twins (both ART and normally conceived) show significantly more symptoms of depression than fathers of singletons (Vilska et al. 2009). Excessive infant crying (using Wessel's criteria i.e. crying >3 hours for >3 days in the last week) is associated with paternal depressive symptoms (van den Berg et al. 2009). Couple depression is a repeated finding in various studies such that where one partner is depressed there is a heightened risk of depression in the other (Areias et al, 1996, Edhborg et al, 2005, Field et al, 2010). Goodman (2004) found that the prevalence of paternal depression ranged from 1.2 per cent to 25 per cent in various community samples, but that the rates increased from 24 per cent to 50 per cent amongst men whose partners had postpartum depression.

There has also been research into potential interventions. Where infant crying has been a causative factor then Smart and Hiscock (2007) found that education about normal infant behaviours and management strategies helped maternal and paternal mental health. Other recognized interventions might encompass CBT, antidepressants, interpersonal therapy and group therapy.

With regard to other potential mental health problems, the issue of male bereavement is probably under-researched. Bereavement is generally held to be a huge risk factor for depression, but in modern times males may witness traumatic scenes in hospital such as the attempted resuscitation of a newborn or a cherished partner. The risk of these scenarios may be expected by health staff, but to emotionally involved partners and relatives these scenes where highly valued lives are threatened may form the kernels of PTSD memories that are re-experienced for many years or complicated bereavement reactions. The undoubted advantages and disadvantages of allowing relatives to witness such resuscitations and the ethical issues involved are outside the scope of this chapter.

Puerperal psychosis

Postpartum psychosis (or puerperal psychosis) is a rare occurrence affecting less than 1 in 1,000 women (Terp and Mortensen 1998). The psychosis develops within days of giving birth. It is important to exclude and treat physical causes such as uterine infection, chest infection, or urinary tract infection, which might be accompanied by fever, rigors and signs of physical illness. Presentations may include mania or schizophreniform psychosis, with hallucinations and delusions. Once physical causes have been excluded treatment would be dictated by the severity of the condition and any risks of suicide or danger to the infant. Admission could be considered, if necessary requiring detention under a Mental Health Act, such as the UK Mental Health Act (2007). As presentations are relatively early and often seen after first pregnancies there may be a chance that these are present and detected in the maternity unit. If so a hospital liaison psychiatrist may be asked to assess the woman. In the UK, the community midwife or health visitor would need to alert the GP to access secondary care. In some areas a direct referral to community mental health care may be possible if the facility is available. Mother and Baby units are, in this day and age, still depressingly scarce (approx. 12 in the UK) leading to the trauma of separation of mother and family whilst mental illness is resolving with treatment. Treatments may include antipsychotic drugs (such as quetiapine) or mood stabilisers (such as valproate), with due care and attention as to whether the mother is still breast feeding. The mother and baby unit should be able to make an assessment of any current and on-going risks to the baby and hopefully work towards fostering and strengthening the relationship between mother and baby as the mother's illness resolves. In addition, a family-centred care approach is which fathers and other family members are involved is encouraged once the mother's illness is improving. This form of psychosis is a more likely scenario than an all-new sudden psychosis postpartum. See psychosis case scenario below.

Psychosis: a case scenario

Gill had a history of schizoaffective disorder. She was 28 and had been intermittently ill since the age of 18 when she had run away to London and worked for a time in the sex industry. She had been diagnosed with a 'drug-induced psychosis' when she was 20, but since then had been admitted three times under section 3 of the Mental Health Act. Over the past eight years she had been out of hospital for only three. For the last two years she had been living in a flat and had a boyfriend staying with her, who was also a service user. She had been maintained on depot injections of risperidone and on oral sodium valproate. She had wanted a child, however, and stopped her medication. A few months later she became pregnant. She was managing off medication for six months when her partner left her; thereafter she started to become chaotic in her behaviour, dancing in the street in the early hours of the morning and singing songs about the Virgin Mary.

Gill was admitted to a mixed acute psychiatric ward, on another section 3 but was assaulted by a male and felt intimidated and fearful for her baby, which she insisted was an 'immaculate conception'. She said she was hearing the voices of the Virgin Mary and of her husband Joseph talking to her (second person auditory hallucinations) and that they told her to be 'joyous' and 'to stay awake and refuse the devil's medication' (command hallucinations). She became agitated and upset when staff challenged her ideas, and when a member of staff tried to give her some diazepam to calm her she assaulted the nurse with a chair, breaking her jaw. Gill was subsequently admitted to an all-female psychiatric intensive care unit. Initially, staff attempted to manage her without medication, but Gill was highly disturbed and not sleeping. There was discussion about the risks posed by any rapid tranquilisation or regular antipsychotic to the baby (in the second trimester now), but it was felt that the mother's mental health needs and physical risks to the baby of violence outweighed these risks and medication was administered. There was a gradual response over the next few weeks, but Gill's insight was so poor that she was adamant she would discontinue medication as soon as she was discharged.

As Gill approached the delivery date the consultant psychiatrist, key nurse and community care co-ordinator from the psychiatric team met with Gill's consultant obstetrician, hospital midwife and the specialist mental health midwife to formulate a birth plan with Gill as a team. The consultant psychiatrist began work with the Mother and Baby Unit consultant to see whether Gill might be considered for a place following the birth of her baby. This follow up care was agreed. Gill remained in the Mother & Baby Unit (MBU) for 8 weeks and was then supported by the community mental health care team and a specialist Health Visitor.

Medication and breastfeeding

We also need to bear in mind that following birth, babies may encounter any drugs that are secreted in breast milk. Manufacturers usually suggest that women taking psychotropic medication should avoid breastfeeding, and gathering research evidence on medication from breastfeeding mothers is difficult. Recent reviews have suggested that some SSRI antidepressants (but not fluoxetine) and Nortiptyline (a tricyclic antidepressant) may be relatively safe in breastfeeding mothers (Devanzo et al. 2011). However, lithium, nefazodone and doxepin should be avoided.

Conclusions

Most women experience pregnancy, childbirth and early motherhood without mental health problems. However, there is evidence to suggest that approximately one in seven women will experience a mental health problem in pregnancy or following birth. It is vitally important to meet the needs of these expectant and newly delivered mothers who either already have on-going mental health issues or are at risk of developing and experiencing them during pregnancy, childbirth and following birth. There is good evidence that a befriending approach and social support is beneficial to both pregnant women and newly delivered mothers. Local peer support is highly valued and appears to be a buffer against developing poor mental health. Trusting relationships are developed and this type of local support encourages and enables pregnant women and mothers to disclose their anxieties and fears. This also reduces the risk of feeling alone and being isolated within the local community. Health professionals need to work alongside these local community befrienders and offer support and help when the need arises.

Women who have an existing mental illness are at increased risk of relapse during pregnancy and after giving birth, therefore, pre-conceptual counselling and care is recommended. Health professionals need to be alert and continually assess these at-risk women and work collaboratively with the mental health team and other professionals to meet the needs of individual women.

The recognition of mild to moderate mental health problems such as, anxiety and stress, panic symptoms, baby blues, antenatal depression, postnatal depression (including paternal), eating disorders, substance misuse and severe mental health conditions such as puerperal psychosis, schizophrenia and bipolar disorder should be included in continual professional education.

Health professionals can help alleviate postnatal family mental health morbidity by addressing the issue of paternal depression. Recognising depression in fathers and enquiring about their own past history of depression and current symptoms may be worthwhile. In view of the repeated finding regarding couple or dyadic depression it would be good practice to screen the father for depression as well. For whatever reasons, including ignorance or overt sexism, male postnatal depression has been neglected in terms of recognition, treatment and research. It is time to address this neglected area to reduce morbidity in fathers and to prevent any adverse impact on the couple's relationship and their child's development. This will assist to tackle the novel concept of 'couple depression'.

Improved communication between health professionals and others is essential to meet the needs of women with mental health issues. Referrals and requests for support and specialised care must be followed up to ensure that women's needs are addressed effectively.

Reflective exercise

- Can you describe and discuss the risk factors that can predispose pregnant women and new mothers to mental health problems?
- What positive and negative influences can families have upon a pregnant woman and a new mother's mental health and well-being?
- Describe how birth trauma can affect a new mother's mental health and well-being.
- Can you consider why it is difficult for health professionals to identify postnatal depression in new mothers and also new fathers?
- Describe how being from a CALD background can contribute to the likelihood of a pregnant woman becoming anxious and stressed during pregnancy and then following the birth of her baby.

References

Andersen LB, Melvaer LB, Videbech P, Lamont RF, Joergensen JS (2012) Risk factors for developing post-traumatic stress disorder following childbirth: a systematic review. *Acta Obstet Gynecol Scand* 91(11): 1261–72. doi: 10.1111/j.1600-0412.2012.01476.x.

Andersson L, Sundstrom-Poromaa I, Wulff M, Astrom M, Bixo M (2004) Neonatal outcome following maternal antenatal depression and anxiety: a population-based study. *American Journal of Epidemiology* 159: 872–81.

APA (2012) *HIV and Aids*. American Psychiatric Association. 1000 Wilson Boulevard Suite 1825 Arlington, VA 22209. www.psychiatry.org/hiv-and-aids (viewed 14/06/13).

Areias ME, Kumar R, Barros H, Figueiredo E (1996) Correlates of postnatal depression in mothers and fathers. *British Journal of Psychiatry* 169(1): 36–41.

Ayers S, Pickering A (2001) Do women get post-traumatic stress disorder as a result of childbirth? A prospective study of incidence. *Birth* 28: 111–18.

Bailham D, Joseph S (2003) Post-traumatic stress following childbirth: a review of the emerging literature and directions for research and practice. *Psychology, Health and Medicine* 8: 159–68.

Bandelow B, Sojka F, Broocks A, Hajak G, Bleich S, Ruther A (2006) Panic disorder during pregnancy and postpartum period. *European Psychiatry* 1: 495–500.

Beard JL, Hendricks MK, Perez EM, Murray-Kolb LE, Berg A, Vernon-Feagans L, Irlam J, Isaacs W, Sive A, Tomlinson M (Feb, 2005) Maternal iron deficiency anemia affects postpartum emotions and cognition. *Journal of Nutrition* 135(2): 267–72.

Beck CT (2004) Post-traumatic stress disorder due to childbirth: the aftermath. *Nursing Research* 53(4): 216–24.

Beck CT (2001) Predictors of postnatal depression: an update. *Nursing Research* 50 (5): 275–85.

Bennett HA, Boon HS, Romans SE, Grootendorst P (2007) Becoming the best mom that I can: women's experiences of managing depression during pregnancy: a qualitative study. *BMC Women's Health* 7: 13. doi:10.1186/1472-6874-7-13. www.biomedcentral.com/1472-6874/7/13 (viewed 02/07/12).

Bergman K, Sarkar P, O'Connor TG, Modi N, Glover V (2007) Maternal stress during pregnancy predicts cognitive ability and fearfulness in infancy. *Journal of American Academy of Child and Adolescent Psychiatry* 46(11): 1454–63.

Blackmore ER, Cote-Arsenault D, Tang W, Glover V, Evans J, Golding J, O'Connor TG (2011) Previous prenatal loss as a predictor of perinatal depression and anxiety. *British Journal of Psychiatry* 198(5): 373–8.

Busfield J (2010) Gender and mental health. In Kuhlmann E, Annandale E (eds) *The Palgrave Handbook of Gender and Healthcare.* Houndmills: Palgrave Macmillan.

Chaudron LH, Nirodi N (2010) The obsessive-compulsive spectrum in the perinatal period: a prospective pilot study. *Archives of Women's Mental Health* 13(5): 403–10.

Clatworthy J (2012) The effectiveness of antenatal interventions to prevent postnatal depression in high-risk women. *Journal of Affective Disorders* 137(1–3): 25–34. www.sciencedirect.com/science/article/pii/S0165032711000838.

CMACE (2011) *Saving Mothers' Lives: reviewing maternal deaths to make motherhood safer: 2006–2008.* The Eighth Report on Confidential Enquiries into Maternal Deaths in the United Kingdom. Centre for Maternal and Child Enquiries. BJOG 118 (Suppl. 1): 1–203.

Cox JL, Holden JM, Sagovsky R. (1987) Detection of postnatal depression: development of the 10-item Edinburgh Postnatal Depression Scale. *British Journal of Psychotherapy* 150: 782–6.

Darcy JM, Grzywacz JG, Stephens RL, Leng I, Clinch CR, Arcury TA (2011) Maternal depressive symptomatology: 16-month follow-up of infant and maternal health-related quality of life. *Journal of the American Board of Family Medicine* 24(3): 249–57.

Deave T, Heron J, Evans J, Emond A (2008) The impact of maternal depression in pregnancy on early child development. *British Journal of Obstetrics and Gynaecology* 115: 1043–51.

Edhborg M, Matthiesen AS, Lundh W, Widström AM (2005) Some early indicators for depressive symptoms and bonding 2 months postpartum: a study of new mothers and fathers. *Archives of Women's Mental Health* 8(4): 221–31.

Emerson WR (1998) Birth trauma: the psychological effects of obstetrical interventions. *Journal of Prenatal, Perinatal Psychology & Health* 13(1): 11–44.

Ensor J (2013) Woman with severe mental disorder given right to have abortion by judge, *Daily Telegraph,* 21 May 2013. www.telegraph.co.uk/news/uknews/law-and-order/10072388/Woman-with-severe-mental-disorder-given-right-to-have-abortion-by-judge.html (viewed 21/02/15).

Escriba-Aguir V, Artazcoz L (2011) Gender differences in postpartum depression: a longitudinal cohort study. *Journal of Epidemiology & Community Health* 65(4): 320–6.

Ferketich SL, Mercer RT (1995) Predictors of role competence for experienced and inexperienced fathers. *Nursing Research* 44(20): 89–95.

Field T, Diego M, Hernandez-Reif M, Figueiredo B, Deeds O, Contogeorgos J, Ascencio A (2010) Prenatal paternal depression. *Infant Behavior and Development* 29(4): 579–83.

Fisher J, Cabral de Mello M, Patel V, Rahman A, Tran T, Holton S, Holmes W (2012) Prevalence and determinants of common perinatal mental disorders in women in low and lower-middle-income countries: a systematic review. *Bulletin of the World Health Organization* 90: 139–49. doi: 10.2471/BLT.11.091850.

Flach C, Leese M, Heron J, Evans J, Feder G, Sharp D, Howard L (2011), Antenatal domestic violence, maternal mental health and subsequent child behaviour: a cohort study. BJOG: An International Journal of Obstetrics & Gynaecology118: 1383–91. doi: 10.1111/j.1471-0528.2011.03040.

Forray A, Focseneanu M, Pittman B, McDougle CJ, Epperson CN (2010) Onset and exacerbation of obsessive-compulsive disorder in pregnancy and the postpartum period. *Journal of Clinical Psychiatry* 71(8): 1061–8.

Furber CM, Garrod D, Maloney E, Lovell K, McGowan L (2009) A qualitative study of mild to moderate psychological distress during pregnancy. *International Journal of Nursing Studies* 46: 669–77.

Garabedian, MJ, Lain KY, Hansen WF, Garcia LS, Williams CM, Crofford LJ (Mar. 2011) Violence against women and postpartum depression. *Journal of Women's Health* 20(3): 447–53.

Gattrell C (2005) *Hard Labour: the sociology of parenthood.* Maidenhead: Open University Press.

Gavron H (1968) *The Captive Wife.* Harmondsworth: Penguin.

Gaynes BN, Gavin N, Meltzer-Brody S, Lohr KN, Swinson T, Gartlehner G, Brody S, Miller WC (2005) *Perinatal Depression: prevalence, screening accuracy, and screening outcomes summary.* Rockville, MD: Agency for Healthcare Research and Quality. U.S. Dept. of Health and Human Services.

Gieleghum A, Mittelstaedt ME, Bulik CM (2002) Eating disorders and childbearing: concealment and consequences. *Birth* 29(3): 182–91.

Gjerdingen D, Fontaine P, Crow S, McGovern P, Center B, Miner M (2009) Predictors of mothers' post-partum body dissatisfaction. *Women & Health* 49(6): 491–504.

Goodman JH (2004) Paternal postpartum depression, its relationship to maternal postpartum depression and implications for family health. *Journal of Advanced Nursing* 45(1): 26–35.

Grandey M, Cresswell T, Duerden J, Mannion K (2002) *Drug Misuse in Pregnancy in the Northern and Yorkshire Region*. Stockton-on-Tees: Wolfson Research Institute, University of Durham.

Hans S (1999) Demographic and psychosocial characteristics of substance-abusing pregnant women. *Clinics in Perinatology* 26: 55–74.

Harris J (2012) History of homebirth. In: Steen M (ed.), *Supporting Women to Give Birth at Home: a practical guide for midwives*. London: Routledge, Ch. 1 pp. 1–13.

Hegde S, Latha KS, Bhat SM, Sharma PSVN, Kamath A, Shetty AK (2012) Postpartum depression: prevalence and associated factors among women in India. *Journal of Women's Health, Issues and Care* 1: 1. doi: 10.4172/2325-9795.1000101.

Holloway S (2013) Resilience in mind – early action for mental health. *Community Links*. www.community-links.org/linksuk/?p=3910 (viewed 13/06/13).

Hudson JI, Hirip E, Pope HG Jr, Kessler RC (2007) The prevalence and correlates of eating disorders in the national comorbidity survey replication. *Biological Psychiatry* 61(3): 348–58.

IAPT (Improving Access to Psychological Therapies) (2009) *Perinatal: positive practice guide*. London: Department of Health. www.iapt.nhs.uk/silo/files/perinatal-positive-practice-guide.pdf (accessed 01/09/15).

Iles J, Slade P, Spiby H (May, 2011) Posttraumatic stress symptoms and postpartum depression in couples after childbirth: the role of partner support and attachment. *Journal of Anxiety Disorders* 25(4): 520–30.

Johnson AR, Edwin S, Joachim N, Mathew G, Ajay S, Joseph B (2015) Postnatal depression among women availing maternal health services in a rural hospital in South India. *Pak J Med Sci* 31(2): doi: dx.doi.org/

Johnson Z, Molloy B, Scallon E et al. (2000) Community Mothers' Programme – seven-year follow up of a randomised controlled trial of non-professional intervention in parenting. *Journal of Public Health Medicine* 22(3): 337–42.

Kingdon C (2009) *Sociology for Midwives*. London: Quay Books.

Lavender V (2007) Body image: change, dissatisfaction and disturbance. In: Price S (ed.), *Mental Health in Pregnancy and Childbirth*. Edinburgh: Churchill Livingstone, pp. 123–46.

Leeds L, Hargreaves I (2008) The psychological consequences of childbirth. *Journal of Reproductive and Infant Psychology* 26(2): 108–22.

Lindgren K (2001) Relationships among maternal-fetal attachment, prenatal depression, and health practice in pregnancy. *Research in Nursing & Health* 24: 203–17.

Little L, Lowkes E (2000) Critical issues in the care of pregnant women with eating disorders and the impact on their children. *Journal of Midwifery & Women's Health* 454: 301–7.

Lord C, Rieder A, Hall GBC, Soares CN, Steiner M (2011) Piloting the perinatal obsessive-compulsive scale (POCS): development and validation. *Journal of Anxiety Disorders* 25(8): 1079–84.

Luecken LJ, Lin B, Coburn SS, MacKinnon DP, Gonzales NA, Crnic KA (2013) Prenatal stress, partner support, and infant cortisol reactivity in low-income Mexican American families. *Psychoneuroendocrinology* 38(12): 3092–101.

Melender H (2002) Experiences of fears associated with pregnancy and childbirth: a study of 329 women. *Birth* 27(3): 101–11.

Milgrom J, Schembri C, Ericksen J, Ross J, Gemmill AW (May, 2011) Towards parenthood: an antenatal intervention to reduce depression, anxiety and parenting difficulties. *Journal of Affective Disorders* 130(3): 385–94.

Miller, T. (2007) Is this what motherhood is all about? Weaving experiences and discourse through transition to first-time motherhood. *Gender & Society* 21(3): 337–58.

Mitchell AM, Bulik CM (2006) Eating disorders and women's health: an update. *Journal of Midwifery and Women's Health* 51(3): 193–201.

Molloy M (2007) Volunteering as a Community Mother – a pathway to lifelong learning. *Community Practitioner* 80(5): 28–32.

Morrell CJ, Ricketts T, Tudor K, Williams C, Curran J, Barkham M (2011) Training health visitors in cognitive behavioural and person-centred approaches for depression in postnatal women as part of a cluster randomised trial and economic evaluation in primary care: the PoNDER trial. *Primary Health Care Research & Development* 12(1): 11–20.

Murphy DJ (2003) Women's views on the impact of operative delivery in the second stage of labour: qualitative interview study. *British Medical Journal* 327(7424): 1132.

National Treatment Agency for Substance Misuse (2010) *Women in Drug Treatment: what the latest figures reveal*. London: NTASM.

Newnham EC (2014) Birth control: power/knowledge in the politics of birth. *Health Sociology Review* 23(3): 254–68.

NICE (2004) *Eating Disorders: core interventions in the treatment and management of anorexia nervosa, bulimia nervosa and related eating disorders*. NICE Clinical Guideline 9. London: National Institute for Clinical Excellence. ISBN 1-84257-496-7. www.nice.org.uk/CG009Niceguideline (viewed 01/03/12).

NICE (2007a) *Mental Health Problems during Pregnancy and after Giving Birth*. NICE Clinical Guideline 45. London: National Institute for Health and Clinical Excellence.

NICE (2007b) *Intrapartum Care*. NICE Clinical Guideline 55. London: National Institute for Health and Clinical Excellence.

NICE (2008) *Antenatal Care: routine care for the healthy pregnant woman*. NICE Clinical Guideline 62. London: National Institute for Health and Care Excellence. www.nice.org.uk/cg62 (viewed 21/02/15).

Nilsson E, Lichtenstein P, Cnattingius S, Murray RM, Hultman CM (2002) Women with schizophrenia: pregnancy outcome and infant death among their offspring. *Schizophrenia Research* 58(2/3): 221–9.

Oakley A (1979) *From Here to Maternity: becoming a mother*. Harmondsworth: Penguin.

Paulson JF, Keefe HA, Leiferman J (2009) Early parental depression and child language development. *Journal of Child Psychology and Psychiatry & Allied Disciplines* 50(3): 254-62.

Ramchandani PG, Stein A, O'Connor TG, Heron J, Murray L, Evans J (2008) Depression in men in the postnatal period and later child psychopathology: a population cohort study. *Journal of the American Academy of Child & Adolescent Psychiatry* 47(4): 390–8.

Ramchandani P, Stein A, Evans J, O'Connor T (2005) Paternal depression in the postnatal period and child development: a prospective population study. *Lancet* 365(9478): 2201–5.

Ramnero J, Ost L-G, (2007) Panic and avoidance in panic disorder with agoraphobia: clinical relevance of change in different aspects of the disorder. *Journal of Behavior Therapy & Experimental Psychiatry* 38: 29–39.

Raymond JE (2009) 'Creating a safety net': women's experiences of antenatal depression and their identification of helpful community support and services during pregnancy. *Midwifery* 25(1): 39–49.

RCOG (2011) *Statement on Draft NICE Guidelines. Caesarean Section Guidelines*. www.rcog.org.uk/what-we-do/campaigning-and-opinions/statement/rcog-statement-draft-nice-caesarean-section-guidelines (viewed 01/03/12).

Robertson E, Grace S, Wallington T, Stewart DE (2004) Antenatal risk factors for postpartum depression: a synthesis of recent literature. *General Hospital Psychiatry* 26: 289–95.

Robinson M, Steen M, Robertson S, Raine G (2014) *Evaluation of the Local Mind Resilience Programme. Final report*. London: Mind.

Rubertsson C, Waldenstrom U, Wickberg B (2003) Depressive mood in early pregnancy: prevalence and women at risk in a national Swedish sample. *Journal of Reproductive and Infant Psychology* 21(2): 113–23.

Sanders LB (2006) Assessing and managing women with depression: a midwifery perspective. *Journal of Midwifery and Women's Health* 51: 185–92.

Schatz DB, Hsaio MC, Liu CY (2012) Antenatal depression in East Asia: a review of the literature. *Psychiatry Investigation* 9(2).

Shaban Z, Dolatian M, Shams J, Alavi-Majd H, Mahmoodi Z, Sajjadi H (2013) Post-traumatic stress disorder (PTSD) following childbirth: prevalence and contributing factors. *Iranian Red Crescent Medical Journal* 15(3): 177–82. www.ncbi.nlm.nih.gov/pmc/articles/PMC3745743/ (viewed 21/02/15).

Sherr L, Dave S, Lucas P, Senior R, Nazareth I (2006) A feasibility study on recruiting fathers of young children to examine the impact of paternal depression on child development. *Child Psychiatry & Human Development* 36(3): 295–309.

Skari H, Skredne M, Malt U, Dalholt M, Ostensen AB, Egeland T, Emblem R (2002) Comparative levels of psychological distress, stress symptoms, depression and anxiety after childbirth a prospective population based study of mothers and fathers. *BJOG: An International Journal of Obstetrics and Gynaecology* 109(10): 1154–63.

Smart J, Hiscock H (2007) Early infant crying and sleeping problems: a pilot study of impact on parental well-being and parent-endorsed strategies for management. *Journal of Paediatrics and Child Health* 43(4): 284–90.

Soares CN, Zitek B (July 2008) Reproductive hormone sensitivity and risk for depression across the female life cycle: a continuum of vulnerability? *J Psychiatry Neurosci* 33(4): 331–43.

Sockol LE, Epperson CN, Barber JP (2011) A meta-analysis of treatments for perinatal depression. *Clinical Psychology Review* 31(5): 839–49.

Soet JE, Brack GA Dilorio C (2003) Prevalence and predictors of women's experience of psychological trauma during childbirth. *Birth* 30: 36–46.

Stapleton LRT, Schetter CD, Westling E, Rini C, Glynn LM, Hobel CJ, Sandman CA (2012) Perceived partner support in pregnancy predicts lower maternal and infant distress. *Journal of Family Psychology* 26(3): 453. www.ncbi.nlm.nih.gov/pmc/articles/PMC3992993/ (viewed 01/09/15).

Steen M (2011) *Pregnancy and Birth: everything you need to know.* London: Dorling Kindersley.

Steen M (2009) When food becomes the enemy: eating disorders. *Midwives* 12(2): 30–1.

Steen M (2007) Wellbeing and beyond. *RCM Midwives Journal* 10(3): 116–19.

Steen M, Jones K (2012) Supporting homebirth. In: Steen M (ed.), *Supporting Women to Give Birth at Home: a practical guide for midwives.* London: Routledge. Ch. 4 pp. 81–121.

Steen M, Jones A (2013) Maternal mental health: stigma and shame. *The Practising Midwife* 16(6): 5.

Steen M, Steen S (2014) Striving for better maternal mental health. *The Practising Midwife.* 17(3): 11–14.

Steen M, Jones A, Woodworth B (2013) Anxiety, bonding and attachment during pregnancy, the transition to parenthood and psychotherapy. *British Journal of Midwifery* 21(12): 844–50.

Terp IM, Mortensen PB (1998) Post-partum psychoses: clinical diagnoses and relative risk of admission after parturition. *British Journal of Psychiatry* 172: 521–6.

Tham V, Ryding EL, Christensson K (2010) Experience of support among mothers with and without post-traumatic stress symptoms following emergency caesarean section. *Sexual & Reproductive Healthcare : Official Journal of the Swedish Association of Midwives* 1(4): 175–80.

Thompson M, Kingree J (1998) The frequency and impact of violent trauma among pregnant substance abusers. *Addictive Behaviors* 23: 257–62.

Tucker L (2003) Fear factors: everyone reacts to fear differently. Scientists are beginning to understand why. *Science World* 7 February, 14–15.

Valentine, Jeanette M. Rodriguez, Michael A. Lapeyrouse, Lisa M. Zhang, Muyu (Apr 2011) Recent intimate partner violence as a prenatal predictor of maternal depression in the first year postpartum among Latinas. *Archives of Women's Mental Health* 14(2): 135–43.

Van Bussell J, Spitz B, Demyttenaere K, (2006) Women's mental health before, during, and after pregnancy: a population-based controlled cohort study. *Birth* 33(4): 297–302.

Van den Berg MP, van der Ende J, Crignen AAM, Jaddoe VWV, Moll HA, Mackenbach JP, Hofman A, Hengeveld MW, Tiemeier H, Verhulst FC (2009) Paternal depressive symptoms during pregnancy are related to excessive infant crying. *Pediatrics* 124(1): e96–103.

Vasconcelos MS, Sampaio AS, Hounie AG, Akkerman F, Curi M, Lopes AC, Miguel EC (2007) Prenatal, perinatal, and postnatal risk factors in obsessive-compulsive disorder. *Biological Psychiatry* 61(3): 301–7.

Vilska S, Unkila-Kallio L, Punamäki RL, Poikkeus P, Repokari L, Sinkkonen J, Tiitinen A, Tulppala, M. (2009) Mental health of mothers and fathers of twins conceived via assisted reproduction treatment: a one year prospective study. *Human Reproduction* 24(2): 367–77.

Wolfe BE (2005) Reproductive health in women with eating disorders. *J Obstet Gynecol Neonatal Nurse* 34(2): 255–63.

Workhouse, The (2012) *Liverpool Workhouse*. www.workhouses.org.uk/Liverpool/ (viewed 20/07/12).

Yu Y, Zhang S, Wang G et al. (2013) The combined association of psychosocial stress and chronic hypertension with pre-eclampsia. *American Journal of Obstetrics & Gynecology* 209(5): 438.e1–438.e12.

5 Mental health during childhood

Monika Ferguson, Alison Owen Traynor and Nicholas Procter

An introduction to mental health during childhood

Most children experience good mental health. However, it is estimated that between 10 per cent and 20 per cent of the world's children and adolescents experience at least one form of mental illness (World Health Organisation [WHO] 2014a). It is becoming increasingly recognised that experiences early in life direct the nature and course of mental health and illness in subsequent years, with an estimated 50 per cent of mental illnesses in adults beginning before the age of 14 (WHO 2013). Childhood is a critical period in an individual's development and there is evidence to suggest that various negative, stressful and dysfunctional experiences early in life can have a cumulative influence on impairment to brain structures and functions (Anda et al. 2006), and may contribute to diminished mental health. As such, a global focus is being placed on the importance of promoting mental health in childhood and taking an early intervention and preventative approach to reduce mental illness across the lifespan (WHO 2013). Information and evidence about the burden and onset, risk factors, assessment and treatment, and clinical practice guidelines for common mental health issues in young people feature more prominently over the past 10 to 15 years. There has also been an increase in accessibility of existing research about prevention and treatment of mental health and substance use issues in young people (headspace 2014).

This chapter will focus on what it means to experience mental health and wellbeing in child-hood (birth to 14 years) and why this is important. It will also outline some of the common mental health conditions in childhood, particularly anxiety and depression, as well as trauma-related and neurological conditions. It will explore some of the factors that can contribute to and protect against mental health problems and mental illness. In particular, the chapter will focus on the important role of early attachment relationships and environments as both positive and negative influences on child mental health. It will explore the impact of living with mental illness on children and their families, as well as highlight some of the ways that we can work towards promoting mental health among children. Case studies will be included to offer insight into some children's experiences with mental health concerns, as well as the experiences of their families and support networks.

This chapter will consider:

- The importance of the family context for the development of mentally healthy children;
- Factors within various environments (home, school and broader society) which can influence a child's mental health;
- The range of common mental health conditions experienced by children;
- The importance of early intervention approaches to promote children's mental health and reduce the development of mental health conditions.

Children and mental health

Mental health and wellbeing in childhood

In adulthood, mental health is a fluctuating state and can be seen as a measure of how well a person can cope with day-to-day challenges and bounce back from difficulties they may encounter. When considering children, mental health and wellbeing are thought to include the individual's ability to develop psychologically, physically, emotionally, intellectually and socially. Consideration is also given to their ability to develop, engage in and enjoy personal relationships with their family, relatives and peers, whilst exploring and learning (Zero to Three 2014). Other elements important for child mental health and wellbeing include the development of a positive sense of identity, and the ability to manage thoughts and emotions (WHO 2013).

It is now widely recognised that positive early interpersonal environments (particularly those with parents and caregivers) are vital for the development of a child's mental health and wellbeing. The family environment is the place in which the child's development first begins, where children learn to model the behaviour and reactions of their parents/caregivers, learn to cope with events and emotions, and is where they are (hopefully) provided with support to develop and explore the world. Critical for the developing child is the knowledge of a parent or significant attachment figure who is there to hold and comfort them at times of emotional difficulty or challenge. A supportive environment for learning can build self-esteem and self-worth as children learn to develop new skills and behaviours and to express emotions. In essence, the family environment provides a child with a physical, neurocognitive and social-emotional bedrock for healthy development through childhood and into adulthood (Sawyer et al. 2014).

One key theory for understanding the development of the early relationships formed between a child and significant others is attachment theory. Developed by John Bowlby, attachment theory suggests that:

> what is believed to be essential for mental health is that the infant and young child should experience a warm, intimate and continuous relationship with his mother (or permanent mother-substitute) in which it finds both satisfaction and enjoyment.
>
> (Bowlby 1952, p. 11)

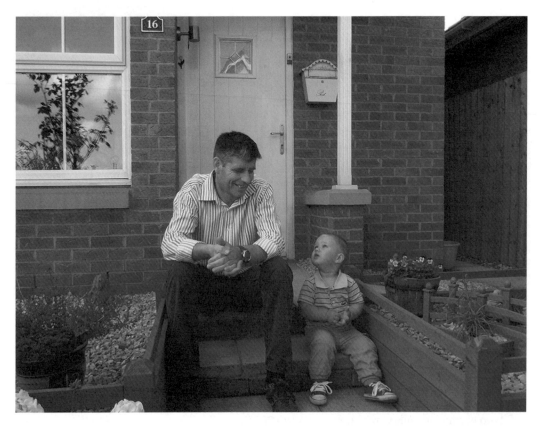

Figure 5.1 A grandfather bonding with his grandson

Today, attachment is more broadly considered to occur with other important caregivers, not just the mother, however the key elements of the theory remain. According to attachment theory, early attachments are often formalised at approximately six to nine months of age, and can be seen when an infant becomes aware of the absence of their primary caregiver and fearful of strangers. Children are thought to develop one of four types of attachment to another person, and they may experience multiple forms of attachment with different adults. These four types of attachment and the caregiving styles associated with these are shown in Figure 5.2.

Caregiving style	Attachment style
Sensitive and loving	Secure
Insensitive and rejecting	Insecure-avoidant
Insensitive and inconsistent	Insecure-resistant
Atypical	Insecure-disorganised

Figure 5.2 Caregiving styles and type of attachment formed

Source: Adapted from Daniel, Wassell and Gilligan 1999.

Secure attachment is considered optimal for positive child mental health. Such relationships with parents, caregivers and other important adults (e.g. grandparents) are characterised by warmth, responsiveness and trust; these provide the child with a template for future relationships, and provide a sense of security and safety (KidsMatter 2014a). These relationships emerge from a nurturing, predictable and stable environment, with adults who respond to the physical, social and emotional needs of the child. In a consistently safe environment children can feel confident to explore their surroundings, to try new things and to feel supported as they attempt new skills. It also encourages children to trust that help will be available if needed. These early relationships form the foundation for relationships later in life. A lack of these positive early relationships can result in children having difficulties in self-regulation, capacity to form future relationships, and management of feelings and behaviour, which can subsequently lead to poor mental health. In particular, the first three years are seen as a vital period for caregivers to build children's emotional and social foundations. Evidence from neuroscience suggests that brain development (particularly the connections between brain cells and synapses) is strengthened by experience (Smith and Allen 2008). For example, the more positive stimuli an infant is given, the better their brain development will be (Smith and Allen 2008).

In addition to attachment, there are a number of influential theories that seek to explain the psycho-social, cognitive and emotional development of children, proposing how they develop knowledge, learn, think and make sense of the world around them. These theories help us identify some of the specific stages and influencing factors in a child's emotional development, social interaction and intellectual development. Whilst not applicable to all cultures, Erikson's stages of psychosocial development offer an aged-based guide. It consists of key 'crises' at each stage and associated developmental tasks; when a crisis is not resolved and the developmental task is not achieved, social and emotional problems may begin to emerge (Eddy 2013). These crises and developmental tasks are shown in Table 5.1.

In contrast to those children who develop positive mental health and wellbeing, others experience mental health problems across a range of domains. According to the United Kingdom's National Service Framework for Children Young People and Maternity Services (Department of Health 2004), 'mental health problems may be reflected in difficulties and/or disabilities in the realm of personal relationships, psychological development, the capacity for play and learning and in distress and maladaptive behaviour' (p. 44). Examples of indicators of wellbeing and poor mental health at different childhood stages can be seen in Table 5.2.

Unlike adults, children, especially infants and the very young, will not be able to verbalise how they feel and may express psychological distress through the presentation of somatic symptoms. Some children are admitted to hospital with a mental health problem when they are presenting a physical illness with real symptoms, such as abdominal pain, headaches, tiredness and limb pain. A literature review identifying risk factors for somatic symptoms in children highlights the prevalence of this phenomenon (Banks and Bevan 2014). This is considered to be a misunderstood and little explained area of child health where children can be wrongly diagnosed. Practitioners need to aware that, for some children, psychological distress and emotional conflict are communicated through physical symptoms.

Collaborative multi-agency and robust partnership working is essential to coordinate services to meet the child and family's needs across the lifespan. It is also very important that a holistic assessment has been made to ensure the individual needs have been identified as there may be more

Table 5.1 Erikson's five stages of psychosocial development and the
associated crises and developmental tasks

Developmental stage	Psychosocial crisis	Developmental task
Infancy	Trust vs. mistrust	Attachment to parent – if successful the individual will be able to form trusting and healthy relationships throughout his or her lifetime
Early childhood	Autonomy vs. shame and doubt	Basic self-control and confidence in environmental exploration – if successful the individual will be able to cultivate self-confidence and independence
Late childhood	Initiative vs. guilt	Sense of purpose – successful resolution results in self-directedness in activities
School age	Industry vs. Inferiority	Competence in tasks – if successful the individual will be able to feel pride in accomplishing his or her work and not feel comparison to others
Adolescence	Identity vs. role confusion	Formation of identity – individuals who are successful at this development stage achieve a sense of identity and confidence about who they are that later enables them to develop intimacy

Source: Adapted from Eddy 2013.

than one problem which will require more than one service. A child who presents with behavioural problems in the classroom or at home may need to have a hearing test to rule out hearing problems, which may have been the root cause of the behaviour. A child who presents with physical symptoms with no medical diagnosis may have an emotional or mental health problem.

Common mental illness/mental health difficulties in childhood

Similarly to adults, children experience fluctuations in their mental health; this is normal and not necessarily indicative of mental illness. However, some children do experience mental illness, or the early signs of an illness which may develop later in life. Although some occasional feelings of upset, despair and worry are all part of child development, the diagnosis of a mental health condition can occur when these feelings and symptoms are prolonged, are beyond that which is considered typical for the individual child's current level of development, and interfere with normal daily life. Children are also susceptible to the same mental illnesses as adults. What differs is the way that children experience these and the way that these are expressed within the child's developmental stage. Additionally, mental illness in children may be more difficult to identify. This difficulty can be attributed in part due to stages of early development meaning that expression will vary. While many conditions share similar features, the developmental stage of the child must be taken into account. Adding to this complexity is that young children do not have the same potential to communicate their feelings, thoughts and emotions in the way as adults do. For this reason, understanding the state of a child's mental health (and the potential presence of a mental illness)

Table 5.2 Examples of indicators of wellbeing and poor mental health in infants, toddlers and pre-schoolers, and school-aged children*

Age range	Indicators of wellbeing	Indicators of poor mental health
Infants (0–18 months)	- alert, relaxed, maintains eye contact, smiles - babbles and smiles - predictable eating and sleeping cycles - enjoys social play (e.g. peek-a-boo) - spends significant time familiarising with body (e.g. sucking own fingers) - engages, disengages, and re-engages with parents/carers - become upset after separation from parent/caregiver but is easily comforted on return - starts and seeks interaction with parent/caregiver	- chronic sleeping or feeding disturbances - excessive crying and difficult to comfort - appears wary or frightened - appears overly quiet, passive or disinterested in surroundings - disinterested in interacting with people - failure to reach developmental milestones - not easily comforted after separation and return of caregiver - lack of gestures (e.g. pointing) to communicate
Toddlers and pre-school children (18 months–5 years)	- engages in pretend play with others - uses words or gestures to express feelings - indicates desire for comfort (e.g. sit on a lap) - recovers from anger - cooperates with others	- limited interest in environment and/or people - indiscriminate affection through displays of affection to strangers - inconsistent sleep pattern - displays limited emotions - hypervigilance, apprehension, anxiousness - angry or aggressive behaviour - failure to seek comfort from caregiver - unable to calm self and manage emotions
School children (5–14 years)	- plays and interacts fairly with peers (takes turns, listens to others, helps others) - communicates and interacts effectively with others - complies with instructions - trusts others - able to manage own feelings and emotions - demonstrates interest in trying new things - persists with new/challenging activities (e.g. problem solving) - enjoys attending school	- unexplained and frequent tantrums - unusual fears - sleep difficulties - feelings of sadness and hopelessness - avoidance of friends and family - refusal to attend school - difficulty getting along with peers - hyperactivity - disinterest in school/decline in school performance - aggressive reactions - concentration difficulties - unexplained changes in behaviour

Note: *A number of these indicators may be symptoms of physical ill health (e.g. excessive crying in infants may represent teething difficulties; difficulty concentrating in school age children may represent vision or hearing difficulties) and therefore it is important to take an holistic approach to consider these symptoms in the context of other factors in the child's life.

Source: Adapted from Cousins 2013 and KidsMatter 2014b.

requires thorough communication with, and input from, key people in the child's life (e.g. parents, caregivers, grandparents, teachers), as well as collateral information and observation of their behaviour and reactions. Assessment should also be tailored to the developmental age and culture of the child. This can be achieved through interactive play and/or drawing activities, often occurring in a non-clinical environment.

Rates of mental illness can be more difficult to determine than they are in adults. Sometimes, this can be because children may experience the early signs of mental illness long before a condition is diagnosed, meaning that rates are often underreported. A survey of the mental health of children and young people (aged 5–16 years) in Great Britain carried out in 2004 provides some indication of the rates of mental illness (Green et al. 2005). The data indicate that mental health problems influence 10.4 per cent of boys and 5.9 per cent of girls in the 5–10 age range, and 12.8 per cent of boys and 9.7 per cent of girls in the 11–15 year range. Additionally, one in ten of the total sample had a clinically diagnosed mental health disorder. In the United States, this rate increases to one in five children and adolescents (Kataoka, Zhang and Wells 2002). These differences may be due to the way that mental health and mental illness are classified and measured. This section will consider some of the more common mental illnesses experienced by children, including: anxiety, depression, trauma and stressor-related disorders, and neurodevelopmental disorders. Some children also engage in suicidal and self-harming behaviours, and this too will be considered.

Anxiety

Anxiety is the most common mental health problem affecting children and young people, and it has many contributing causes, including recent traumatic events (e.g. the loss of a loved one) as well as personality traits and temperament (e.g. shyness). Anxiety disorders share the common features of excessive fear (emotional response to real or perceived imminent threat), anxiety (anticipation of future threat) and related behavioural disturbances (American Psychiatric Association [APA] 2013). Experiencing some fearfulness and anxiousness is common as children respond to changes in the environment and over time learn to cope with new feelings as part of their growth and development (KidsMatter 2014b). In some cases, these experiences are more extreme and children can show a disproportionate and persistent amount of fear. Common symptoms of anxiety include fear and avoidance of particular issues or situations; physical symptoms (such as headaches or stomach aches) prior to certain events/scenarios; school refusal, sleeping problems, including nightmares, trouble falling asleep without a parent nearby; lots of worries and need for reassurance (KidsMatter 2014b). In very young children (aged 3–5 years), some of the more common symptoms involve fears about physical injury (the dark, spiders), social fears (playing with other children or meeting new people), separation (sleeping alone or being away from home) (KidsMatter 2014b) and constantly seeking reassurance. Younger children may not be able to verbalise anxieties but instead may exhibit physical symptoms and complain of pain (e.g. headache, stomach ache); they may also vomit and soil themselves.

Separation anxiety disorder

Separation anxiety is characterised by the experience of excessive fear and/or anxiety related to being separated from home or an attachment figure (APA 2013). Some children may respond to this by becoming extremely upset during times of separation, whereas others may express anger toward the person who is trying to 'take them away' (KidsMatter 2014b). Other children may respond with complaints of physical symptoms, such as stomach aches. It is important to consider typical attachment development here – we would expect a young baby to cry when his/her parent leaves the room, but we would not usually expect this of a school-aged child. This might also involve excessive worry about the imagined loss of, or harm to, an attachment figure.

Selective mutism

Selective mutism refers to an experience where a child consistently fails to speak in situations where they would typically be expected to speak (such as at school) (APA 2013). This can be confusing, as the child may speak in other situations, such as with other children. Other means to communicate may also be used, including pointing or grunting.

Specific phobia

Some children experience specific phobia, which refers to fear and/or anxiousness toward certain objects or stimuli (e.g. certain animals, heights, etc.). It also usually results in avoidance of that stimulus (APA 2013). This experience may be expressed through behaviours such as crying, tantrums, freezing or clinging to parents/attachment figures.

Social anxiety/social phobia

Some children may also experience social anxiety, referring to fear and/or anxiousness about, or avoidance, of social interactions/situations (APA 2013). Usually, this relates to concerns about the possibility of being scrutinised by others. This is often experienced more commonly by older children who are approaching their teens, but can be seen in younger children.

Depression

The onset of depression is usually most likely to occur in the teenage years, rather than during early childhood; however, it can be experienced by, or show early origins in, younger children. Typically, it is characterised by a depressed mood and loss of interest and/or pleasure in a child's usual activities. These feelings of sadness in young children may be externalised and manifest as poor behaviour, including showing anger, irritability and smearing faeces. Other symptoms include alterations in appetite, sleep, psychomotor activity, as well as difficulty concentrating and thinking. Other feelings may also include guilt and emptiness. More so than adults, depression in children may be expressed more as irritability rather than sadness (APA 2013). Thoughts of suicide and death may also be experienced. There are various risk and contributing factors for depression, including genetic inheritance, personality/temperament, and recent upsetting or unsettling experiences.

Trauma and stressor-related conditions

The early experience of trauma, such as neglect or violence, can contribute to the experience of trauma and stressor-related conditions (APA 2013).

Post traumatic stress disorder

Post traumatic stress disorder is the most commonly experienced of trauma and stressor-related conditions. Typically, it is a response occurring after real or threatened death, injury or violence (either to the child or to someone important in the child's life) (APA 2013). The event often appears frequently in symptoms, such as distressing dreams of the event, flashbacks and re-enactment of the event (or aspects of the event) in play or drawings. Some children might also display changes in mood and avoidant behaviour. Others will react with hyperactivity, poor concentration, aggression and antisocial behaviour, which can result in a misdiagnosis of attention deficit hyperactivity disorder (KidsMatter 2014b).

Reactive attachment disorder and disinhibited social engagement disorder

Although rare, there are some conditions which result from serious neglect in the early childhood years when some children have been provided with limited opportunities to develop attachment. These include reactive attachment disorder and disinhibited social engagement disorder, both of which can only be diagnosed after the developmental age of 9 months (and usually before 5 years of age), when children have the developmental capacity to form attachments (APA 2013). Reactive attachment disorder is characterised by inappropriate attachment behaviours, such as a child rarely turning to an attachment figure for comfort, and lack of response to comfort (APA 2013). In contrast, disinhibited social engagement disorder is characterised by inappropriate and overly familiar behaviour with people considered to be strangers to a child (APA 2013). These conditions may also co-occur with other developmental delays associated with social neglect, such as cognitive and language impairment.

Neurodevelopmental disorders

Neurodevelopmental disorders usually emerge in the developmental period, usually early in development, often as result of impaired brain development. These conditions contribute to deficits in a child's personal, social, academic or occupational functioning (APA 2013). Two of the more common neurodevelopmental disorders are autism spectrum disorder and attention deficit hyperactivity disorder. In contrast to anxiety and depression, which may only occur once or fluctuate throughout the lifespan, neurodevelopmental disorders and/or their symptoms are more likely to persist.

Autism spectrum disorder

Autism spectrum disorder is more common among boys than girls and is characterised by deficits in social communication and social interaction across various contexts. Examples include troubles with social-emotional reciprocity (that is, the child's ability to engage with others and share feelings); lack of, or developmentally delayed, speech; impaired use of language; troubles with non-verbal communication (e.g. eye contact); and difficulty with developing, maintaining and understanding relationships (APA 2013). Many children experiencing this condition may also engage in restricted, repetitive patterns of behaviour, activities or interests, such as repetitively lining up pencils or repeating certain words.

Attention deficit hyperactivity disorder

In the UK, attention deficit hyperactivity disorder is the most common behavioural disorder, with figures suggesting if affects around 2–5 per cent of school-aged children and young people, and is more commonly diagnosed in boys than girls. This condition is typically characterised by inattention (wandering off task), disorganisation, and/or hyperactivity (excessive motor activity) / impulsivity (hasty actions) (APA 2013). What this means is that the child often has difficulty staying 'on-task', may appear to not be listening and may lose materials they are given. They may also appear 'fidgety' and unable to 'wait their turn'. The course of this condition is different for each child; however, when it is first diagnosed in the pre-school years it tends to be chronic and severe (Riddle et al. 2013).

Conduct disorders/oppositional defiant disorder

Children will present with a persistent repetitive pattern of high risk behaviours which can be described as 'not sticking to the rules' including aggressive behaviour towards people or animals. In the younger child, features of oppositional defiant disorder are more likely, such as non-compliance, lack of self-regulation, and persistent hostile behaviour.

Suicide and self-harm behaviour

Although suicide and self-harm are behaviours, not mental illnesses, they are often associated with the experience of mental illness or diminished mental health (APA 2013). While reported rates of suicide in young children indicate that this is rare, the impacts of suicide can be devastating for the individual's family and community. Little is known about rates of suicide and self-harm in very young children, and what is known tends to suggest lower rates of these behaviours than in adolescents. According to the WHO (2014b), global rates of suicide are lowest in those under 15 years of age, but the figures are still concerning. For example, in Australia between 2007 and 2011, 53 of the 11,600 recorded suicides occurred in people aged 5–14 years; no records of suicide in children aged <5 years were found. Of the 53, 17 (32 per cent) were of Aboriginal and Torres Strait Islander Australians (Australian Bureau of Statistics 2013). Serious self-harming behaviours (such as overdoses or cutting, and head-banging, hitting or self-scratching in younger children) can be an indicator of mental illness and should alert to the need for intervention. A recent report by the Australian Human Rights Commission (2014) found between 2007–2008 and 2012–2013, there were over 18,000 hospitalisations in Australia for intentional self-harm by children aged 3–17 years. Alarmingly, many more occurrences will not require hospitalisation, meaning that these figures are likely to be an underestimation of actual self-harm rates.

Cautions when diagnosing mental illness in children

While the previously described diagnoses can be important for directing treatment and early intervention approaches, many children may experience some of the symptoms of a mental illness and therefore diagnosis should be undertaken with caution. Recently, Jureidini (2014) has argued that, in today's society, those involved in the care of children are quick to label signs of a child's distress (e.g. sadness, anger, fear), and that this can be damaging as it does not provide opportunity for the child to learn to cope with and manage these feelings. Instead, Jureidini (2014) suggests that distressed and upset children need empathy aimed towards helping and supporting them to manage, survive and benefit from sharing uncomfortable feelings. In this way, it is parents, teachers and health professionals who have a central role in providing the time environment to facilitate this process, rather than focusing on their own concerns regarding what a child is experiencing.

Another concern is the prescription of medication, which often follows from a mental illness diagnosis. For example, antidepressant use in children is on the rise (Mitchell et al. 2014). While doctors are prescribing more mental health medications for children and young people, what is less clear is the reasons for this. The overall upward trends in the prescribing of psychotropic medications has been attributed in part to a greater public awareness of mental illness and subsequent help-seeking behaviour (Partridge, Lucke and Hall 2014), as well as haste to apply and psychiatric label to ordinary, healthy but distressing feelings (Jureidini 2014).

Influences on mental health/illness in childhood

It should now be clear that children can experience a range of mental health conditions. However, many will progress through childhood experiencing positive mental health. Just as for adults, there are various risk and protective influences operating at different levels which can help us to understand why some children experience mental illness and others do not. Risk factors refer to those exposures or circumstances which can increase the likelihood of mental illness, whereas protective factors refer to those which not only decrease the likelihood of mental illness, but may also reduce the impact of mental illness. These influences can be understood to occur within different domains (the individual, family, peers/school, life events, and society) and are summarised in Figure 5.3. Again, like adults, not all children are influenced by these risk and protective factors in the same way, if at all, and a range of factors can predict symptoms of poor mental health (Bayer et al. 2011). There is also thought to be a dose-response relationship between level of exposure to risk factors and later mental illness, suggesting a cumulative effect of risk factors in the early years, with exposure to a greater number of risk factors associated with a greater chance of mental health problems and mental illness later in life (Sabates and Dex 2012).

Child/individual influences

A range of individual influences are linked to mental health outcomes. Some of these are considered risk factors; for example, a shy temperament may lead to internalising (Karevold et al. 2009), and pre-birth complications may lead to impaired cognitive development. Poor physical health can also be a risk factor, with higher rates of both internalising and externalising problems being found in children who experience a chronic physical illness. Internalising may result from factors such as lack of perceived control over the physical condition, lack of opportunities for positive activities, and peer rejection, whereas externalising problems may result from affected brain function and frustration (Bayer et al. 2011).

Domain	Influence
Individual	Complications during birth and early infancy Temperament Self-esteem Coping style Outlook on life Attachment to parents Achieving developmental milestones Resilience
Family	Family disharmony Parenting style Parental relationships/family structure Attachment Parental mental illness/substance abuse Sibling mental/physical illness/disability
Peers/school	Sense of belonging/connectedness Bullying (including cyber bullying) Academic success/failure School attendance Connection between family and school
Life events	School transition Death of a loved one Emotional trauma Violence/abuse (physical, sexual, psychological)
Society	Discrimination Isolation SES/disadvantage

Figure 5.3 Influences on children's mental health across different domains

Other individual factors are protective. Resilience is perhaps the most widely discussed and researched individual protective factor. Resilience refers to those innate qualities of an individual (such as behavioural and emotional self-regulation) that allow them to overcome adversities (Kieling et al. 2011). Various other factors have been found to contribute to resilience building, such as supportive and responsive parenting, and parental education and mental health (Kieling et al. 2011). Individual factors can also influence protective factors in other domains. For example, a study of low-income mothers found that those whose children demonstrated traits of social competence were more likely to have increased parental involvement and appropriate monitoring of their children (Barbot et al. 2014). In turn, this could contribute to a more positive parent–child relationship, which could protect against later mental illness.

Family influences

As established earlier in this chapter, attachment figures and positive relationships within the family are considered central to a child developing positive mental health and a sense of wellbeing. Of the range of family factors essential for development, parenting style has received considerable attention and has been established to have an influence on child mental health. A recent longitudinal study of Australian children found harsh discipline to be a strong and consistent predictor of both internalising and externalising symptoms for children aged 4–5 and 8–9) (Bayer et al. 2011). Similarly, overinvolved/protective parenting predicted internalising symptoms among the younger cohort (from birth to 4–5yr follow-up) (Bayer et al. 2011). Parenting styles characterised by warmth or support were not associated with these symptoms. Certain factors can influence parenting style. For example, one study of low-income mothers found that maternal stress is strongly related to negative parenting (high rejection, low parental control and involvement), and that maternal stress is associated with child internalising and externalising problems (Barbot et al. 2014).

Family structure and harmony has also received attention. Today, it is common for children to live within varied family structures, including two biological parents, adoptive parents, single parents, same-sex parents, and step/cohabitating families. It has been suggested that although certain family structures do not cause poor mental health, there are some factors associated with certain structures which might. For example, a large study of children in the US found that victimisation (including maltreatment, assault, property crime and witnessing family violence) of children was more commonly experienced by children from single parent or step/cohabitating families, compared to those with two biological/adoptive parents. Further, this was found to be associated with high parental conflict, drug/alcohol problems, family adversity and community disorder (Turner et al. 2013). In a longitudinal study, higher rates of depression, antisocial behaviour and hyperactivity were found among children whose parents had divorced, and this was attributed to the socio-economic disadvantage being higher among those families (Strohschein 2012). However, not all children in these situations will experience diminished mental health and this may be attributed to individual protective factors (e.g. resilience) and other family factors (e.g. secure attachment with one of their caregivers/other important adult influences).

Case Study 5.1

Molly is a 4 year old girl. She has been living in an adoptive home for the past six months; prior to this time, she spent the last two years in two different foster home placements. For the first two years of her life, Molly suffered severe neglect while living with her birth mother. Her mother also drank alcohol heavily during her pregnancy.

Recently, Molly was referred to the Child and Adolescent Mental Health Service (CAMHS) by her social worker, Steven. Steven has known Molly since she was 9 months old, when her family was subject to a safeguarding investigation due to neglect and concerns of substance misuse. Both Steven and Molly's adoptive mother, Pam, were worried about the challenging behaviour Molly was exhibiting. Pam described frequent and intense angry outbursts, and explained that Molly had been resisting physical closeness, despite previously having been quite cuddly. Pam also noticed that Molly rarely made eye contact, and that the children she was in contact with found her too boisterous and did not want to play with her.

Intervention from CAMHS first involved careful assessment of Molly's needs and behaviour, through consultation with Molly and her adoptive family. A particular focus was placed on her attachment relationships. Through dolls and stories, the CAMHS worker sought to understand how Molly saw herself, her family, friends and relationships with others. The complex nature of the difficulties experienced during Molly's first years of life was also explored, along with the disruption she experienced during her foster care placements. Consideration was given to multiple explanations for Molly's current behaviour, including that her mother's alcohol use during pregnancy may have been responsible for Molly's behaviour and possible learning difficulties. Molly was diagnosed with an attachment disorder and a care plan was developed.

In addition to individual play therapy for Molly, a central component of Molly's care plan was education and assistance in the form of family therapy, provided by a specialist CAMHS worker who was experienced in working with traumatised children. The purpose of this approach was to support Molly's adoptive parents to better understand attachment disorder and to develop skills to alleviate Molly's and their distress. Assessment was also made of the adoptive parents' abilities, knowledge and needs. Molly's parents learnt new management strategies, such as the importance of consistent approaches and reactions to Molly's behavioural outbursts. Their ability to cope and support Molly was improved by their increasing knowledge and understanding of attachment disorders. As they began to understand the reasoning behind Molly's behaviour, they began to see the behaviour as the problem, not Molly. They were also encouraged to meet with other carers who had similar experiences. This, along with regular contact with experienced CAMHS, helped to improve their engagement and parenting of Molly.

Findings of Molly's assessment were also shared with others responsible for Molly's care, such as early education, health and medical services. This was achieved through close liaison and information sharing between the CAMHS worker, Molly's social worker, and these services. This contributed to a multi-agency approach to Molly's care.

Peer/school influences

Outside of the time spent with their families, children also spend a significant amount of time among their peers, in settings such as child-care, pre-school and school. Peers are highly important for multiple reasons – they allow opportunities for children to develop and expand the social skills they are acquiring at home, to engage in cooperative play, and to develop their language and other forms of communication. These activities set the scene for the development of strong friendships, which is important as positive peer relationships are known to be an important protective factor against mental illness. However, negative peer relationships can also be a notable risk factor. For example, a large study of 5–7 year old children found that those who were bullied experienced more internalising problems. These children were also unhappier at school (Arseneault et al. 2006). This is likely to have flow-on effects, such as difficulty forming peer relationships and friendships, and being unwilling or unable to attend school (which influences opportunities for learning and educational attainment).

Life events

Certain life events can influence a child's mental health. The exposure to multiple forms of victimisation (e.g. sexual assault, maltreatment, witnessing family violence, and other major violent exposure) has been found to significantly contribute to depression, anger and aggression. More exposure to victimisation has been found for those children who are part of a racial or ethnic minority, a low-income household, whose parents have a lower level of education, and single/stepparent households (Turner, Finkelhor and Ormrod 2006). The way that a child deals with these events and the impact that this has on their mental health can be influenced by the previously discussed risk and protective factors. For example, a study of children involved in the 2010 Chilean earthquake found that, of those who reported symptoms of post traumatic stress disorder, symptoms were more pronounced for those who experienced conflict with their caregiver and/or those whose caregiver was unavailable to discuss the earthquake (Garfin et al. 2014). Similarly, a review of the mental health of displaced and refugee children found, as might be expected, exposure to violence was a notable risk factor, whereas social support was a key protective factor upon resettlement in high-income countries (Fazel et al. 2012).

Societal influences

Societal influences refer to factors such as socio-economic status and advantage/disadvantage which are pre-determined (often before a child is born). A notable emphasis has been placed on understanding how these factors contribute to increased risk of mental illness. One longitudinal study of the influence of poverty found current level of poverty to be associated with externalising symptoms, but persistent poverty to be linked to internalising symptoms (McLeod and Shanahan 1993). The influence of poverty on mental health can be understood from a number of perspectives (Yoshikawa, Aber and Beardslee 2012). For example, poverty can influence parental stress, mood and conflict, which in turn can influence their parenting behaviours, which may contribute to child distress. The unemployment and/or job instability associated with poverty also influences a child's access to resources necessary for learning and development. These factors may subsequently influence a child's access to mental health services (if required) and hinder opportunities for early intervention.

Living with poor mental health

Experiencing poor mental health and/or a mental illness can have a profound impact on a child's life, influencing their ability to flourish, develop and reach their potential across various life domains. As will be explored in further chapters of this book, many risk factors and mental illnesses have their origins in childhood, which stresses the importance of understanding the influence of poor mental health and how to promote positive mental health early in life.

Reduced mental health can influence a child's functioning and development, impacting upon a range of areas, including their behaviour, emotions, thoughts, social relationships and learning (KidsMatter 2014b). Often, difficulties can be seen in more than one of these areas and the relationship between them can be bi-directional. As discussed earlier in this chapter, many mental health conditions are characterised by the presence of internalising or externalising behaviour, which influences how a child interacts with the world around them. Internalising behaviour can impact a child's ability to engage with others, whereas externalising behaviour can result in socially inappropriate and/or disruptive behaviour. We also saw that symptoms can influence a child's emotions – that is, the way they express or manage their feelings. Reduced mental health can impact a child's thoughts, including negative thoughts about themselves (e.g. 'nobody likes me') or about others (e.g. worrying thoughts about potential harm to a loved one). These thoughts can prevent children from interacting with others and engaging in activities, which may reduce opportunities for social development and other aspects of development (e.g. a child may avoid playing on equipment in the school yard, which is beneficial for developing gross motor skills) and health (e.g. physical activity has known consequences for mental health). As such, social relationships can be hindered. Children may have difficulty playing with others, understanding social cues and behaving in a socially appropriate manner. With peers being an important influence during the early years, and friendship being particularly important in adolescence, struggles in this domain can have long-lasting impacts. Finally, learning – that is, the ability to take in, understand and recall information, as well as communicate and interact with others and use physical skills – can also be influenced. For example, the symptoms of a mental health condition may reduce a child's ability to pay attention and stay focussed. These latter two domains are particularly important and warrant further attention, along with the impacts on the child's family.

Impacts on friendships and social development

Poor mental health can influence a child's ability to trust others, particularly in the form of building friendships. For example, internalising symptoms mean that children experiencing distress or discomfort can be shy and easily upset, whereas externalising symptoms mean that children can be loud and difficult to follow. Additionally, some of the mental health conditions described on pages 92–97 of this chapter are specifically characterised by difficulties in relationship forming, or social skills. For example, a study of children (aged 4–17 years) diagnosed with autism spectrum disorder found that severity of the condition was associated with lower numbers and quality of reciprocal friendships (Mazurek and Kanne 2010). With positive friendships considered to be important for social development and a protective factor against poor mental health, this is concerning.

Further, the experience of a mental health condition can result in a vulnerability to bullying and peer-victimisation. One study of 13 year olds found higher rates of bullying for those diagnosed with autism spectrum disorder compared to both their typically developing peers and peers diagnosed with an intellectual disability. The bullying was chronic, largely verbal and had a profound emotional impact (Turner, Finkelhor and Ormrod 2010). Similar findings have been made for children experiencing internalising and externalising problems, with internalising children being perceived as 'weak' and 'easy targets', whereas externalising children may be more likely to be perceived as 'picking fights' and be bullied as a result. This can have some longer-term consequences. For example, a longitudinal study of children diagnosed with attention deficit hyperactivity disorder found that peer rejection in childhood predicted anxiety in adolescence (Mrug et al. 2012).

A consequence of difficulties in forming friendships and/or with bullying is the resulting exclusion from social activities. Social activities provide important opportunities for children to develop social skills, as well as to further develop friendships and gain social support (which are known protective factors). These experiences can also influence a child's willingness to attend school and ability to pay attention in class. Again, this can compound and exacerbate the experience of mental illness.

Impacts on education attendance and learning

Reduced school attendance can be a consequence for some children experiencing a mental health condition, particularly depression and separation anxiety (Egger, Costello and Angold 2003). This has obvious consequences for opportunities to engage in learning, as well as social interactions with peers. Similarly, school performance can be diminished (Owens et al. 2012), and this can be attributed to a number of factors, such as the inability to concentrate and a lack of confidence to ask questions during class. This can be more pronounced for children experiencing neurodevelopmental disorders. For example, experiencing attention deficit hyperactivity disorder can influence the acquisition of basic academic skills and school readiness (e.g. attention capacity and interacting with peers) during pre-school (Daley and Birchwood 2010). Similarly, a study of children aged 6–11 years found links between anxious, withdrawn and depression symptoms, and intellectual function, language, visual construction skills, attention, processing speed and academic skills (Lundy et al. 2010).

Impacts on the child's family

The importance of family and early interpersonal relationships was established earlier in the chapter, and it is important to recognise the impact that a child's poor mental health can have on the relationships they develop within their family system (Herring et al. 2006). For example, parents may find it difficult to connect with a child who expresses internalising symptoms, or become frustrated with a child who expresses externalising symptoms. In turn, this can make it more difficult to form a bond with their child (a known protective factor). It is also important to recognise that parenting a child experiencing a mental illness can also have significant consequences on parents/caregivers, such as stress and disrupted marital functioning (Johnston and Mash 2001). Similarly, there may be impacts for siblings of the child, such as increased susceptibility to behavioural problems and difficulties adjusting to stressors resulting from the child's mental health condition (Petalas et al. 2012). This highlights the importance of interventions and treatment approaches which take a whole-of-family approach.

Mental health promotion/supports

To reduce the aforementioned impacts of poor mental health, there is a range of ways that the mental health of children can be promoted and supported. Globally, it is accepted that an early intervention approach is most successful for reducing the longer-term impacts of mental illness, with the WHO (2013) highlighting the importance that must be placed on early intervention and mental health promotion, as well efforts to reduce risk factors and enhance resilience. The WHO (2013) also suggests that the focus of these approaches should be on evidence-based psychosocial interventions within the community, rather than pharmacological interventions. Therefore, although some children will require medical assistance to minimise the symptoms of their mental illness (e.g. to treat the hyperactivity symptoms of attention deficit hyperactivity disorder), we have focussed here on early intervention approaches.

There are a number of settings in which early intervention approaches can occur, particularly within the community, in child-care centres and schools, as well as online. These mental health promotion initiatives can be both universal – that is, targeted at all children, or selective and indicated – that is, targeted at children who are known to be at risk of developing mental health problems (Kieling et al. 2011). These early interventions sit within a systems approach, which emphasises the importance of understanding and addressing a child's mental health within the context of the systems they are part of (e.g. family, school, community and society). An awareness of the range of services available is important in order for health professionals to be able to offer support to parents, caregivers, and others who play an important role in a child's health and wellbeing.

Support for parents and caregivers

With parents and caregivers recognised as a primary influence on a child's development, interventions directed at supporting these individuals have been explored. A review of the literature on parent/caregiver support interventions identified the importance of initiatives such as those which aim to improve parent–child connection/attachment at birth (e.g. during the peri-natal phase), as well as those in early childhood, such as enhanced caregiver sensitivity and attunement, parenting programs for specific childhood behaviour, as well as targeted programs for high risk groups (such as to improve parental mental health, reduce physical and emotional abuse), and home visit programs (Stewart-Brown and Schrader-McMillan 2011). Support and education can also be targeted toward parents of children with diagnosed mental illness. For example, one study showed that a 20-week program for parents of children diagnosed with autism spectrum disorder resulted in improvements in the children's adaptive behaviour (communication and social skills) and autism symptoms at a 6-month follow-up, and that education and behaviour management was better than education and counselling (Tonge et al. 2014). In another example, the 12-session CALM (Coaching Approach behaviour and Leading by Modeling) program for parents and their 3–8 year old children experiencing a range of anxiety conditions was associated with diagnostic and functional improvements (Comer et al. 2012).

Case Study 5.2

Belinda is a single mother to her six year old daughter, Maddy. She is also the victim of domestic violence. Her pregnancy was difficult; she often experienced nausea and spot bleeding, and she was required to have an emergency Caesarean Section. When Maddy was born, Belinda was unable to breast feed her. Maddy was a very colicky baby, often crying and difficult to settle. Belinda never felt connected with Maddy; instead, she often felt detached and disengaged. She is not close to her family and so has no additional supports.

After two years of being unhappy and engaging in increased alcohol use to mask the verbal and domestic abuse she was subjected to, Belinda left her de facto partner. She went to the GP who commenced her on antidepressants. Around this time, behavioural problems in the form of tantrums emerged with Maddy. Belinda did not feel that Maddy liked her. Belinda decided to attend a community clinic at the local children's centre. Staff at the clinic established that Maddy was aggressive, showing signs of developmental delay, poor attachment, and minimal bonding with Belinda. At their suggestion, Belinda participated in a six-week parenting course. Initially, this made Belinda feel more like a 'bad mother' as she felt embarrassed by Maddy's behaviour, and realised how extensive her daughter's difficulties were. Over time, Belinda was able to more fully engage in the parenting course, making a new friendship network. Belinda continued to struggle with increased alcohol use. However, this too mellowed as her social networks and connectedness with Maddy increased. She began to feel more in control of her relationship with Maddy.

(Nicholas Procter)

School-based interventions

Given that children spend a significant proportion of their daily life in early childhood in education and school settings, it is not surprising that there is considerable evidence to suggest that these can serve as important environments for mental health promotion and resilience development (Weare and Nind 2011). This can be particularly important for those children whose home environments may result in increased risk for mental illness (e.g. lack of supportive parenting, low SES, etc.), or who have difficulty accessing services (e.g. due to parental disinterest or lack of financial access to resources) (Weare and Nind 2011).

A large study of school-based programs (from kindergarten to high school) found evidence for the success of these programs in increasing social behaviour and academic performance (Durlak et al. 2011). Researchers have also identified a number of successful features of school-based programs, including: effective teaching skills of those implementing the intervention, a focus on positive mental health, striking a balance between universal and targeted approaches, starting early and continuing with older children, and programs being of longer duration and set within a whole of school approach (Weare and Nind 2011). Other programs include school-based social-emotional learning programs. While some researchers suggest that such programs can be effectively delivered by teachers, without outside assistance, others suggest that more targeted interventions, such as those made to specifically reduce anxiety, are more effective when conducted by health professionals (Stallard et al. 2014). Moreover, research has stressed the importance of interventions which not only focus on the individual child, but which involve how children respond to their peers who are experiencing a mental health condition. For example, one study tested the role of school-based social skills interventions for high functioning children with autism in mainstream schooling; particularly, it explored the influence of training for these children, compared to training for their peers (Kasari et al. 2012). The study found that increases in social involvement were most pronounced with peer training, highlighting the importance of a whole-of-school approach.

In Australia, a leading example of a school-based initiative is KidsMatter, a partnership between schools, the Australian government and health services (KidsMatter, 2014c). The program aims to improve connectedness with families, to support the parenting role and to enhance family networks, by connecting families with services. It not only provides a framework and resources for educating people (parents, caregivers, child-care workers, teachers) about child mental health, but it also provides programs for a range of mental health aspects, from belonging and inclusion, to establishing positive relationships for children, to programs for parents, carers and families to support their child's mental health and wellbeing and to support those who are showing early signs of mental health difficulties. An evaluation of the KidsMatter Early Childhood program found that, although many of the children were mentally healthy, of those who showed early signs of mental health difficulties, 1 in 6 were no longer experiencing these at the end of the program (two years later) (Vasilevski and Cavanagh 2013). In addition, there were positive impacts on families. At the end of the program, family understanding of child mental health issues had increased and parents/caregivers also felt more able to support their child's emotional and social development. Teachers also reported similar gains.

Online supports

With ever-expanding technology, children are becoming proficient with the use of electronic devices and the internet (Holloway, Green and Livingstone 2013), and there is the potential for online resources to promote positive mental health (Burns et al. 2010). For example, initiatives such as Kids Helpline

(Kids Helpline 2014) in Australia and ChildLine (ChildLine 2014) in the UK, not only offer children a free service to talk (either over the phone or online) about the problems they are experiencing, but also contain online platforms with resources tailored to help children learn about mental illness. Beyond this, they also provide information for children about how to take care of their own physical and mental health (e.g. tips for exercise and dealing with negative emotions) as well as resources to have fun, such as online games, puzzles and pictures. They also offer stories on topics that might be influencing a child's mental health, such as the addition of a new family member (adult or child), peer pressure, blended families, how to make friends and deal with bullying, etc. as well as tips for coping when times are tough. Resources such as these could be a useful way for children to learn the skills to actively explore the notion of mental health and to take control of their own mental health. Similarly, such resources are also available for parents (e.g. Kids Matter 2014c in Australia).

Child and adolescent mental health services

While early intervention and prevention programs may be effective, a number of children suspected of experiencing a mental health concern can be referred to child and adolescent mental health services (CAMHS). These are offered in a number of countries worldwide and are usually funded by public mental health services. CAMHS services are staffed by a range of health and mental health professionals (e.g. nurses, social workers and psychologists) and provide a variety of services, including the assessment and treatment of mental illness, and individual and family counselling/therapy. They can also provide and/or deliver some of the previously mentioned community early mental health promotion and parenting programs. Usually, access to these services is by referral from another health care worker (e.g. GP or school counsellor). Engaging children and families with CAMHS can be difficult when there are negative perceptions and prejudice which will reduce the likelihood of those who need help or advice approaching their GP, health visitor, school nurse or accepting a referral to this service (National Child and Maternal Health Intelligence Network 2014).

Case Study 5.3

Jason is an 11 year old boy who was referred to his local child and adolescent mental health service (CAMHS) on the recommendation of his school teacher for behavioural management issues at school. His teacher reported incidences of aggression – both physical and verbal – in the playground and classroom, refusal to do written tasks, and running away from class. Other forms of antisocial behaviour were also reported, such as threatened and actual hitting of other children, as well as stealing other children's belongings and food.

During an initial consultation with the CAMHS worker, an extended assessment history was taken and a sustained history of domestic violence was revealed. Jason's father had an alcohol and illicit substance use problem. When drinking, his father was verbally abusive and threatening towards Jason, his mother and his siblings (an older brother and younger sister). The children have all witnessed their father assault their mother when drunk. There have also been financial struggles, with both parents experiencing patches of unemployment.

(continued)

(continued)

The parenting styles Jason experienced were markedly different. His mother was passive and she often spent her time at home in a distant, non-engaged manner; there were no rules or routines at home when she was in charge. In contrast, Jason's father enforced strict and punitive rules when he is in charge. The children were frightened of him.

The CAMHS worker established a multifaceted treatment plan for Jason: liaison is provided to support the school; individual therapy to address emotional regulation for Jason; parenting support for both parents; and family therapy. Initial improvement was seen following the build-up of a positive parenting relationship between the parents and the children. This took the form of individual and combined family sessions, incorporating a boundary setting activity.

The same kind of behavioural management strategies used in the school were adopted at home. For Jason, close liaison between school, mental health team and family brought consistent approaches to behaviour management and psychoeducation. Jason and his siblings responded well to alternative parenting options, positive feedback and a more settled form of parental engagement. There was a discerning move away from an inconsistent, threatening, invalidating and fearful home environment to one which was more settled and consistent.

Conclusion

Most children will progress through childhood without developing a mental health condition. However, others will experience fluctuations in their mental health as they develop and mature, and sometimes these experiences will lead to poorer mental health in childhood. For some children, these experiences will lead to a mental health condition later in life. It is vital that we understand how to recognise symptoms of reduced mental health among children, as these differ from what we see in adults. In particular, signs of internalising and externalising can be indicators of poor mental health. This understanding can be enhanced by knowledge of behaviours that are developmentally appropriate. It is also vital that we continue to understand and emphasise the importance of early family environments and how to encourage these environments to be as positive and supportive of optimal child development as possible. Promoting mental health in childhood should not focus solely on preventing mental illness; rather, the focus should be placed on encouraging healthy, resilient children who are able engage in positive interactions with others and their environment.

Reflective exercise

- Look at how families interact in your surroundings; why do you think the family context is important for the development of a child's mental health and wellbeing? What have you observed that supports your thinking?
- Caution should always be taken when diagnosing a child's mental health condition; describe some factors that should be considered when making a diagnosis. What evidence have you found to support these factors?

- Talk to your colleagues about how living with a mental illness might influence the life of a child and those around them. Is there a consensus view? Is the view negative or positive? What are the most common responses and why?
- Children will present mental health difficulties in a multitude of different ways; how would you differentiate and observe the differences between internalising and externalising expressions of mental health problems in children? What evidence would support your observations?

References

American Psychiatric Association (APA) 2013, *Diagnostic and statistical manual of mental disorders: DSM-5*, 5th edn, APA, Arlington, Va.

Anda, RF, Felitti, VJ, Bremner, JD, Walker, JD, Whitfield, C, Perry, BD, Dube, SR and Giles, WH 2006, 'The enduring effects of abuse and related adverse experiences in childhood. A convergence of evidence from neurobiology and epidemiology', *European Archives of Psychiatry and Clinical Neuroscience*, vol. 256, no. 3, pp. 174–186.

Arseneault, L, Walsh, E, Trzesniewski, K, Newcombe, R, Caspi, A and Moffitt, TE 2006, 'Bullying victimization uniquely contributes to adjustment problems in young children: a nationally representative cohort study', *Pediatrics*, vol. 118, no. 1, pp. 130–138.

Australian Bureau of Statistics (ABS) 2013, *Causes of death, Australia, 2011*, cat. no. 3303.0, ABS, Canberra.

Australian Human Rights Commission 2014, *Children's rights report 2014*, Australian Human Rights Commission, Canberra.

Banks, K and Bevan, A 2014, 'Predictors for somatic symptoms in children', *Nursing Children and Young People*, vol. 26, no. 1, pp. 16–20.

Barbot, B, Crossman, E, Hunter, SR, Grigorenko, EL and Luthar, SS 2014, 'Reciprocal influences between maternal parenting and child adjustment in a high-risk population: A 5-year cross-lagged analysis of bidirectional effects', *American Journal of Orthopsychiatry*, vol. 84, no. 5, pp. 567–580.

Bayer, JK, Ukoumunne, OC, Lucas, N, Wake, M, Scalzo, K and Nicholson, JM 2011, 'Risk factors for childhood mental health symptoms: National longitudinal study of Australian children', *Pediatrics*, vol. 128, no. 4, e865–879.

Bowlby, J 1952, *Maternal care and mental health*, World Health Organization, Geneva.

Burns, JM, Davenport, TA, Durkin, LA, Luscombe, GM and Hickie, IB 2010, 'The internet as a setting for mental health service utilisation by young people', *Medical Journal of Australia*, vol. 192, no. 11, S22.

ChildLine 2014, *ChildLine*, viewed 20 November 2014, <www.childline.org.uk/Pages/Home.aspx>.

Comer, JS, Puliafico, AC, Aschenbrand, SG, McKnight, K, Robin, JA, Goldfine, ME and Albano, AM 2012, 'A pilot feasibility evaluation of the CALM Program for anxiety disorders in early childhood', *Journal of Anxiety Disorders*, vol. 26, no. 1, pp. 40–49.

Cousins, J 2013, 'Assessing and responding to infant mental health needs', *Community Practitioner*, vol. 86, no. 8, pp. 33–36.

Daley, D and Birchwood, J 2010, 'ADHD and academic performance: Why does ADHD impact on academic performance and what can be done to support ADHD children in the classroom?', *Child: Care, Health and Development*, vol. 36, no. 4, pp. 455–464.

Daniel, B, Wassell, S and Gilligan, R 1999, *Child development for child care and protection workers*, Jessica Kingsley, London.

Department of Health 2004, *National service framework for children, young people and maternity services core standards*, Department of Health, London.

Department of Health 2014, *Closing the gap: Priorities for essential change in mental health*, Department of Health, London.

Durlak, JA, Weissberg, RP, Dymnicki, AB, Taylor, RD and Schellinger, KB 2011, 'The impact of enhancing students' social and emotional learning: A meta-analysis of school-based universal interventions', *Child Development,* vol. 82, no. 1, pp. 405–432.

Eddy, LL 2013, *Caring for children with special healthcare needs and their families: A handbook for healthcare professionals*, Wiley-Blackwell, Oxford.

Egger, HL, Costello, JE and Angold, A 2003, 'School refusal and psychiatric disorders: a community study', *Journal of the American Academy of Child and Adolescent Psychiatry*, vol. 42, no. 7, pp. 797–807.

Fazel, M, Reed, RV, Panter-Brick, C and Stein, A 2012, 'Mental health of displaced and refugee children resettled in high-income countries: Risk and protective factors', *The Lancet*, vol. 379, no. 9812, pp. 266–282.

Garfin, DR, Silver, RC, Gil-Rivas, V, Guzmán, J, Murphy, JM, Cova, F, Rincón, PP, Squicciarini, AM, George, M and Guzmán, MP 2014, 'Children's reactions to the 2010 Chilean earthquake: The role of trauma exposure, family context, and school-based mental health programming', *Psychological Trauma: Theory, Research, Practice, and Policy*, vol. 6, no. 5, pp. 563–573.

Green, H, McGinnity, A, Meltzer, H, Ford, T and Goodman, R 2005, *Mental health of children and young people in Great Britain, 2004*, Palgrave Macmillan, Basingstoke.

headspace 2014, *headspace: National Youth Mental Health Foundation*, viewed 5 December, 2014, <www.headspace.org.au/>.

Herring, S, Gray, K, Taffe, J, Tonge, B, Sweeney, D and Einfeld, S 2006, 'Behaviour and emotional problems in toddlers with pervasive developmental disorders and developmental delay: Associations with parental mental health and family functioning', *Journal of Intellectual Disability Research*, vol. 50, no. 12, pp. 874–882.

Holloway, D, Green, L and Livingstone, S 2013, *Zero to eight. Young children and their internet use*, EU Kids Online, London School of Economics, London.

Johnston, C and Mash, EJ 2001, 'Families of children with attention-deficit/hyperactivity disorder: Review and recommendations for future research', *Clinical Child and Family Psychology Review*, vol. 4, no. 3, pp. 183–207.

Jureidini, J 2014, 'Let children cry', *Medical Journal of Australia*, vol. 201, no. 10, pp. 612–613.

Karevold, E, Røysamb, E, Ystrom, E and Mathiesen, KS 2009, 'Predictors and pathways from infancy to symptoms of anxiety and depression in early adolescence', *Developmental Psychology*, vol. 45, no. 4, pp. 1051–1060.

Kasari, C, Rotheram-Fuller, E, Locke, J and Gulsrud, A 2012, 'Making the connection: Randomized controlled trial of social skills at school for children with autism spectrum disorders', *Journal of Child Psychology and Psychiatry*, vol. 53, no. 4, pp. 431–439.

Kataoka, SH, Zhang, L and Wells, KB 2002, 'Unmet need for mental health care among U.S. children: Variation by ethnicity and insurance status', *American Journal of Psychiatry*, vol. 159, no. 9, pp. 1548–1555.

Kids Helpline 2014, *Kids Helpline*, viewed 20 October 2014, <www.kidshelp.com.au/>.

KidsMatter 2014a, *Fact sheet – Healthy relationships and families*, Commonwealth of Australia, Canberra.

KidsMatter 2014b, *KidsMatter early childhood. Early childhood mental health: An introduction*, Commonwealth of Australia, Canberra.

KidsMatter 2014c, *KidsMatter early childhood*, viewed 20 October 2014, <www.kidsmatter.edu.au/early-childhood>.

Kieling, C, Baker-Henningham, H, Belfer, M, Conti, G, Ertem, I, Omigbodun, O, Rohde, LA, Srinath, S, Ulkuer, N and Rahman, A 2011, 'Child and adolescent mental health worldwide: Evidence for action', *The Lancet*, vol. 378, no. 9801, pp. 1515–1525.

Lundy, SM, Silva, GE, Kaemingk, KL, Goodwin, JL and Quan, SF 2010, 'Cognitive functioning and academic performance in elementary school children with anxious/depressed and withdrawn symptoms', *The Open Pediatric Medicine Journal,* vol. 4, doi: 10.2174/1874309901004010001.

Mazurek, MO and Kanne, SM 2010, 'Friendship and internalizing symptoms among children and adolescents with ASD', *Journal of Autism and Developmental Disorders*, vol. 40, no. 12, pp. 1512–1520.

McLeod, JD and Shanahan, MJ 1993, 'Poverty, parenting, and children's mental health', *American Sociological Review*, vol. 58, no. 3, pp. 351–366.

Mitchell, A, Davies, M, Cassesse, C and Curran, R 2014, 'Antidepressant use in children, adolescents and young adults: 10 years after the food and drug administration black box warning', *The Journal for Nurse Practitioners*, vol. 10, no. 3, pp. 149–156.

Mrug, S, Molina, BSG, Hoza, B, Gerdes, AC, Hinshaw, SP, Hechtman, L and Arnold, LE 2012, 'Peer rejection and friendships in children with attention-deficit/hyperactivity disorder: Contributions to long-term outcomes', *Journal of Abnormal Child Psychology,* vol. 40, no. 6, pp. 1013–1026.

National Child and Maternal Health Intelligence Network 2014, *Language and definition of mental health*, viewed 20 October 2014, <www.chimat.org.uk/tacklingstigma/language>.

Owens, M, Stevenson, J, Hadwin, JA and Norgate, R 2012, 'Anxiety and depression in academic performance: An exploration of the mediating factors of worry and working memory', *School Psychology International,* vol. 33, no. 4, pp. 433–449.

Partridge, B, Lucke, J and Hall, W 2014, 'Over-diagnosed and over-treated: A survey of Australian public attitudes towards the acceptability of drug treatment for depression and ADHD', *BMC Psychiatry*, vol. 14, no. 74, doi:10.1186/1471-244X-14-74.

Petalas, MA, Hastings, RP, Nash, S, Hall, LM, Joannidi, H and Dowey, A 2012, 'Psychological adjustment and sibling relationships in siblings of children with autism spectrum disorders: Environmental stressors and the broad autism phenotype', *Research in Autism Spectrum Disorders,* vol. 6, no. 1, pp. 546–555.

Riddle, MA, Yershova, K, Lazzaretto, D, Paykina, N, Yenokyan, G, Greenhill, L, Abikoff, H, Vitiello, B, Wignal, T, McCracken, JT, Kollins, SH, Murray, DW, Wigal, S, Kastelic, E, McGough, JJ, dosReis, S, Bauzó-Rosario, A, Stehli, A and Posner, K 2013, 'The preschool attention-deficit/hyperactivity disorder treatment study (PATS) 6-year follow-up', *Journal of the American Academy of Child and Adolescent Psychiatry*, vol. 52, no. 3, pp. 264–278.

Sabates, R and Dex, S 2012, *Multiple risk factors in young children's development. CLS Cohort Studies Working Paper 2012/1,* Centre for Longitudinal Studies, London.

Sawyer, A, Gialamas, A, Pearce, A, Sawyer, MG and Lynch, J 2014, *Five by five: A supporting systems framework for child health and development.* University of Adelaide, School of Population Health, Adelaide.

Smith, D and Allen, G 2008, *Early intervention: Good parents, great kids, better citizens*, Centre for Social Justice and the Smith Institute, London.

Stallard, P, Skryabina, E, Taylor, G, Phillips, R, Daniels, H, Anderson, R and Simpson, N 2014, 'Classroom-based cognitive behaviour therapy (FRIENDS): A cluster randomised controlled trial to Prevent Anxiety in Children through Education in Schools (PACES)', *The Lancet Psychiatry*, vol. 1, no. 3, pp. 185–192.

Stewart-Brown, SL and Schrader-Mcmillan, A 2011, 'Parenting for mental health: What does the evidence say we need to do? Report of Workpackage 2 of the DataPrev project', *Health Promotion International*, vol. 26, no. S1, pp. i10–i28.

Strohschein, L 2012, 'Parental divorce and child mental health: Accounting for predisruption differences', *Journal of Divorce and Remarriage*, vol. 53, no. 6, pp. 489–502.

Tonge, B, Brereton, A, Kiomall, M, Mackinnon, A and Rinehart, NJ 2014, 'A randomised group comparison controlled trial of "preschoolers with autism": A parent education and skills training intervention for young children with autistic disorder', *Autism,* vol. 18, no. 2, pp. 166–177.

Turner, HA, Finkelhor, D and Ormrod, R 2006, 'The effect of lifetime victimization on the mental health of children and adolescents', *Social Science and Medicine*, vol. 62, no. 1, pp. 13–27.

Turner, HA, Finkelhor, D and Ormrod, R 2010, 'Child mental health problems as risk factors for victimization', *Child Maltreatment,* vol. 15, no. 2, pp. 132–143.

Turner, HA, Finkelhor, D, Hamby, SL and Shattuck, A 2013, 'Family structure, victimization, and child mental health in a nationally representative sample', *Social Science and Medicine*, vol. 87, pp. 39–51.

Vasilevski, V and Cavanagh, S 2013, 'Striking improvements in children's mental health: KidsMatter in early childhood education and care services', *InPsych: The bulletin of The Australian Psychological Society Limited*, pp. 22–25.

Weare, K and Nind, M 2011, 'Mental health promotion and problem prevention in schools: What does the evidence say?', *Health Promotion International*, vol. 26, no. S1, pp. i29–i69.

WHO (World Health Organisation) 2013, *Mental health action plan 2013–2020*, WHO, Geneva.

WHO 2014a, *Child and adolescent mental health*, viewed 20 October 2014, <www.who.int/mental_health/maternal-child/child_adolescent/en/>.

WHO 2014b, *Preventing suicide: A global imperative*, WHO, Geneva.

Yoshikawa, H, Aber, JL and Beardslee, WR 2012, 'The effects of poverty on the mental, emotional, and behavioral health of children and youth: Implications for prevention', *American Psychologist*, vol. 67, no. 4, pp. 272–284.

Zero to Three 2014, *Early childhood mental health*, viewed 5 November 2014, <www.zerotothree.org/child-development/early-childhood-mental-health/>.

6 Adolescence and young adult mental health

Scott Steen

Introduction

This chapter will focus specifically on the mental health of adolescents and young adults, as well as consider how it can impact on an individual in later life. It will introduce the reader to concepts and theories relating to adolescent mental health and the development of services within the UK, over the latter part of the twentieth century, the behavioural, emotional and physiological changes that can occur during this period and how they interact with one another will also be discussed. A section considering the role and influence of family, friends and peers on adolescent mental health is also presented. The chapter will conclude by exploring a number of mental health problems that may emerge during this stage.

The reader will be introduced to contemporary research that seeks to evaluate and understand the nature of a young person's mental health. It will also aim to identify how health professionals, parents, educators and support workers can each play a role in promoting positive mental health in adolescence. Case scenarios have been selected to assist the reader in understanding the benefits of intervening and promoting positive mental health during this stage. The terms *adolescent*, *young adult* and *young person* are used interchangeably and defining this stage is discussed within the text. Much of the research discussed is with reference to a UK setting, although other international research is specified accordingly.

> No adolescent ever wants to be understood, which is why they complain about being misunderstood all the time.
>
> (Stephen Fry, 2003)

This chapter will consider:

- How to recognise the risk of mental health problems in adolescents and young adults;
- The important role health professionals and support workers can play when giving care and support to adolescents and young adults;
- The importance of promoting positive mental health and wellbeing to adolescents and young adults;
- How to recognise vulnerable adolescents and young adults;
- How adolescents and young adults with mental health problems can be at an increased risk of problems later on in life.

Adolescence and young adult mental health

Adolescence is derived from the Latin word '*adolescere*', which means 'grow to maturity'. It is a stage of development that is defined by the pubertal transition into adulthood, involving biological, psychological and social changes (Alsaker, 1995). The period of adolescence is a fluid concept and one which is known to change across time and culture (Coleman, 2011; Eveleth and Tanner, 1976; Himes, 2006; Tanner, 1981). It is a period that is often associated with the teenage years, but its onset and duration can last anywhere between the ages of 7 to 25 years old (Johnson et al., 2011). Adolescence is often a time that is associated with affirming one's identity, the development of more complex social and sexual relationships, increased autonomy and independence, and increased educational and occupational demands (Coleman, 2011; Goldin and Katz, 2009; Hill, 1983). From a biological standpoint, the physiological changes that occur in both genders with the onset of puberty greatly alter individuals' body shape and size, reproductive related physiology and brain development. It is often a period that is characterised as the transition from childhood to adulthood and from school into work.

The nature of adolescence has evolved over the last century, particularly in the Western world. Compulsory education, restrictions on child labour, the complexities of an industrialised and technologically advancing state, increased prosperity, cultural migration, improved media and information distribution, as well as increased liberalisation and civil rights are just a handful of factors that have all contributed in defining a change of what adolescence means (Gillibrand et al., 2011, p. 358). Goldin and Katz (2009) point out that the longer-term consequences of academic success in recent history means there is an added pressure at this stage to achieve, potentially leading to greater anxiety and stress. Disruptions during this stage, by way of poor mental health, could therefore have considerable ramifications.

Early theories and concepts

The concept that adolescence is one of increased conflict and inner turmoil is as old as Ancient Greek thinking (Coleman, 2011). Leading theories of adolescent development over the past century also reflect this idea. Granville Stanley Hall proposed that the period of adolescence is one of "storm and stress" (Hall, 1904 as cited in Arnett, 1999). Arnett (2006) discusses how Hall's view of adolescence was generally one of increased behavioural and emotional turmoil brought about by dramatic and unpredictable growth spurts. Erikson's (1968) Theory of Psychosocial Development describes a crisis in identity at this stage due to a young person's emerging identity being at odds and in conflict with the role expectations of others. Likewise, Anna Freud describes an imbalance of the id and ego during adolescent development (Muss, 1988). One final theory worthy of note is David Elkind's (1967) Egocentrism in Adolescence. Elkind characterised adolescence by a number of cognitive distortions that develop from the newfound ability to formulate a hypothetical perspective. He argued that an adolescent can be made to feel as though they are under constant scrutiny due to perceiving themselves as being on a kind of 'social stage' with an 'imaginary audience'. They may also experience feelings of isolation, believing their abilities and experiences to be unique to everyone else's, a concept which Elkind coined 'personal fable'.

The reason these theories have been selected and highlighted here is that they describe adolescence as being a troubled and turbulent transition. However, developments in the latter part of the twentieth century served to challenge these concepts. During the 1960s and 1970s, empirical evidence began to emerge that suggested the majority of adolescents coped with stressful life events in a resilient way and that relationships with their family and peers were generally positive (Coleman, 2011, p. 15). From the 1960s to the 1980s, there was a demand for research that sought to understand the aetiology of disorders in young people, attracting health professionals from various specialities (Hersov, 1986). In more recent decades, efforts have been made to prioritise the investigation and delivery of prevention and intervention programmes (Cottrell and Kraam, 2005). Today it is now generally recognised that many mental health problems originate in childhood and adolescence (Heginbotham and Williams, 2005).

Service provision and development

Government strategies within the UK and internationally have emphasised a multidisciplinary approach to caring and supporting young people (Department of Health, 2004; EC Directorate-General for Health and Consumer Protection, 2006; U.S. Department of Health and Human Services, 1999). However, the fragmentation in services may serve as a barrier when accessing care; a young person's mental healthcare needs are often dealt with in less well equipped settings such as schools, the home, primary care, youth justice and welfare services (Corcoran, 2011, p. 190). Nonetheless, many of the presenting issues that can occur during this stage can be managed in primary care without the need to refer to specialist services (Dogra et al., 2009, p. 31). The development in service provision for children and young people parallels many of the changes in adult mental healthcare, changes which seek to provide greater community-based services as opposed to inpatient care. Evidence from the US highlights this trend with hospitalisation length of stays for young people falling significantly from 44.05 days to 10.7 days on average, from 1991 to 2008 (Meagher et al., 2013).

The UK Child and Adolescent Mental Health Services (CAMHS) is a specialist NHS service for young people's mental healthcare. In an attempt to review and offer a strategic framework for the organisation of CAMHS, the *Together We Stand* (Health Advisory Service, 1995) and *The Health of the Nation: Child and Adolescent Mental Health Services* (Department of Health, 1995) policy documents were developed in order to help audit and benchmark services. The policy split care into four tiers, of universal, specialist, multidisciplinary and inpatient care, with each tier determined by the severity of an individual's mental health condition. However this approach has been criticised for promoting a hierarchical system of care, when in fact it is argued that CAMHS professionals should be working across all tiers (Richardson et al., 2010). The number of nurses working within CAMHS has increased rapidly over the last two decades and their roles have broadened. This broadening of roles now means that nurses are increasingly involved in designing and managing services as well as delivering them (Townley and Williams, 2009). CAMHS professionals provide a range of psychotherapeutic interventions and deal in a range of multi-agency working. However it is a specialism that is often little understood by service-users, professionals and commissioners alike (Richardson et al., 2010). Other European countries also tend to provide separate specialist clinics for child and adolescent mental healthcare, but still place great emphasis on preventative approaches (Jané-Llopis and Anderson, 2006).

We will now take a brief look at the changes that occur during adolescence in terms of development and its potential impact on young person's mental wellbeing.

Brain and physiological development

As mentioned previously, one of the defining characteristics of adolescence is marked by the onset and ongoing development in puberty. The factors that affect pubertal onset can be complex and multifaceted, determined by a person's genes, environment and lifestyle (Alsaker and Flammer, 2006). Physical and bodily changes that occur during this stage can have an impact on a young person's identity, sociability and self-esteem (Bearman et al., 2006; Chen and Jackson, 2012; Dawson and Dellavalle, 2013; Laursen and Hartl, 2013; Wertheim et al., 2009; Westwood and Pinzon, 2008). These will be explored in further detail in subsequent sections, but for now it is worth considering the development of the brain during adolescence.

The development of the brain and connections between brain regions during adolescence can be defined as being one of immense change (Dahl and Spear, 2004; Fair et al., 2009; Kelly et al., 2009; Lenroot and Giedd, 2010; Paus, 2010; Steinberg, 2008; Supekar et al., 2009). By way of synaptic pruning, the brain facilitates the neural structure to develop more efficient, focused and specialised systems (Fair et al., 2008, 2009; Luna et al., 2010). Pruning refers to the overall reduction of the neuronal and synaptic connections within the brain. This process is important in facilitating 'top-down' executive thinking over 'bottom-up' reactive thinking (Casey et al., 2008; Ernst et al., 2005; Hwang et al., 2010). It is thought to be critical in the processes of learning and can be influenced by factors in the environment (Craik and Bialystock, 2006).

Changes in particular regions of the brain have also been found to develop at a different rate (Blakemore, 2012). These include the prefrontal cortex and limbic system, which have been found to undergo developmental transformations across a range of species during the period of adolescence (Spear, 2000). The prefrontal cortex is thought to be critical in the processes of higher-order executive functioning and abstract thought, and therefore may play a role in harm-avoidant behaviours. This region has been found to mature more gradually than other areas of the brain in adolescence (Bava and Tapert, 2010). The difference in maturing rate of certain regions means that other more developed regions, such as that of the limbic system, may dominate emotional processing. The result of this could manifest in impaired decision-making and a susceptibility for reward seeking (Dahl and Spear, 2004; Ernst et al., 2005; Eshel et al., 2007; Galvan et al., 2006; Steinberg, 2008). Reward seeking can be thought of as a motivated behaviour for pursuing exciting experiences and has been shown to peak in the middle teenage years, between 13 and 16 years of age (Steinberg, 2008). Ernst et al. (2009) suggest this may be based on an evolutionarily beneficial principle. They point out that the process would allow adolescents to explore social contact beyond the family unit and thus help enhance genetic diversity. This may also help to explain the social behaviour seen during adolescence, which aligns itself with an increase towards peer orientation (Forbes and Dahl, 2010; Steinberg and Morris, 2001). Cognitive development in adolescence allows thought processing to become more abstract and analytical. The growing independence that emerges during this stage aligns itself well with these ongoing brain developments.

Changes to sleeping patterns

It is worth briefly considering the changes to sleeping patterns that are known to occur during adolescence. The deregulation of circadian rhythms is common during this stage (Dahl and Lewin, 2002; Hansen et al., 2005) and may result in potential maladaptive sleeping patterns such as day-time sleepiness (Feinberg and Campbell, 2010). When compared with children or adults, adolescent groups appear to exhibit a shift in the release and levels of melatonin (a hormone linked with sleep) by as much as two hours (Carskadon et al., 2004; Taylor et al., 2005). Harris, Qualter and Robinson (2013) found that dysfunctional sleep in pre-adolescents (8–11 years) could lead to decreases in social interaction, further impacting on sleep. This growing cycle may then lead to irritability and social withdrawal, potentially exacerbating feelings of social isolation. Less sleep in adolescence has been associated with poorer academic performance and an increased likelihood of depressive symptoms being reported, even when controlling for other socio-demographics (Gau et al., 2004; Ohida et al., 2004; Pagel et al., 2007; Roberts et al., 2009;). A possible explanation for this could be the ongoing developments in the brain discussed above that may also influence the complex interaction of circadian, social and other factors (Feinberg and Campbell, 2010). Other exacerbating factors might include the modern availability of media such as television and the Internet (Cain and Gradisar, 2010; Punamäki et al., 2007; Van den Bulck, 2004). Therefore, attitudes towards the sleeping patterns of adolescents are important and appreciating the impact of sleep deprivation on behaviour and cognition may be helpful in raising awareness of this. Reacting positively to the general functioning and patterns of sleep in this age group is necessary to reduce stress and discord with other age groups that may not share the same patterns.

Recognising vulnerable adolescents

It is important to recognise that many adolescents will have a positive mental health status during these years (Coleman, 2011). Although many adolescents can be resilient to the effects of mental health problems and stressful life events, there are a number of young people who can go on to develop behavioural, emotional or neurodevelopmental disorders. The study of adolescence demands research that integrates biology, context and psychological development (Steinberg and Morris, 2001). Additional stressors in the environment (family or illness-related) may have a notice-able impact on adolescents whose brain development is still ongoing (Jehta and Segalowitz, 2012, p. 21). Moreover, genetic expression has been found to increase over time, between the ages of 13 and 35 years, increasing the heritability impact of mental health problems (Bergen et al., 2007).

The emergence of a lifetime risk for psychopathology has been found to peak at age 14, with over half of mental health disorders starting by this age (Kessler et al., 2005, 2007; Maughan and Kim-Cohen, 2005). Current estimates within England suggest that around 1 per cent of 5–16 year olds exhibit a clinically recognisable mental health problem (Green et al., 2005). A three-year fol-low-up survey to this study, conducted in 2007, involving 67 per cent of the original sample (5,364 of 7,977), found that 30 per cent of those who had an emotional disorder in the original survey were still experiencing it in the follow-up (Parry-Langdon, 2008). Estimates from the US for the prevalence of disorders causing severe impairment and/or distress in 13–18 year olds (n=10,123) is approximately 22.2 per cent (Merikangas et al., 2011). Epidemiological evidence from international sources suggests that longer periods of depressive and anxiety-related symptoms during adolescence are associated with the emergence of a disorder in later life (Fergusson et al., 2005; Kessler et al., 2005, 2012; Maughan and Kim-Cohen, 2005; Patton et al., 2014).

Untreated mental health problems during this period can lead to a number of poor outcomes such as family conflict, poor physical health, anti-social behaviours including crime and a decline in academic performance (Rutter and Smith, 1995). Estimates from national and international surveys report low numbers of young people accessing treatment, with only around a quarter of those with a diagnosable mental health problem receiving treatment (Burnett-Zeigler et al., 2012; Green et al., 2005; Ma et al., 2005; Meltzer et al., 2003; Merikangas et al., 2011, 2103; Mojtabai, 2006; Patel et al., 2007). Despite a large proportion of mental health problems presenting in adolescence, treatment tends not to occur until a number of years later (Kessler et al., 2007). Moreover, the costs associated with untreated mental health problems in adolescence can be substantial for both the individual and society (McCrone et al., 2008). The Kennedy Review (2010), on evaluating children and young people's NHS services, pointed out that adolescents can often be thought of as the 'forgotten group' in healthcare. The overriding stigma and common misunderstandings surrounding mental illness within this group may mean that cases often go unnoticed and consequently untreated. Recognising vulnerable adolescents early is crucial in preventing these onsets, therefore making it a fundamental part of any health professionals' work.

On the individual level, risk factors for experiencing poor mental health during adolescence have been found to include a low IQ, learning disability, shifts in pubertal timing, communication difficulties, a difficult temperament, physical or neurological illness, especially if chronic, poor educational performance and low self-esteem (Dogra et al., 2009; Mental Health Foundation, 2004). It should also be noted that the opposite of these risk factors might serve as protective factors.

Young people with a learning or physical disability, especially if severe, are at an increased risk of reporting emotional distress, developing a mental health problem and attempting to commit suicide (Einfeld et al., 2011; Emerson, 2003; Emerson et al., 2009; Honey et al., 2011; Svetaz et al., 2000). In the UK, up to 10 per cent of children are affected by learning difficulties, which have an impact on their mental health and subsequent academic performance (Foresight, 2008). These are similar to levels found in the US with a 9.7 per cent estimated prevalence rate (Altarac and Saroha, 2007).

Family, friends and peer influence upon adolescent mental health

Adolescence defines a period of growing independence from parents, carers and family. The family can be thought of to include anyone involved in nurturing a young person's developmental and emotional needs, which would encompass their parents, step-parents, carers, siblings, grandparents, close friends and family friends (Dogra et al., 2009). The risk factors associated with the onset of a mental health problem in adolescence can be multiple and complex. A young person's development does not occur in isolation. Their development is influenced by the social context surrounding them, particularly the family context (Das Gupta and Frake, 2009). Likewise, different types of problems, whether they are behavioural, emotional or neurodevelopmental, will each have their separate origins and it is difficult to pinpoint an exact cause. There still remains debate around which factors are more prominent in the development of certain disorders. It is useful, however, to consider certain risk factors so these can be more readily identified and an adolescent can be offered the appropriate care and support. This will also potentially serve to reduce the development and impact of persistent mental health problems into adulthood.

The impact of parental influence still appears to be prominent during this stage of life (Cottrell et al., 2007). Positive family and peer relationships can provide a safeguard for an adolescent who may have experienced a negative and/or stressful life event (Petersen et al., 1993). This might be difficult to maintain as conflict between parents and adolescents are known to increase during this stage of life (Steinberg and Morris, 2001). This is of interest as the perceived rejection of parents has been associated with increased rates of depression in adolescents (Stice et al., 2004). Likewise, poorer outcomes have been associated in children with mothers who are clinically depressed (Knapp et al., 2011) (see Chapter 4 for more discussion). Other indicators in the family context have been found to precipitate the onset of a mental health problem. These can include: parental separation or divorce (Patton et al., 2014), low level of parental education, a single parent household and a female gender (Rushton et al., 2002; Yaroslavsky et al., 2013), as well as being brought up in families of low socio-economic status and larger family units (Surgeon General's Office, 2001). Young people living in the poorest households bracket have been found to be three times more likely to develop a mental health problem than compared with those in the upper groups (Green et al., 2005). This highlights the role that social disadvantage may play in young people's mental health.

The absence of a father, but not mother, has also been associated with an earlier onset of puberty in both male and female adolescents (Bogaert, 2005, 2008), as has increased family conflict (Belsky et al., 2007, 2010). This suggests the home environment and personal experiences are important for the expression of pubertal maturation. Other risk factors of note can include: persistent parental conflict, family breakdown, poor parental attachment, inconsistent or unclear boundaries and discipline, rejecting or aggressive family relationships, failure to adapt, abusive parents, chronic parental illness, psychopathology, criminality, alcoholism and death or loss (Dogra et al., 2009, p. 36).

A relationship in which both parent and adolescent are willing to cooperate may improve a young person's resilience and support their mental wellbeing (Kerr et al., 2008). It is important to recognise that the relationship is likely to be two-directional and the young person can have just as much influence on the adult as the other way round (Schaffer, 2006). A family with a core set of values that are made clear and consistent, and one that reacts to adversity or major life events in a flexible and responsive manner, is likely to make the young person more resilient. Yap et al. (2014a) looked into the evidence on modifiable parental factors influencing anxiety and depression in 12–18 year olds. They drew on a meta-analysis involving 111 studies. The review found that the risk for anxiety and depression-related symptoms being reported was associated with a lower level of perceived warmth from parents, higher inter-parental conflict, over-involvement and aversiveness. Lower levels of autonomy granting and high parental monitoring increased the risk for depression, but not anxiety. The review involved a robust design but its findings are limited in its generalisability across cultures and an increased number of studies looking into associations with depression. Nonetheless, it does illustrate the impact parents can still have in adolescence. Their parenting style is important to consider, given that parental monitoring in itself may be beneficial but an authoritarian style might not be.

A follow-up Delphi study was conducted with 27 international experts who agreed on 90 strategies (>90 per cent expert consensus), categorised under 11 sub-headings, for parents to use in their approach toward parenting (Yap et al., 2014b). The toolkit highlights the importance of paren-tal/carer involvement in an adolescent's life that seeks to gradually enhance the young person's autonomy as they grow older. This may include the setting of clear boundaries without being too overbearing. Another strategy is to ensure the parent/carer does not attribute self-blame in the event of a mental health problem emerging. A young person can develop a mental health problem in a happy, well-adjusted family. It is beneficial for the parent/carers to recognise, adapt and support the individual to lessen their suffering if so. For other sources that might be helpful in supporting resilience building in both children and adolescence see 'The Five Ways to Wellbeing', developed by the UK Government Office for Science (Foresight Project, 2008) and McDougall et al. (2010).

Influence of siblings

Meta-analytical evidence of cross-sectional data found small to moderate effect sizes (−0.12 to 0.28) related to a young person's mental health and the quality of the relationship with their sibling (Buist et al., 2013). As it is cross-sectional, it is not possible to determine which direction the effect occurs, although it is likely to be two-directional. Sibling conflict was significant in the develop-ment of behavioural and emotional problems, potentially through social learning. In addition, the presence of a sibling has been associated with a later onset in the timing of puberty in females, as marked by age of first menarche (Bogaert, 2008; Matchock and Susman, 2006; Milne and Judge, 2010). Relationships within the family, between siblings, parents and the extended family, can all impact on each other. Balancing conflict between each member is a concern for both the individual and family and may be necessary for a health professional to consider in the presence of mental health problems.

Differences in gender

With respect to gender, it would seem that females are more likely to present with emotional prob-lems, such as mood, anxiety, as well as eating disorders, whereas males are more likely to present with behavioural and neurodevelopmental problems, such as conduct disorder, attention deficit hyperactivity disorder and autism (Green et al., 2005; Kessler et al., 2012; Merikangas et al., 2011). Moreover, girls are more likely to be admitted to hospital for self-harm or attempted suicide (ONS, 2014), but there are more instances of death from suicide in boys (Hagell et al., 2013). See Chapters 7 and 8 for further discussions on gender differences in adults.

Differences in age

It is also worth noting inter-age differences of mental wellbeing during adolescence. Evidence from the US found the median age of onset for certain mental health conditions differed across a sam-ple of 13–18 year olds (n=10,123) (Merikangas et al., 2011). It was found that anxiety disorders emerged around 6 years old, whereas behavioural and mood disorders emerged around 11 and 13 years old respectively. This trend matches other evidence collected by West and Sweeting (2003) who found mood disorders increased in mid-adolescence, largely due to increases in female reports. The trend in age and emergence of certain conditions, as well as their interaction with other factors, helps to highlight the complex nature of mental health in adolescents and is worth considering when approaching this subject.

Influence of culture, religion and ethnic origin

Cultural context is important when considering mental health problems as certain societies, ethnic groups and customs foster behaviours that could be viewed differently in another society (Dogra et al., 2009). Cross-cultural comparisons are therefore difficult as cultural conceptualisation of what constitutes a disorder may vary. Likewise, existing mental illness constructs are noticeably Westernised. There are also certain disorders that appear to be more prevalent in certain parts of the world such as the emergence of eating disorder in the Western world (Bordo, 2013; Levine and Smolak, 2010; Swanson et al., 2012). Across Asian countries, those who are mentally ill are commonly believed to be dangerous.. This can then lead to social distancing behaviours and isolation from the community, which can in turn create a consequence for potential marriage partners, thus also stigmatising the family (Lauber and Rössler, 2007; Ng, 1997; Yang et al., 2007). In addition, young refugees or asylum seekers are at an increased risk of developing mental health problems. This is due to potentially experiencing or witnessing traumas, as well as having to acclimatise to a new culture (Dogra et al., 2009, p. 121). Discrimination against and social exclusion of those in a minority ethnic status can have deleterious effects on an individual's mental health and wellbeing (Dinos, 2014). Societal pressures to conform to expectations from the family, peers and communities may be different to what a young person desires, which could also present issues. See Chapters 2 and 3 for further discussion of cultural, religious and ethnic minority influences

Experiencing abuse and maltreatment

Abuse and experience with violence during childhood and adolescence are known to be risk factors for poor mental health (Sansone et al., 2005). Increases in rates of anxiety, depression and suicidal ideation have been linked to early experiences of abuse (physical and/or sexual), parental neglect or exposure to violence (Brodsky and Stanley, 2008; Ward et al., 2001). UK epidemiological data on severe child maltreatment, defined as severe physical, sexual and emotional abuse by any adult, report exposure to such victimisation to be approximately 18.6 per cent for 11–17 year olds (19 per cent female; 18.2 per cent male), rising to 25.3 per cent in 18–24 year olds (30.6 per cent females; 20.3 per cent males). For younger children, maltreatment is more likely to come from adults known to the child, such as relatives, neighbours or family friends, whereas with older groups, the most likely perpetrator tend to be unknown to the victim, or strangers (Radford et al., 2011). Young people exposed to family adversity or who have a pre-existing mental health problem and experience bullying should be given a high priority in the provision of interventions as these are the ones most likely to self-harm (Fisher et al., 2012). There is evidence to suggest that patterns of sexual abuse can also differ, with males more likely to be abused by people from outside the family, whereas females are more at risk of intra-familial abuse (Rogers and Pilgrim, 2010).

Peer influence upon adolescent mental health

Peer relationships are where many adolescents learn about themselves, others and the world. A strong social support is crucial for managing conflict and stressful life events. Social relationships are integral to all age groups but require notable attention during the adolescent period. In Western countries, a young person's primary confidant is thought to shift from parents towards close peers from ages 12–14 years onwards (Dogra et al., 2009, p. 110). It has been reported that young people experiencing mental health problems or engaging in harmful risk behaviours are likely to influence others to do the same and this can also impact on the individual to repeatedly commit this behaviour (Coleman, 2011, pp. 180–181). However, having peers who conform to more conventional attitudes and behaviours, such as alcohol use, may serve to act as a protective factor against abuse (Corte and Sommers, 2005). Aikins et al. (2005) recognise that peer relationships offer a platform for social learning and a source of support in adolescence.

Adolescents tend to be considered more sociable than children are and more sensitive to their acceptance or rejection by peers (Steinberg and Morris, 2001). Adolescent girls may also be more sensitive to this as they have been found to invest more into relationships (Girgus and Nolen-Hoeksema, 2006, as cited in Corcoran, 2011, p. 144). Peer rejection can lead to increased rates of anxiety and depression (Litwack et al., 2010; Masten et al., 2009, 2012). This may be mediated in part by increasingly sensitive and active regions of the brain (Masten et al., 2009, 2010, 2012). Attempting to conform and fit within a group enhances the impact of peer influence and may make an individual more susceptible to peer pressure. Behavioural risks in early developing females have been attributed to the influence from older teens in their social group (Cavanagh, 2004). Moreover, in areas of increased deprivation, violence committed by young males has been linked to friendships involving older peers (Harding, 2009). The varied rates of development and intense changes adolescents undergo during this period may mean that some are introduced to certain types of potentially harmful behaviours, or complex social and sexual relations, earlier than most. If this is the case then an individual may incur greater detriment to their health, wellbeing, sociability and academic or work-related performance.

Enabling a young person to identify the influence of their social peers and their influence on others could help to improve self-awareness. By encouraging an individual to seek out and build on the more positive relationships, and clarify their identity among peers, separating out the behaviour of the group and themselves, may help to boost a young person's self-efficacy. Peers and social networks are clearly important for this age group and the influence of their peers bears consideration (Figure 6.1).

Influence of pubertal timing

Pubertal timing refers to the onset of puberty and its progress in development compared with same-sex or similar-aged peers. Adolescents vary discernibly in their timing at onset of puberty. The extent of this variance has been associated with an increased risk of mental health problems, including depressive symptoms (Benoit et al., 2013; Ge et al., 2003; Michaud et al., 2006), anxiety-related issues (Kaltiala-Heino et al., 2003; Zehr et al., 2007), conduct and problem behaviours (Burt et al., 2006; Celio et al., 2006), negative self-body image (McCabe and Ricciardelli, 2004), disordered

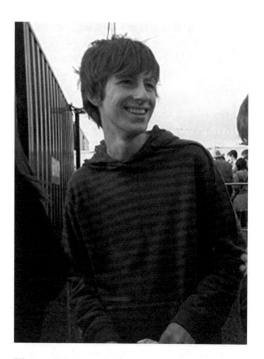

Figure 6.1 Developing a young person's self-efficacy and self-awareness is important

eating patterns (Striegel-Moore et al., 2001; Zehr et al., 2007), and drug and alcohol abuse (Biehl et al., 2007; Bratberg et al., 2007), among others. Social and environmental factors such as the adolescent peer group (Cavanagh, 2004), parenting styles and relationships (Arim and Shapka, 2008), romantic partners (Halpern et al., 2007; Natsuaki et al., 2009) and stressful life events (Ge et al., 2001) have all been found to moderate the effects of pubertal timing on mental health. The detrimental effects of pubertal timing may be mediated by complex interactions between childhood experiences and adolescents' interpersonal relationships, such as a stressful family context (Benoit et al., 2013). Furthermore, the psychological outcomes of pubertal timing have been found to persist into young adulthood (Graber et al., 2004; Zehr et al., 2007). However, for many this impact may reduce once a person reaches the onset of puberty and maturing into adulthood (Coleman, 2011, p. 34).

For females, early maturation among peers has been associated with reductions in perceived popularity, inner turmoil and may exhibit increased bodily dissatisfaction (Alsaker and Flammer, 2006; Benoit et al., 2013; Graber et al., 2006; Moore and Rosenthal, 2006). On the other hand, for males, the earlier onset of puberty may lead to more positive consequences, such as increased self-confidence, popularity, greater athletic and academic ability, as well as the social advantages of a more mature physical appearance (Benoit et al., 2013; Moore and Rosenthal, 2006). In this regard, later maturing males may be at risk (Conley and Rudolph, 2009; Moore and Rosenthal, 2006; Siegel et al., 1999). The deviance hypothesis proposes that those adolescents who are maturing earlier or later than what is expected or socially and culturally accepted are more vulnerable to psychological maladjustments, as they do not fit with the peer trajectory of change (Petersen and Crockett, 1985; Simmons and Blyth, 1987; Susman et al., 2003). Supporting adolescents during this period is crucial, as is ensuring the provision of sufficient information to this group about the variance in pubertal maturation.

Influence of media and social media

It is worthwhile reflecting on the role of the media and the rise in technology that is now in use among adolescents. The rate of change in technology and the power of the Internet are redefining social communication. For adolescents, the dramatic increase in mobile phones, the ubiquity of online social networks and the availability of information sharing are forging each generation in stark contrast to previous ones. The utility of online resources opens up access to global information, educational resources, entertainment, activism and resources for advice, as well as sharing experiences with others. On the other hand, it does present a number of risks such as access to illegal content, biased information or misinformation, on-site advertising, abuse, cyber-bullying, possible grooming by strangers and invasion of privacy (Livingstone, 2009). Moves should be made to enable and encourage the opportunities that the age of the Internet offers, whilst attempting to reduce the exposure to the additive risks it introduces. An open and transparent discussion on these matters is important so that adolescents are aware of the benefits and risks.

Social networking sites have increased in popularity over the last decade, particularly among adolescents. A survey looking into access to social networking sites involving 12–17 year olds (n=802) found rates to be increasing year on year, as was the amount of information this group shared online. Almost half of the respondents admitted to logging on to a social networking site daily and their experiences were mostly positive (Madden et al., 2013). Qualitative evidence involving 92 college students in the US found the reasons for the use of Facebook centred mainly on communication, particularly with those who were not immediately accessible geographically (Pempek et al., 2009). Nonetheless, it is generally recognised that people become more disinhibited online, making the sending of negative comments more likely as opposed to in the real world (Suler, 2004). Dutch adolescents aged 10 to 19 years receiving mainly negative comments and feedback online were more likely to report lower self-esteem and mental wellbeing (Valkenburg et al., 2006). Poor-quality interactions online have also been associated with higher levels of depressive symptoms being reported (Davila et al., 2012; Selfhout et al., 2009). Social networks open up a new aspect of human communication and may be a helpful resource for many young people in times of social isolation. However, careful monitoring and educating young people on the risks of social networks may lessen the dangers associated with them.

In the US, adolescents aged 14–17 years old send and receive on average 60 text messages a day, with older adolescent girls sending the most at almost 100 or more daily (Lenhart et al., 2010). These rates are similar to those found in the UK (Livingstone et al., 2014). Such activity presents new phenomena to explore, such as the emergence of 'sexting', which involves the act of sending sexually explicit images or messages to others by mobile phone. Evidence is still emerging on the effects of this although evidence from the US has found an association between sexting and sexual behaviours, substance use, excessive time spent texting and other health risk behaviours, including suicidal ideation, in 12–18 year olds (n=1,289) (Dake et al., 2012). Many young people do not perceive sexting to be a 'big deal' (Lenhart, 2009). Attention is now gathering in response to the legal issues surrounding the age gap in some sexters (Calvert, 2009; Corbett, 2009; House of Commons Health Committee, 2014). Educating young people on the risks associated with this practice is critical and must be done in a non-judgmental and respectful manner. Further research is also needed to keep pace with the changes in technology and its effect on social interactions for young people.

Internet use may lead to depressive symptoms in adolescents who exhibit and report poor friendship quality (Selfhout et al., 2009). Likewise prolonged periods of time engaged in video games have also been linked to impact on a young person's attention skills, emotional response, risk-taking behaviour and academic performance (Beullens et al., 2011; Gentile, 2009; Hull et al., 2012; Wang and Dey, 2009). Certain personality traits can predict increased hostility in gaming such as an increased neuroticism and decreased level of agreeableness and conscientiousness (Markey and Markey, 2010). On the other hand there are also notable benefits of gaming uncovered by research such as improved eye-hand coordination in a virtual surgery task (Rosser et al., 2007), improved contrast sensitivity functioning in the eye (Li et al., 2009), as well as reducing depressive symptoms through playing a game orientated towards destroying negative thoughts (Merry et al., 2012b). A prolonged period of anything is likely to have a detrimental impact on an individual. Balancing the amount of exposure a young person has by limiting screen time will likely be beneficial.

The availability of the Internet opens up the possibility of accessing cognitive behavioural therapy (CBT), self-help, support groups, or other related psychotherapeutic interventions online (Andersson and Cuijpers, 2009; Foroushani et al., 2011; Grover et al., 2011; Richardson et al., 2010). This may be helpful in overcoming the stigma associated with mental health problems, the low rate of adolescents seeking or accessing treatment and improving access as the therapist support required is reduced. Spence et al. (2011) separated 115 adolescents (12–18 year olds) into three groups consisting of a course of online CBT programme, face-to-face CBT and a waiting list control for the treatment of a range of anxiety disorders. After 12 weeks of treatment, there were no significant differences between the online and face-to-face course of therapy but both were more effective than the control group ($p<0.05$) and effects were maintained at 12-month follow-up. Satisfaction among adolescent users of computerised CBT programmes tends to be high but the rates of dropout are also noticeably high (Richardson et al., 2010). Online therapy programmes may hold promise but more research is needed to explore who is likely to benefit most.

Health professionals are in a key position to educate families about the complexities of the digital world, both in its risks and benefits (O'Keeffe and Clarke-Pearson, 2011). Encouraging open discussion between adolescents and their parents as well as encouraging parents to become better educated about the technology their children are using could be useful.

Bullying and cyber-bullying

Bullying can take on many forms but it is usually a behaviour that is defined by the use of threat, intimidation, coercion or force for the purposes of aggressively dominating or terrorising another individual. The behaviour is often repeated and may take on forms involving physical violence, name-calling, teasing, the spreading of rumours and/or cyber-bullying. Cyber-bullying involves the use of the technology to repeatedly harass and bully others. Online harassment has been associated with increased rates of depressive symptoms (Ybarra and Mitchell, 2004). In 2010, 16 per cent of UK children reported being bullied, with 8 per cent saying they were bullied via the Internet. This had reversed in 2013, showing cyber-bullying was now more common than face-to-face bullying (12 per cent vs. 9 per cent) (Livingstone et al., 2014).

A UK national survey involving 1,843 adolescent respondents reported that 22.4 per cent of participants reported being bullied on a daily basis and 57 per cent of those reportedly being bullied were dissatisfied with support services on offer (Ditch the Label, 2013). The toll taken on victims could be detrimental to both their physical and mental health. Indeed, meta-analytical evidence suggests strong links between peer victimisation and the onset of common mental health problems and psychosomatic problems (Gini and Pozzoli, 2009; Hawker and Boulton, 2000). Other meta-analytical evidence, involving 34 studies (n=284,375) analysing peer victimisation in relation to suicidal ideation, as well as 9 studies (N=70,102) looking directly into its association with bullying, found a significant relationship between bullying and suicidal ideation (van Geel et al., 2014). However, bullying alone does not tend to lead to suicide as evidence from the US suggests only a small percentage (around 3.2 per cent) of adolescent suicide specifically listed bullying as a precipitating factor (n=1,046). The factors leading to suicide are likely to be multiple (Karch et al., 2013). For example, young people who are identified as being homosexual or bisexual appear to be at an increased risk of being bullied, performing self-harming behaviour and attempting to commit suicide (Berlan et al., 2010). Bullying may not help in reducing the onset of a mental health problem and young people with a pre-existing condition may be at further risk of being bullied.

There is also evidence to suggest that bullying affects not only the victim, but also the bully and those observing, as they are then more likely to go on to develop mental health problems of their own (Gini and Pozzoli, 2009; Wolke et al., 2013). Bullies may use bullying tactics to achieve a higher social status or dominance over another (Scholte and van Aken, 2013). Efforts should be made to provide prevention and intervention programmes on the effects of bullying and aim to support young people who are victimised by it. Minimising the emotional impact of peer victimisation is critical to combat this association. Programmes that seek to enhance cognitive behavioural skills and educate adolescents in judging social situations and the harmful effects of bullying may be helpful at improving this occurrence (Coleman, 2011, p. 186–187). The coordination of educators, parents and health professionals may be necessary, as is attempting to reinforce each party's approachability for adolescents facing victimisation.

Schools and the role of educators

The school setting has been recognised as being a useful resource for the prevention of mental health problems and the promotion of positive mental wellbeing (Masia-Warner et al., 2006). School-based intervention programmes that are included as a component of the school-based curriculum may also be helpful in overcoming stigma and transportation difficulties, and reducing costs and offering a familiar setting (Barrett and Pahl, 2006; Farrell and Barrett, 2007; Masia-Warner et al., 2006). Moreover, the school environment may reinforce learning as it is a setting which reflects this (Rambaldo et al., 2001). Relationships with teachers have been shown to be a significant factor in school satisfaction of early adolescents (Booth and Sheehan, 2008). School-based programmes that attempt to focus on and tackle bullying have been found to improve mental wellbeing and academic performance (Durlak et al., 2011). Meta-analytical evidence has shown these programmes to be effective in reducing anxiety and depression-related symptoms (Corrieri et al., 2013; Neil and Christensen, 2009). However, rolling out prevention programmes in school such as that for depression may be premature, as evidence exists to demonstrate no observable beneficial impact and may in fact produce harmful repercussions, increasing the reporting of depressive symptoms (Stallard et al., 2012). School nurses are well placed to deal with the complexity of issues that adolescents may present and may offer them a non-judgmental, impartial resource. Nevertheless, evidence suggests that this workforce may not feel equipped to deal with these issues due to a lack of insight or additional training (Haddad et al., 2010). More research and training is needed in this area but the support and collaboration of educators, healthcare professionals, parents or carers could prove to be an invaluable resource.

Role of the health professional

Health professionals in specialist services are involved in a diverse range of interventions in various capacities and settings. This can involve a range of individuals, such as a young child, or older adolescent, as well as their families and educators. Nurses involved in these services can provide general care for young people or specialised care for specific mental health problems such as managing self-harm (Dogra and Leighton, 2009, p. 3). Chronic mental health problems are usually dealt with in primary care and within the community. Approachability is key and attempting to offer a non-biased, non-judgmental, warm and comforting setting may encourage an adolescent to open up more. Health professionals and educators should not feel inhibited in discussing mental health problems with adolescents as many difficulties will remain undisclosed and may deteriorate if not identified. Taking on board notable risk factors and consulting the relevant diagnostic manuals and treatment guidelines will help build knowledge for improving mental wellbeing in this age group.

As a health professional and educator, it is not always feasible to promise confidentiality. The young person can be supported by limited confidentiality, but when a risk to themselves or others is evident then the professional in question has a duty to take action. Making this explicit from the outset will ensure clarity and understanding, as well as preserving a young person's trust in professionals, both now and in the future (Dogra et al., 2008). Ongoing risk in the cases of chronic mental health conditions may require a named professional. It is good practice to propose and make clear the structure of any intervention, clarifying your own understanding of what is being discussed, setting boundaries and ensuring careful planning and focus throughout. Across adolescence there are a wide spectrum of behaviours, with many balancing childhood tendencies and emerging adult responsibilities. Likewise, their literary, emotional and behavioural competency may be still developing; therefore clarifying your own understanding can be a useful tool. The use of listening, reflection, attentiveness and sensitivity, as well as attending to how they express themselves in body language and tone, is equally important. As with all approaches make sure not to trivialise a young person's issues and it is important to take steps to ensure you do not pass judgment.

Treatments for mental health problems

The evidence base for young people and their mental health has steadily increased over the last decade, although debate still exists around the uncertainties of available psychotherapeutic interventions within this age group. Treatments tend to combine several approaches consisting of a pharmacological, psychological and family and community component (Fonagy et al., 2002). In place of generic psychological interventions, treatments are becoming increasingly specialised and formulated (AACAP, 2007; beyondblue, 2011; Cheung et al., 2007; NICE, 2005). Having clear protocols along with a standardised instrument is useful in helping health professionals to feel more prepared for dealing with mental health problems in adolescents (Taliaferro et al., 2013). For a systematic review of effective treatments of mental health disorders in children and adolescents, consult Cartwright-Hatton et al. (2004) and Tennant et al. (2007).

Psychotherapy

As the importance of early experiences became more widely recognised, the emergence of more specialised psychotherapeutic interventions for young people began to develop. The behaviourist movement on operant and classical conditioning as well as the child-focused work of Donald Meichenbaum and colleagues also served to help develop this field (Weisz and Gray, 2008). Psychological therapies have demonstrated effectiveness for treating mental health problems in this age group (Cartwright-Hatton et al., 2004; Fonagy et al., 2005, pp. 1–41; Kendall, 2011). However, Murray and Cartwright-Hatton (2006) point out that without a robust and extensive training programme put in place the delivery of evidence-based therapies could be ineffectual. Considering this, it is also worth noting that a national survey of UK CAMHS professionals found two-thirds of therapists self-disclosed that they required more training in child-focused CBT (n=538) (Stallard et al., 2007). Other evidence also shares some concern around the apparent shortage of therapists in some areas of England specialising in child and adolescent therapies (Department for Children, Schools and Families, 2008). Recent developments in England have seen the implementation of the Improving Access to Psychological Therapies (IAPT) programme. The IAPT programme is a government-funded initiative first established to provide evidence-based psychotherapeutic interventions to those who would not have had equitable access otherwise (DH, 2008). It has recently widened its scope to include the provision of services for children and adolescents so they too can gain access to evidence-based treatments. The programme has enlisted the workforce of existing CAMHS health professionals and is nearing its final stages of national rollout.

CBT is a form of psychotherapy has been used extensively in treating young people's mental health. The technique aims to alter maladaptive behaviour and repetitive thinking patterns, which serve to sustain the disorder, encouraging the young person to identify unrealistically negative thoughts and challenge these with more positive interpretations (e.g. 'Not everyone likes me, but at least I have some really good friends'). It can be delivered in many forms, and across a range of formats. CBT has demonstrated efficacy in the treatment of anxiety disorders for children and adolescents over no treatment, or treatment-as-usual, although its efficacy long term or as against medication is still limited (Cartwright-Hatton et al., 2004; Cox et al., 2012; Weisz, McCarty and Valeri, 2006).

Medication

Medication prescribing for children and adolescents in the UK remain quite rare, with approximately 7 per cent of those with an emotional disorder and 9 per cent with a conduct disorder taking any form of medication. The main use of psychotropic medication in this age group is usually for hyperkinetic disorders, taken by 43 per cent of young people with these disorders (Green et al., 2005). Rates of antidepressant prescribing for adolescents are also low in the US (Merikangas et al., 2013). Antidepressants have been linked to a decrease in suicide among young people (Isacsson and Rich, 2008). While the use of antidepressants may be effective in the treatment of adult depression, children and adolescents remain under-represented in research (Patel et al., 2007). Moreover, the side effects that can result from medication may make them an unlikely treatment option and other psychotherapeutic interventions are usually opted for, as they are considered to be relatively side effect free.

Family-based interventions

Evidence to support family-based interventions is still emerging. Peer and familial relation-ships should be encouraged to enhance positive processes and seek to minimise threats during this crucial stage of life (Jehta and Segalowitz, 2012, pp. 53–69). The home environment and family setting is where most young people live their lives and considering the family context is necessary in most treatment plans. When assessing for risk in adolescents it is useful to engage all parties including the individual, family, educators and health professionals to help create a shared understanding of potential mental wellbeing difficulties. Working collaboratively with families can help identify unhelpful family patterns without a risk of undermining parental authority and capability in raising their child. Family-based interventions tend to take into account different perspectives, contexts and interpretations and tend to consider the family as being able to find their own resolutions to difficulties. Those administering these interventions will need to meet and discuss with the family about their engagement and suitability, as well as clarify the purpose of the sessions. The purpose of the interventions is to empower families by educating them and providing them with useful problem-solving strategies. It is usually delivered as part of a multi-modal approach in combination with other interventions (Dogra et al., 2009, pp., 234–235).

Resilience building

Intervening at the point of crisis with a psychological treatment is one approach to combatting the incidence of mental health problems in young people. However, Donovan and Spence (2000) argue that the focus should not be on treatment but on prevention. Nonetheless, most prevention programmes may produce only modest effects and be unable to treat a disorder once it develops (Garber, 2006; Horowitz and Garber, 2006; Merry et al., 2012a; Stice et al., 2009). Although there have been many advances in the field of psychological treatment many of those that suffer will not receive treatment or may suffer in silence (see section on Recognising vulnerable adolescents above, pp. 117–118). Those that do receive treatment may not experience any benefit and this could lead them to discontinue prematurely or be referred elsewhere (Farrell and Barrett, 2007). The ineffectiveness of treatment may be the result of it being implemented too late, with the effects of a disorder already having made an impact on an individual's life, both socially and academically

(Donovan and Spence, 2000). Universal programmes attempting to build resilience in young people could be used to enhance general mental wellbeing of at-risk adolescents (Barrett and Turner, 2004; Ng, Ang and Ho, 2012; Oliver et al., 2006). For family, personal and community units, an effective prevention measure is to promote the development of cognitive resilience (Foresight, 2008).

Transitional care

There is a need for effective coordination of those transitioning from child and adolescent services onto adult services, between the ages of 16 and 25 years, in order to address the gaps that can occur. Singh et al. (2010) identified 154 individuals across six UK mental health services transitioning from CAMHS onto adult mental health services over a one-year period. The authors encountered difficulties searching the central CAMHS database and had to rely on clinician recall to identify cases. They found that 64 (42 per cent) individuals did not make the transition to adult services yet were considered eligible for referral. Interview data with 11 randomly selected participants reported poor planning in a majority of cases and continuing parental involvement. Drawing on these findings and other existing evidence, Singh et al. (2010) advise a number of measures to improve the transitionary period. These include: aligning referral thresholds between services, adopting a flexible transition boundary, carefully planning and preparing the individual and services for transition, improving information transfer, managing and reducing multiple transitions, such as between teams in adult services, increasing liaison, and developing an integrated youth mental health programme, as opposed to emphasising silo treatment centres.

Living with poor mental health

This section selects and discusses briefly a select number of mental health problems that can emerge during adolescence. This is by no means an exhaustive list and will provide the reader with only a brief overview of the chosen conditions and available interventions.

Depression

Clinical depression involves feeling sad, down or irritable for at least two weeks, stopping a young person from enjoying things they used to like, or engaging in social activities (Kelly et al., 2013). During this stage, depression has been linked with an increased risk of suicide, reduced educational performance and poorer social relationships (Gibb et al., 2010). It is considered the most prevalent and widely reported mental health problem within this age group, with over a quarter of adolescents reportedly affected by depressive symptoms (Rushton et al., 2002). The World Health Organisation (WHO, 2014) estimated depression to be the top cause of illness and disability in 10–19 year olds worldwide, with suicide reported to be the third main cause of death, behind road traffic accidents and HIV/AIDS (WHO, 2014). In-patient treatment is recommended where there is a high risk of self-harm or suicide. In mild-moderate cases, counselling or psychotherapy is usually recommended to address issues of self-esteem, self-efficacy, relationship management and problem-solving skills. Those who do not respond to these therapies could be considered for medication and more intense psychotherapy. Issues around past experiences may need to be addressed where necessary and the family may also need to be educated (Dogra et al., 2009, pp. 184–185).

Anxiety disorders

An anxiety disorder is usually typified by a heightened and constant state of arousal. This may make daily activities difficult, both inside and outside of school or work (Department for Education, 2014; Kitchener et al., 2013; McLoone et al., 2006). In Great Britain (England, Scotland and Wales) the prevalence rate of anxiety disorders in young people is estimated to be 4.4 per cent (Green et al., 2005). The onset of an anxiety disorder has also been found to emerge earlier than other mood and emotional disorders (Merikangas et al., 2011). If left untreated, this may lead to greater difficulties in late adulthood including an impact on one's career, social circles, more time spent with health-care services and the development of possible comorbidities and substance abuse (Donovan and Spence, 2000; McCrone et al., 2008; Patel et al., 2007; Rapee et al., 2005). In terms of treatment, cognitive therapy is thought to be useful in its symptom reappraisal method. Encouraging the use of self-talk may also be therapeutic for younger adolescents, who use it in their play and problem-solving activities more readily than adults (Dogra et al., 2009, pp. 218–219).

Eating disorders

Dissatisfaction with one's own body and appearance may result in the emergence of an eating disorder. It is well recognised that these types of disorder affect adolescent girls in particular. For example, 40 per cent of all anorexia nervosa cases are made up of girls between 15 and 19 years of age (Bulik et al., 2005; HSCIC, 2013; Micali et al. 2013; Vostanis, 2007). The development of eating disorders is thought to be the result of individuals striving for thinness and is reinforced by culture, particularly in the Western world, as well as portrayals in the media or on social media. Discrepancies between the supposed 'ideal' and the image of one's self may then lead to conflict and anxiety, perhaps leading to dietary action, such as restricting food and purging (Striegel-Moore and Bulik, 2007). An eating disorder may also be an effort to exert control over one's life (Fairburn et al., 2003).

The major physiological changes that occur during puberty may lead young people to become sensitive about their body shape and weight, particularly among girls. This may drive a series of weight-controlling behaviours (Faulkner, 2007). Hereditary and genetic factors may also play a role (Klein and Walsh, 2004). The recovery process for treating eating disorders is known to take a considerable amount of time and effort, meaning that patience and understanding of the condition on a case-by-case basis is crucial. The physical toll taken on an individual because of under-nutrition is also worth considering. Encouraging a regular, well-balanced meal regime, in consultation with a dietician, as well as educating the young person and their family about their condition, is also recommended (Dogra et al., 2009, pp. 192–198).

Eating disorder: a case scenario

Liam was a bright and intelligent boy in the last years of high school when his disordered eating came to the attention of his school. Teachers close to him had noticed he was beginning to look run down and pale, matched with a noticeable loss in weight. Because of his feeling faint and weak from a lack of eating, Liam would often miss class. He also employed a number of behaviours that would hide the fact that he was not eating regularly, such as ensuring he ate in the presence of teachers. After a while, the school became concerned and informed his parents who had been unaware up until that point. Liam feels that his parents had ignored these issues and actively neglected paying attention to the fact that their child had an eating disorder. He describes how everyone around him was concerned, including other people's parents, but he felt no such concern from his own parents.

Liam was referred to an eating disorders unit and put on an urgent list due to the severity of his problem. He also had to be taken out of school. His treatment included a course of one-to-one CBT over a 9-month period. The treatment started out more intensely and gradually decreased in frequency and intensity as the therapy wore on. The therapy involved challenging negative thinking patterns and attempting to uncover where these thoughts were emerging. Liam believes much of his disordered eating patterns stem from the turbulent relationship he has with his father. He remembers from a very young age that his father would often call him 'fat' or 'obese', which led him to think he had to be thin to be good. Once he reached adolescence, he realised he could take more control over this aspect of his life. Unfortunately, his time in therapy reached a poor conclusion when he broke down in tears in response to the notes the therapist had shared with him about his issues. Upon reading them, Liam felt that the therapist had belittled most of his childhood experiences of abuse. He believed the therapist did not pay much attention to these issues and instead was effectively telling him to 'get over it'. As a result, the therapeutic relationship broke down.

During and after this experience, Liam found support and comfort in a close family friend. He described this woman as loving, supportive, caring and, importantly, she imposed no pressure or expectation on him to get better. He also noticed that this sort of love and attention had been missing in the relationship with his parents. Over the course of many months, he began to engage in many activities which involved country walks, social events and regular Sunday dinners. The progress towards regular eating patterns was long and he still is known to have minor relapses, but his health and weight are back to a normal level. Liam now reflects on his eating disorder and points out that once he had a safe base and relationship to build on, he realised that such behaviour was not a worthwhile answer for him anymore.

Conduct disorder and oppositional defiant disorder (ODD)

Conduct disorders are characterised by a repetitive and persistent pattern of behavioural problems which violate the rights and wellbeing of others, or are considered inappropriate for their age. They can either be socialised or unsocialised, depending on how they relate to a peer group. Characteristics are usually typified by aggressive, destructive, bullying, arson, defiant, cruel, repeatedly lying and stealing behaviours. The UK prevalence rate of conduct disorders for 11–16 year olds is estimated to be 6.6 per cent, and higher in males (8.1 per cent) than females (5.1 per cent) (Green et al., 2005). Conduct disorders and ODD are the most common reason why children and adolescents are referred to mental health services in the UK (NICE, 2013). Just under half (43 per cent) of children and young adults who have a conduct disorder have been shown to still have these three years on (Parry-Langdon, 2008). Longitudinal data from the US found an association with ongoing antisocial personality disorders in adulthood in those with a history of conduct disorders in childhood and adolescence (Rowe et al., 2010). Seeking information from teachers about a young person's functioning in school may be helpful in ensuring diagnoses of conduct disorder are not missed (Ford et al., 2003). Multisystemic therapy seeks to identify and break down the context and systems reinforcing a young person's antisocial behaviour and appears to be an effective intervention (Schoenwald et al., 2008). Medication tends to be limited in its effect and should be considered in consultation with a specialist service (Dogra et al., 2009, pp. 155–156).

Alcohol and substance abuse

Alcohol and substance abuse can be harmful for adolescents, threatening their health, wellbeing, sociability, academic performance, athleticism and mood. Survey data suggests alcohol use tends to commence in early adolescence (13–14 year olds) and its rate of use increases markedly, year on year, up until an individual's twenties (Faden, 2006). The latest figures for England report that approximately 52 per cent of 11 to 15 year olds have reportedly tried smoking, alcohol or taken drugs although trends are decreasing (n=7,589 across 254 schools) (Fuller, 2013). According to the Health Survey for England, younger people (16–24 year olds) are more likely to drink heavily on a single occasion than any other age group (Fat and Fuller, 2011). Prolonged alcohol and substance use in adolescence has been linked to a number of risk factors including drink driving, sexual promiscuity, use of illegal substances, increased aggressive behaviour, particularly among males, neurological damage and alcoholism in adulthood (Behrendt et al., 2008; Callaghan et al., 2013; Choo et al., 2008; Corte and Sommers, 2005; Dawson et al., 2007, 2008; Kirby and Barry, 2012; McQueeny et al., 2009; van Gastel et al., 2013). Identifying the direct role substance abuse plays in the impact on adolescents' mental health is difficult as it is often associated with other lifestyle factors which may also be detrimental. Reducing alcohol and substance abuse within this age group may bring about both immediate and future benefits in tackling emerging issues early.

For adolescents, receiving health advice from adults may be hard to accept, as they are part of a culture that places drinking at the centre of many social activities (Coleman, 2011, p. 107). A way to reduce alcohol consumption or substance abuse in adolescents could be achieved by directly challenging common misconceptions about the use of these (Corte and Sommers, 2005). Careful monitoring, rehabilitation programmes, family-based interventions and medically assisted withdrawal or goals towards abstinence may be necessary. It is important to state the harmful effects of abusing these substances without making the individual feel criticised or judged (Dogra et al., 2013, pp. 200–201). Updates on UK NICE guidance (2011) support the continued use of motivational interviewing and family-based interventions. It is worth considering the circumstances or the possibility for an underlying condition that could be triggering their abuse. In these cases, it is important to offer support and seek treatment where possible.

Comorbidity

Whilst this chapter has discussed a limited number of conditions in relation to adolescent mental health, it is important to recognise that these disorders rarely occur in a discrete manner. A major survey for the mental health of children and adolescents in Great Britain found a sizeable proportion of individuals with an emotional disorder also suffered with another clinically recognisable disorder (27 per cent) (Green et al., 2005). Elsewhere, epidemiological data has highlighted a high comorbidity rate among adolescents in those suffering with diagnosable mental health disorders (Angold et al., 1999; Costello et al., 2003, 2006; Merikangas et al., 2011). The abuse of alcohol is common in a number of mental health disorders including anxiety, conduct disorder and depression (Burnett-Zeigler et al., 2012; Corte and Sommers, 2005; Wiesner et al., 2005). Although it is not always possible to ascertain the direction of this relationship, it is likely that one exacerbates the other. The mixture of symptoms included across mental health disorder classifications makes categorisation difficult. Treatment guidelines and diagnostic manuals have clear benefits in assigning appropriate care, but it is worthwhile recognising their limitations.

Asperger's/Attention deficit hyperactivity disorder: a case scenario

Harry has Asperger syndrome and attention deficit hyperactivity disorder, and as a result finds it difficult to stay on task. He is known to have poor relationships with others and states that he has been bullied all of his life. He is, however, very close to his younger brother who suffers with a chronic illness that has led to him frequently visiting hospital. Harry is also small for his age, which means that he has borne the brunt of bullying by his peers more often than not. Due to his autistic symptoms, Harry finds it difficult to understand another person's perspective and may not always know when someone is using humour. This is thought to relate to some of the bullying that he can experience as well as certain difficulties he has in communicating with others. He sometimes takes many comments to heart, finding it difficult to distinguish bullying from teenage banter. Handwriting and presenting in front of others can also be an issue.

Due to the nature of Harry's circumstances, he has been engaged with a number of different treatment packages. He is currently taking fluoxetine (Prozac – an antidepressant) as advised by his doctor. In school, he has received 26 counselling sessions over the course of a 16-month period with his school counsellor. He works exceptionally hard and, on an emotional level, he is a very deep thinker. His attention difficulties require the use of prompts to stay focused and on task. Harry believes the bullying he has received over many years has been a major factor in his feeling so low. His counsellor has worked with him on how to react to the bullying, instead now reporting it to a teacher confidant, rather than retaliating himself. His school counsellor has been using CBT techniques to challenge his negative thinking and encourage a more positive way of thinking about things. This, however, needs ongoing support.

Harry's parents have also been concerned that he is suicidal, which led to his counsellor conducting an assessment for suicidal thoughts and depression. The assessment revealed that although he has been feeling very low, he would never act on his thoughts, and he states that he loves his family too much. His counsellor has offered Harry her email address should he need to contact her, particularly during the holidays, and has provided him with a list of organisations to contact should he need to talk, e.g. ChildLine, Young Minds, Samaritans. This ongoing support is believed to be necessary and efforts will be extended to help Harry with his negative thoughts.

Self-harm and suicide

Self-harming refers to the deliberate harm imposed on oneself, damaging body tissue. The majority of individuals who self-harm are aged between 11 and 25 years old, making it an especially adolescent concern (Mental Health Foundation, 2006). A substantial minority of adolescents self-disclose self-harming behaviours and cases may remain unknown to health professionals or parents (Evans et al., 2005; Meltzer et al., 2001; Moran et al., 2012; Turp, 1999). Denial and secrecy are common and make treatment and identification difficult. Moreover, suicide remains one of the leading causes of death worldwide for this age group (Eaton et al., 2006; Gould et al., 2003; WHO, 2014). Suicidal ideation and self-harming have been found to peak between the ages of 14 and 18 years of age (Hawton et al., 2003, 2012; Husky et al., 2012). Most of these behaviours have been found to resolve spontaneously (Moran et al., 2012) but early detection is crucial in preventing subsequent serious issues developing (Pelkonen and Marttunen, 2003).

When assessing the risk for self-harm or suicide, factors to be aware of are: the presence of a mental health disorder and/or alcohol or substance abuse, previous self-harming or suicidal behaviour, living in a deprived area, disruptive family-environmental factors such as parental psychopathology, bereavement, childhood maltreatment, social isolation and/or poor academic performance (Evans et al., 2005; Hawton and James, 2005; Madge et al., 2008; Moran et al., 2012; Pelkonen and Marttunen, 2003; Skegg, 2005). In terms of the gender divide, it is usually reported that more females tend to self-harm and attempt suicide (ONS, 2014), whereas more males die from suicide (Hagell et al., 2013). Suicidal contagion relates to the phenomenon that someone may be more likely to attempt to commit suicide if they identify with someone who has committed suicide, either close to them, or portrayed in the media, and it is known to be common among adolescent groups (Pirkis and Nordentoft, 2011; Swanson and Colman, 2013). Understanding and tackling these risks has important clinical implications (Hawton et al., 2012). Suicide at any age can be difficult for anyone close to the individual. Its impact on family, peers, and society is far-reaching, and attempts to reduce its prevalence, particularly in young people, should be a priority of any health service and community.

Being aware of a young person's history with other services will give a good indication as to their risk. It is okay to ask someone if they are feeling suicidal. This will not plant the idea in their head, but you may be able to show your genuine concern. Professionals should aim to offer a calm and non-judgmental approach to care, overcoming potential complex emotions that can result and polarise professionals' views about self-harm or suicide (Wood, 2009). Educating health professionals and restricting access to lethal means may also help in preventing suicide and self-harm (Mann et al., 2005).

Conclusions

Although the period of adolescence is one of immense change brought about by the onset of puberty and social context, many adolescents experience their transition into adulthood without ever developing a mental health problem. However, evidence suggests that the majority of mental health problems during the life course emerge during this stage. Identifying the risk factors associated with poor mental health is vital in delivering care for this age group and preventing further onsets into adulthood. There appears to be a great deal of unmet need, and research is still in its infancy around how best to care for adolescents with poor mental health. Family-based interventions appear to be an effective intervention and involving and appreciating the family context is important when devising a care plan. Educating adolescents and their parents on the benefits of a positive mental wellbeing could also prove invaluable.

Schools and the role of educators are in a useful position to promote wellbeing and also to identify risks and provide support, although evidence is still developing. The ongoing developments that occur during this stage, both physiologically and socially, have an important bearing on adolescent mental health. The rise in technology could serve to both improve access and care for young people with poor mental health but their use needs to be monitored. Likewise, the role of peer influence can be both positive and negative and efforts should be made to lessen the impact of negative peer pressure and bullying during this stage.

Promoting resilience and ensuring the right access to care is available for this often forgotten age group are also important, particularly in transitionary care. The study of adolescent mental health demands research that integrates biology, context and psychological development. Likewise, the risks associated with poor mental health can often be complex and multi-faceted. Appreciating a young person's autonomy and educating them on the benefits of maintaining health and wellbeing and being aware of physical, emotional and behavioural risks and the care available to them could serve to empower them, and reduce the impact of mental health problems during this crucial stage.

Reflective exercise

- What are the main changes that occur during puberty, and how might this impact on an individual's mental health?
- How might the family and social context influence the development of a young person's mental health?
- What effects does the timing of puberty have on the mental wellbeing of an adolescent, for both males and females?
- What are the benefits and risks associated with the increase in the availability of technology and access to the Internet for adolescents?
- What interventions are available to young people presenting with a mental health problem?

References

AACAP. (2007). Practice parameter for the assessment and treatment of children and adolescents with depressive disorders. *Journal of American Academy of Child and Adolescent Psychiatry*, *46*(11).

Aikins, J. W., Bierman, K. L., and Parker, J. G. (2005). Navigating the transition to junior high school: The influence of pre-transition friendship and self-system characteristics. *Social Development*, *14*(1), 42–60.

Alsaker, F. D. (1995). Is puberty a critical period for socialization? *Journal of Adolescence*, *18*(4), 427–444.

Alsaker, F. D., and Flammer, A. (2006). Pubertal maturation. In Jackson, S., and Goossens, L. (Eds.), *Handbook of adolescent development*. New York: Psychology Press.

Altarac, M., and Saroha, E. (2007). Lifetime prevalence of learning disability among US children. *Pediatrics*, *119*(1), 77–83.

Andersson, G., and Cuijpers, P. (2009). Internet-based and other computerized psychological treatments for adult depression: A meta-analysis. *Cognitive Behaviour Therapy*, *38*(4), 196–205.

Angold, A., Costello, E. J., and Erkanli, A. (1999). Comorbidity. *Journal of Child Psychology and Psychiatry*, *40*(1), 57–87.

Arim, R. G., and Shapka, J. D. (2008). The impact of pubertal timing and parental control on adolescent problem behaviors. *Journal of Youth and Adolescence*, *37*(4), 445–455.

Arnett, J. J. (1999). Adolescent storm and stress, reconsidered. *American Psychologist*, *54*(5), 317.

Arnett, J. J. (2006). G. Stanley Hall's Adolescence: Brilliance and nonsense. *History of Psychology*, *9*(3), 186.

Barrett, P. M., and Pahl, K. M. (2006). School-based intervention: Examining a universal approach to anxiety management. *Australian Journal of Guidance and Counselling*, *16*(1), 55–75.

Barrett, P. M., and Turner, C. M. (2004). Prevention of childhood anxiety and depression. In Barrett, P. and Ollendick, T. H. (Eds.), *Handbook of interventions that work with children and adolescents*. Chichester: Wiley (429–474).

Bava, S., and Tapert, S. F. (2010). Adolescent brain development and the risk for alcohol and other drug problems. *Neuropsychology Review*, *20*(4), 398–413.

Bearman, S. K., Presnell, K., Martinez, E., and Stice, E. (2006). The skinny on body dissatisfaction: A longitudinal study of adolescent girls and boys. *Journal of Youth and Adolescence*, *35*(2), 217–229.

Behrendt, S., Wittchen, H. U., Höfler, M., Lieb, R., Low, N. C. P., Rehm, J., and Beesdo, K. (2008). Risk and speed of transitions to first alcohol dependence symptoms in adolescents: a 10-year longitudinal community study in Germany. *Addiction*, *103*(10), 1638–1647.

Belsky, J., Steinberg, L. D., Houts, R. M., Friedman, S. L., DeHart, G., Cauffman, E., . . . and Susman, E. (2007). Family rearing antecedents of pubertal timing. *Child Development*, *78*(4), 1302–1321.

Belsky, J., Steinberg, L., Houts, R. M., and Halpern-Felsher, B. L. (2010). The development of reproductive strategy in females: Early maternal harshness→ earlier menarche→ increased sexual risk taking. *Developmental Psychology*, *46*(1), 120.

Benoit, A., Lacourse, E., and Claes, M. (2013). Pubertal timing and depressive symptoms in late adolescence: The moderating role of individual, peer, and parental factors. *Development and Psychopathology*, *25*(2), 455–471.

Bergen, S. E., Gardner, C. O., and Kendler, K. S. (2007). Age-related changes in heritability of behavioral phenotypes over adolescence and young adulthood: A meta-analysis. *Twin Research and Human Genetics*, *10*(3), 423–433.

Berlan, E. D., Corliss, H. L., Field, A. E., Goodman, E., and Bryn Austin, S. (2010). Sexual orientation and bullying among adolescents in the growing up today study. *Journal of Adolescent Health*, *46*(4), 366–371.

Beullens, K., Roe, K., and Van den Bulck, J. (2011). Excellent gamer, excellent driver? The impact of adolescents' video game playing on driving behavior: A two-wave panel study. *Accident Analysis and Prevention*, *43*(1), 58–65.

beyondblue. (2011). *Clinical practice guidelines for depression and related disorders – anxiety, bipolar disorder and puerperal psychosis – in the perinatal period. A guideline for primary care health professionals.* Melbourne: beyondblue: the national depression initiative.

Biehl, M. C., Natsuaki, M. N., and Ge, X. (2007). The influence of pubertal timing on alcohol use and heavy drinking trajectories. *Journal of Youth and Adolescence, 36*(2), 153–167.

Blakemore, S. J. (2012). Imaging brain development: The adolescent brain. *Neuroimage, 61*(2), 397–406.

Bogaert, A. F. (2005). Age at puberty and father absence in a national probability sample. *Journal of Adolescence, 28*(4), 541–546.

Bogaert, A. F. (2008). Menarche and father absence in a national probability sample. *Journal of Biosocial Science, 40*(4), 623–636.

Booth, M. Z., and Sheehan, H. C. (2008). Perceptions of people and place: Young adolescents' interpretation of their schools in the United States and the United Kingdom. *Journal of Adolescent Research, 23*(6), 722–744.

Bordo, S. (2013). Not just 'a white girl's thing': The changing face of food and body image problems. In Counihan, C., and Van Esterik, P. (Eds.), *Food and culture: A reader.* New York: Routledge.

Bratberg, G. H., Nilsen, T. I., Holmen, T. L., and Vatten, L. J. (2007). Perceived pubertal timing, pubertal status and the prevalence of alcohol drinking and cigarette smoking in early and late adolescence: A population based study of 8950 Norwegian boys and girls. *Acta Paediatrica, 96*(2), 292–295.

Brodsky, B. S., and Stanley, B. (2008). Adverse childhood experiences and suicidal behavior. *Psychiatric Clinics of North America, 31*(2), 223–235.

Buist, K. L., Deković, M., and Prinzie, P. (2013). Sibling relationship quality and psychopathology of children and adolescents: A meta-analysis. *Clinical Psychology Review, 33*(1), 97–106.

Bulik, C. M., Reba, L., Siega-Riz, A. M., and Reichborn-Kjennerud, T. (2005). Anorexia nervosa: Definition, epidemiology, and cycle of risk. *International Journal of Eating Disorders, 37*(S1), S2–S9.

Burnett-Zeigler, I., Walton, M. A., Ilgen, M., Barry, K. L., Chermack, S. T., Zucker, R. A., . . . and Blow, F. C. (2012). Prevalence and correlates of mental health problems and treatment among adolescents seen in primary care. *Journal of Adolescent Health, 50*(6), 559–564.

Burt, S. A., McGue, M., DeMarte, J. A., Krueger, R. F., and Iacono, W. G. (2006). Timing of menarche and the origins of conduct disorder. *Archives of General Psychiatry, 63*(8), 890–896.

Cain, N., and Gradisar, M. (2010). Electronic media use and sleep in school-aged children and adolescents: A review. *Sleep Medicine, 11*(8), 735–742.

Callaghan, R. C., Gatley, J. M., Veldhuizen, S., Lev-Ran, S., Mann, R., and Asbridge, M. (2013). Alcohol- or drug-use disorders and motor vehicle accident mortality: A retrospective cohort study. *Accident Analysis and Prevention, 53*, 149–155.

Calvert, C. (2009). Sex, cell phones, privacy, and the first amendment: When children become child pornographers and the Lolita effect undermines the law. *CommLaw Conspectus: Journal of Communications Law and Policy, 18*, 1–65.

Carskadon, M. A., Acebo, C., and Jenni, O. G. (2004). Regulation of adolescent sleep: Implications for behavior. *Annals of the New York Academy of Sciences, 1021*(1), 276–291.

Cartwright-Hatton, S., Roberts, C., Chitsabesan, P., Fothergill, C., and Harrington, R. (2004). Systematic review of the efficacy of cognitive behaviour therapies for childhood and adolescent anxiety disorders. *British Journal of Clinical Psychology, 43*(4), 421–436.

Casey, B. J., Jones, R. M., and Hare, T. A. (2008). The adolescent brain. *Annals of the New York Academy of Sciences, 1124*(1), 111–126.

Cavanagh, S. E. (2004). The sexual debut of girls in early adolescence: The intersection of race, pubertal timing, and friendship group characteristics. *Journal of Research on Adolescence, 14*(3), 285–312.

Celio, M., Karnik, N. S., and Steiner, H. (2006). Early maturation as a risk factor for aggression and delinquency in adolescent girls: A review. *International Journal of Clinical Practice, 60*(10), 1254–1262.

Chen, H., and Jackson, T. (2012). Gender and age group differences in mass media and interpersonal influences on body dissatisfaction among Chinese adolescents. *Sex roles*, *66*(1–2), 3–20.

Cheung, A. H., Zuckerbrot, R. A., Jensen, P. S., Ghalib, K., Laraque, D., and Stein, R. E. (2007). Guidelines for adolescent depression in primary care (GLAD-PC): II. Treatment and ongoing management. *Pediatrics*, *120*(5), e1313–e1326.

Choo, T., Roh, S., and Robinson, M. (2008). Assessing the "Gateway Hypothesis" among middle and high school students in Tennessee. *Journal of Drug Issues*, *38*(2), 467–492.

Coleman, J. C. (2011). *The nature of adolescence* (4th ed.). New York: Psychology Press.

Conley, C. S., and Rudolph, K. D. (2009). The emerging sex difference in adolescent depression: Interacting contributions of puberty and peer stress. *Development and Psychopathology*, *21*(2), 593–620.

Corbett, D. (2009). Let's talk about sext: The challenge of finding the right legal response to teenage practice of 'sexting'. *Journal of Internet Law*, *13*(6), 3–8.

Corcoran, J. (2011). *Mental health treatment for children and adolescents*. New York: Oxford University Press.

Corrieri, S., Heider, D., Conrad, I., Blume, A., König, H. H., and Riedel-Heller, S. G. (2013). School-based prevention programs for depression and anxiety in adolescence: A systematic review. *Health Promotion International*, dat001.

Corte, C. M., and Sommers, M. S. (2005). Alcohol and risky behaviors. *Annual Review of Nursing Research*, *23*(1), 327–360.

Costello, E. J., Mustillo, S., Erkanli, A., Keeler, G., and Angold, A. (2003). Prevalence and development of psychiatric disorders in childhood and adolescence. *Archives of General Psychiatry*, *60*(8), 837–844.

Costello, E. J., Foley, D. L., and Angold, A. (2006). 10-year research update review: The epidemiology of child and adolescent psychiatric disorders: II. Developmental epidemiology. *Journal of the American Academy of Child and Adolescent Psychiatry*, *45*(1), 8–25.

Cottrell, D., and Kraam, A. (2005). Growing up? A history of CAMHS (1987–2005). *Child and Adolescent Mental Health*, *10*(3), 111–117.

Cottrell, S. A., Branstetter, S., Cottrell, L., Harris, C. V., Rishel, C., and Stanton, B. F. (2007). Development and validation of a parental monitoring instrument: Measuring how parents monitor adolescents' activities and risk behaviors. *The Family Journal*, *15*(4), 328–335.

Cox, G. R., Callahan, P., Churchill, R., Hunot, V., Merry, S. N., Parker, A. G., Hetrick, S. E. (2012). Psychological therapies versus antidepressant medication, alone and in combination for depression in children and adolescents. Cochrane Database of Systematic Reviews 2012, Issue 11. Art. No.: CD008324. DOI:10.1002/14651858.CD008324.pub2.

Craik, F. I., and Bialystok, E. (2006). Cognition through the lifespan: Mechanisms of change. *Trends in Cognitive Sciences*, *10*(3), 131–138.

Dahl, R. E., and Lewin, D. S. (2002). Pathways to adolescent health sleep regulation and behavior. *Journal of Adolescent Health*, *31*(6), 175–184.

Dahl, R. E., and Spear, L. P. (2004). Adolescent brain development: Vulnerabilities and opportunities. *Annals of the New York Academy of Science.* 1021, 1–22.

Dake, J. A., Price, J. H., Maziarz, L., and Ward, B. (2012). Prevalence and correlates of sexting behavior in adolescents. *American Journal of Sexuality Education*, *7*(1), 1–15.

Das Gupta, P.M. and Frake, C. (2009). The child and the family. In Dogra, N., and Leighton, S. (Eds.), *Nursing in child and adolescent mental health*. Maidenhead: Open University Press.

Davila, J., Hershenberg, R., Feinstein, B. A., Gorman, K., Bhatia, V., and Starr, L. R. (2012). Frequency and quality of social networking among young adults: Associations with depressive symptoms, rumination, and corumination. *Psychology of Popular Media Culture*, *1*(2), 72.

Dawson, A. L., and Dellavalle, R. P. (2013). Acne vulgaris. *British Medical Journal*, *346*(f2634), 1–7.

Dawson, D. A., Goldstein, R. B., and Grant, B. F. (2007). Rates and correlates of relapse among individuals in remission from DSM-IV alcohol dependence: A 3-year follow-up. *Alcoholism: Clinical and Experimental Research*, *31*(12), 2036–2045.

Dawson, D. A., Goldstein, R. B., Patricia Chou, S., June Ruan, W., and Grant, B. F. (2008). Age at first drink and the first incidence of adult-onset DSM-IV alcohol use disorders. *Alcoholism: Clinical and Experimental Research, 32*(12), 2149–2160.

Department for Children, Schools and Families. (2008). *Departmental report 2008*. Public Communications Unit. Norwich: The Stationery Office.

Department for Education. (2014). *Mental health and behaviour in schools. Departmental advice for school staff*. London: Department for Education.

Department of Health. (1995). *The health of the nation handbook: Child and adolescent mental health services*. London: Department of Health.

Department of Health. (2004). *National service framework for children, young people and maternity services*. Core Standards: Best Practice Guidance. London: Department of Health.

Department of Health. (2008). *Improving access to psychological therapies implementation plan: National guidelines for regional delivery*. London: Department of Health.

Dinos, S. (2014). Stigma creating stigma: A vicious circle. *Psychiatric Bulletin, 38*(4), 145–147.

Ditch the Label. (2013). The Annual Cyberbullying Survey 2013. Retrieved from www.ditchthelabel. org/downloads/the-annual-cyberbullying-survey-2013.pdf

Dogra, N., and Leighton, S. (2009). *Nursing in child and adolescent mental health*. Maidenhead: Open University Press.

Dogra, N., Parkin, A., Gale, F. and Frake, C. (2008). *A multidisciplinary handbook of child and adolescent mental health for front-line professionals*. London: Jessica Kingsley Publishers.

Dogra, N., Das Gupta, M., and Leighton, S. (2009). The aetiology of child mental health problems. In Dogra, N., and Leighton, S. (Eds.), *Nursing in child and adolescent mental health*. Maidenhead: Open University Press.

Donovan, C. L., and Spence, S. H. (2000). Prevention of childhood anxiety disorders. *Clinical Psychology Review, 20*(4), 509–531.

Durlak, J. A., Weissberg, R. P., Dymnicki, A. B., Taylor, R. D., and Schellinger, K. B. (2011). The impact of enhancing students' social and emotional learning: A meta-analysis of school-based universal interventions. *Child Development, 82*(1), 405–432.

Eaton, D. K., Kann, L., Kinchen, S., Ross, J., Hawkins, J., Harris, W. A., . . . and Wechsler, H. (2006). Youth risk behavior surveillance – United States, 2005. *Journal of School Health, 76*(7), 353–372.

Einfeld, S. L., Ellis, L. A., and Emerson, E. (2011). Comorbidity of intellectual disability and mental disorder in children and adolescents: A systematic review. *Journal of Intellectual and Developmental Disability, 36*(2), 137–143.

Elkind, D. (1967). Egocentrism in adolescence. *Child Development, 38*(4), 1025–1034.

Emerson, E. (2003). Prevalence of psychiatric disorders in children and adolescents with and without intellectual disability. *Journal of Intellectual Disability Research, 47*(1), 51–58.

Emerson, E., Honey, A., Madden, R., and Llewellyn, G. (2009). The well-being of Australian adolescents and young adults with self-reported long-term health conditions, impairments or disabilities: 2001 and 2006. *Australian Journal of Social Issues, 44*(1), 39–54.

Erikson, E. H. (1968). *Identity: Youth and crisis*. New York: Norton.

Ernst, M., Nelson, E. E., Jazbec, S., McClure, E. B., Monk, C. S., Leibenluft, E., . . . and Pine, D. S. (2005). Amygdala and nucleus accumbens in responses to receipt and omission of gains in adults and adolescents. *Neuroimage, 25*(4), 1279–1291.

Ernst, M., Romeo, R. D., and Andersen, S. L. (2009). Neurobiology of the development of motivated behaviors in adolescence: A window into a neural systems model. *Pharmacology Biochemistry and Behavior, 93*(3), 199–211.

Eshel, N., Nelson, E. E., Blair, R. J., Pine, D. S., and Ernst, M. (2007). Neural substrates of choice selection in adults and adolescents: Development of the ventrolateral prefrontal and anterior cingulate cortices. *Neuropsychologia, 45*(6), 1270–1279.

Evans, E., Hawton, K., and Rodham, K. (2005). In what ways are adolescents who engage in self-harm or experience thoughts of self-harm different in terms of help-seeking, communication and coping strategies? *Journal of Adolescence*, 28(4), 573–587.

Eveleth, P. B., and Tanner, J. M. (1976). *Worldwide variation in human growth*. Cambridge: Cambridge University Press.

Faden, V. B. (2006). Trends in initiation of alcohol use in the United States 1975 to 2003. *Alcoholism: Clinical and Experimental Research*, 30(6), 1011–1022.

Fair, D. A., Cohen, A. L., Dosenbach, N. U., Church, J. A., Miezin, F. M., Barch, D. M., . . . and Schlaggar, B. L. (2008). The maturing architecture of the brain's default network. *Proceedings of the National Academy of Sciences*, 105(10), 4028–4032.

Fair, D. A., Cohen, A. L., Power, J. D., Dosenbach, N. U., Church, J. A., Miezin, F. M., . . . and Petersen, S. E. (2009). Functional brain networks develop from a 'local to distributed' organization. *PLoS Computational Biology*, 5(5), e1000381.

Fairburn, C. G., Cooper, Z., and Shafran, R. (2003). Cognitive behaviour therapy for eating disorders: A 'transdiagnostic' theory and treatment. *Behaviour Research and Therapy*, 41(5), 509–528.

Farrell, L. J., and Barrett, P. M. (2007). Prevention of childhood emotional disorders: Reducing the burden of suffering associated with anxiety and depression. *Child and Adolescent Mental Health*, 12(2), 58–65.

Fat, L. N., and Fuller, E. (2011). Drinking patterns. In *Health Survey England – 2011*. Leeds: Health and Social Care Information Centre.

Faulkner, S. (2007). Eating disorders, diet and body image. In Coleman, J., Hendry, L. and Kloep, M. (Eds.). *Adolescence and health*. Chichester: John Wiley.

Feinberg, I., and Campbell, I. (2010). Sleep and circadian rhythms during adolescence. *Brain and Cognition*, 72(1), 56–65.

Fergusson, D. M., Horwood, L. J., Ridder, E. M., and Beautrais, A. L. (2005). Subthreshold depression in adolescence and mental health outcomes in adulthood. *Archives of General Psychiatry*, 62(1), 66–72.

Fisher, H. L., Moffitt, T. E., Houts, R. M., Belsky, D. W., Arseneault, L., and Caspi, A. (2012). Bullying victimisation and risk of self harm in early adolescence: Longitudinal cohort study. *British Medical Journal*, 344, e2683, 1–9.

Fonagy, P., Target, M., Cottrell, D., Phillips, J., and Kurtz, Z. (2005). *What works for whom. A critical review of treatments for children and adolescents*. New York: The Guilford Press.

Forbes, E. E., and Dahl, R. E. (2010). Pubertal development and behavior: hormonal activation of social and motivational tendencies. *Brain and Cognition*, 72(1), 66–72.

Ford, T., Goodman, R., and Meltzer, H. (2003). The British Child and Adolescent Mental Health Survey 1999: The prevalence of DSM-IV disorders. *Journal of the American Academy of Child and Adolescent Psychiatry*, 42(10), 1203–1211.

Foresight Mental Capital and Wellbeing Project (2008). *Final project report – Executive summary*. London: The Government Office for Science.

Foroushani, P. S., Schneider, J., and Assareh, N. (2011). Meta-review of the effectiveness of computerised CBT in treating depression. *BMC Psychiatry*, 11(1), 131.

Fry, Stephen (2003). *Moab Is My Washpot*. London: Soho Press.

Fuller, E. (2013). *Smoking, drinking and drug use among young people in England in 2012*. Leeds: Health and Social Care Information Centre.

Galvan, A., Hare, T. A., Parra, C. E., Penn, J., Voss, H., Glover, G., and Casey, B. J. (2006). Earlier development of the accumbens relative to orbitofrontal cortex might underlie risk-taking behavior in adolescents. *The Journal of Neuroscience*, 26(25), 6885–6892.

Garber, J. (2006). Depression in children and adolescents: Linking risk research and prevention. *American Journal of Preventive Medicine*, 31(6), 104–125.

Gau, S. S. F., Soong, W. T., and Merikangas, K. R. (2004). Correlates of sleep-wake patterns among children and young adolescents in Taiwan. *Sleep: Journal of Sleep and Sleep Disorders Research*, 26(4): 449–454.

Ge, X., Conger, R. D., and Elder Jr, G. H. (2001). Pubertal transition, stressful life events, and the emergence of gender differences in adolescent depressive symptoms. *Developmental Psychology*, *37*(3), 404.

Ge, X., Kim, I. J., Brody, G. H., Conger, R. D., Simons, R. L., Gibbons, F. X., and Cutrona, C. E. (2003). It's about timing and change: Pubertal transition effects on symptoms of major depression among African American youths. *Developmental Psychology*, *39*(3), 430.

Gentile, D. (2009). Pathological video-game use among youth ages 8 to 18: A national study. *Psychological Science*, *20*(5), 594–602.

Gibb, S. J., Fergusson, D. M., and Horwood, L. J. (2010). Burden of psychiatric disorder in young adulthood and life outcomes at age 30. *The British Journal of Psychiatry*, *197*(2), 122–127.

Gillibrand, R., Lam, V., and O'Donnell, V. L. (2011). *Developmental Psychology*. Harlow: Prentice Hall Pearson Education.

Gini, G., and Pozzoli, T. (2009). Association between bullying and psychosomatic problems: A meta-analysis. *Pediatrics*, *123*(3), 1059–1065.

Goldin, C. D., and Katz, L. F. (2009). *The race between education and technology*. Cambridge, MA: Harvard University Press.

Gould, M. S., Greenberg, T. E. D., Velting, D. M., and Shaffer, D. (2003). Youth suicide risk and preventive interventions: A review of the past 10 years. *Journal of the American Academy of Child and Adolescent Psychiatry*, *42*(4), 386–405.

Graber, J. A., Brooks-Gunn, J., and Warren, M. P. (2006). Pubertal effects on adjustment in girls: Moving from demonstrating effects to identifying pathways. *Journal of Youth and Adolescence*, *35*(3), 391–401.

Graber, J. A., Seeley, J. R., Brooks-Gunn, J., and Lewinsohn, P. M. (2004). Is pubertal timing associated with psychopathology in young adulthood? *Journal of the American Academy of Child and Adolescent Psychiatry*, *43*(6), 718–726.

Green, H., McGinnity, Á., Meltzer, H., Ford, T., and Goodman, R. (2005). *Mental health of children and young people in Great Britain, 2004*. Basingstoke: Palgrave Macmillan.

Grover, M., Naumann, U., Mohammad-Dar, L., Glennon, D., Ringwood, S., Eisler, I., . . . and Schmidt, U. (2011). A randomized controlled trial of an Internet-based cognitive-behavioural skills package for carers of people with anorexia nervosa. *Psychological Medicine*, *41*(12), 2581–2591.

Haddad, M., Butler, G. S., and Tylee, A. (2010). School nurses' involvement, attitudes and training needs for mental health work: A UK-wide cross-sectional study. *Journal of Advanced Nursing*, *66*(11), 2471–2480.

Hagell, A., Coleman, J., and Brooks, F. (2013). *Key data on adolescence 2013*. London: Association for Young People's Health.

Halpern, C. T., Kaestle, C. E., and Hallfors, D. D. (2007). Perceived physical maturity, age of romantic partner, and adolescent risk behavior. *Prevention Science*, *8*(1), 1–10.

Hansen, M., Janssen, I., Schiff, A., Zee, P. C., and Dubocovich, M. L. (2005). The impact of school daily schedule on adolescent sleep. *Pediatrics*, *115*(6), 1555–1561.

Harding, D. J. (2009). Violence, older peers, and the socialization of adolescent boys in disadvantaged neighborhoods. *American Sociological Review*, *74*(3), 445–464.

Harris, R. A., Qualter, P., and Robinson, S. J. (2013). Loneliness trajectories from middle childhood to pre-adolescence: Impact on perceived health and sleep disturbance. *Journal of Adolescence*, *36*(6), 1295–1304.

Hawker, D. S., and Boulton, M. J. (2000). Twenty years' research on peer victimization and psychosocial maladjustment: A meta-analytic review of cross-sectional studies. *Journal of Child Psychology and Psychiatry*, *41*(4), 441–455.

Hawton, K., and James, A. (2005). Suicide and deliberate self harm in young people. *British Medical Journal*, *330*(7496), 891–894.

Hawton, K., Saunders, K. E., and O'Connor, R. C. (2012). Self-harm and suicide in adolescents. *The Lancet*, *379*(9834), 2373–2382.

Hawton, K., Hall, S., Simkin, S., Bale, L., Bond, A., Codd, S., and Stewart, A. (2003). Deliberate self-harm in adolescents: a study of characteristics and trends in Oxford, 1990–2000. *Journal of Child Psychology and Psychiatry*, *44*(8), 1191–1198.

Health Advisory Service (1995). *Together we stand*. London: HMSO.

Heginbotham, C., and Williams, R. (2005). Achieving service development by implementing strategy. In Williams, R. and Kerfoot, M. (Eds.). *Child and adolescent mental health services: Strategy, planning, delivery, and evaluation*. Oxford: Oxford University Press.

Hersov, L. (1986). Child psychiatry in Britain – the last 30 years. *Journal of Child Psychology and Psychiatry*, *27*(6), 781–801.

Hill, J. P. (1983). Early adolescence: A research agenda. *The Journal of Early Adolescence*.

Himes, J. H. (2006). Examining the evidence for recent secular changes in the timing of puberty in US children in light of increases in the prevalence of obesity. *Molecular and Cellular Endocrinology*, 254, 13–21.

Honey, A., Emerson, E., and Llewellyn, G. (2011). The mental health of young people with disabilities: Impact of social conditions. *Social Psychiatry and Psychiatric Epidemiology*, *46*(1), 1–10.

Horowitz, J. L., and Garber, J. (2006). The prevention of depressive symptoms in children and adolescents: A meta-analytic review. *Journal of Consulting and Clinical Psychology*, *74*(3), 401.

House of Commons Health Committee (2014). *Children's and adolescents' mental health and CAMHS Third Report of Session 2014–15*. London: The Stationery Office.

HSCIC. (2013). *Provisional monthly topic of interest: Eating disorders*. Health and Social Care Information Centre. Retrieved from www.hscic.gov.uk/catalogue/PUB13478/prov-mont-hes-admi-outp-ae-April%202013%20to%20October%202013-toi-rep.pdf (accessed 01/09/15).

Hull, J. G., Draghici, A. M., and Sargent, J. D. (2012). A longitudinal study of risk-glorifying video games and reckless driving. *Psychology of Popular Media Culture*, *1*(4), 244.

Husky, M. M., Olfson, M., He, J. P., Nock, M. K., Swanson, S. A., and Merikangas, K. R. (2012). Twelve-month suicidal symptoms and use of services among adolescents: Results from the National Comorbidity Survey. *Psychiatric Services*, *63*(10), 989–996.

Hwang, K., Velanova, K., and Luna, B. (2010). Strengthening of top-down frontal cognitive control networks underlying the development of inhibitory control: A functional magnetic resonance imaging effective connectivity study. *The Journal of Neuroscience*, 30(46), 15535–15545.

Isacsson, G., and Rich, C. (2008). Antidepressant medication prevents suicide: A review of ecological studies. *European Psychiatric Review*, *1*, 24–26.

Jané-Llopis, E., and Anderson, P. (Eds.) (2006). *Mental health promotion and mental disorder prevention across European Member States: A collection of country stories*. Luxembourg: European Communities.

Jehta, M. K., and Segalowitz, S. J. (2012). *Adolescent brain development. implications for behavior*. Waltham, MA: Academic Press.

Johnson, M. K., Crosnoe, R., and Elder, G. H. (2011). Insights on adolescence from a life course perspective. *Journal of Research on Adolescence*, *21*(1), 273–280.

Kaltiala-Heino, R., Kosunen, E., and Rimpelä, M. (2003). Pubertal timing, sexual behaviour and self-reported depression in middle adolescence. *Journal of Adolescence*, *26*(5), 531–545.

Karch, D. L., Logan, J., McDaniel, D. D., Floyd, C. F., and Vagi, K. J. (2013). Precipitating circumstances of suicide among youth aged 10–17 years by sex: Data from the national violent death reporting system, 16 States, 2005–2008. *Journal of Adolescent Health*, *53*(1), S51–S53.

Kelly, A. C., Di Martino, A., Uddin, L. Q., Shehzad, Z., Gee, D. G., Reiss, P. T., . . . and Milham, M. P. (2009). Development of anterior cingulate functional connectivity from late childhood to early adulthood. *Cerebral Cortex*, *19*(3), 640–657.

Kelly, C., Kitchener, B. A., and Jorm, A. F. (2013). *Youth mental health first aid: A manual for adults assisting young people* (3rd ed.). Melbourne: Mental Health First Aid Australia.

Kendall, P. C. (Ed.). (2011). *Child and Adolescent Therapy: Cognitive-Behavioral Procedures*. New York: Guilford Press.

Kennedy, I. (2010). *Getting it right for children and young people. Overcoming cultural barriers in the NHS so as to meet their needs.* A review by Professor Sir Ian Kennedy. Gov.UK, HMSO. Permission: Open Government Licence (OGL).

Kerr, M., Stattin, H., and Pakalniskiene, V. (2008). Parents react to adolescent problem behaviors by worrying more and monitoring less. In Kerr, M., Stattin, H., and Engels, R. C. M. E. *What can parents do?* Chichester: John Wiley (91–112).

Kessler, R. C., Angermeyer, M., Anthony, J. C., de Graaf, R., Demyttenaere, K., Gasquet, I., . . . and Uestuen, T. B. (2007). Lifetime prevalence and age-of-onset distributions of mental disorders in the World Health Organization's World Mental Health Survey Initiative. *World Psychiatry*, *6*(3), 168.

Kessler, R. C., Avenevoli, S., Costello, E. J., Georgiades, K., Green, J. G., Gruber, M. J., . . . and Merikangas, K. R. (2012). Prevalence, persistence, and sociodemographic correlates of DSM-IV disorders in the National Comorbidity Survey Replication Adolescent Supplement. *Archives of General Psychiatry*, *69*(4), 372–380.

Kessler, R. C., Chiu, W. T., Demler, O., and Walters, E. E. (2005). Prevalence, severity, and comorbidity of 12-month DSM-IV disorders in the National Comorbidity Survey Replication. *Archives of General Psychiatry*, *62*(6), 617–627.

Kirby, T., and Barry, A. E. (2012). Alcohol as a gateway drug: A study of US 12th graders. *Journal of School Health*, *82*(8), 371–379.

Klein, D. A., and Walsh, B. T. (2004). Eating disorders: Clinical features and pathophysiology. *Physiology and Behavior*, *81*(2), 359–374.

Knapp, M., McDaid, D., and Parsonage, M. (2011). *Mental health promotion and mental illness prevention: The economic case.* London: Department of Health.

Lauber, C., and Rössler, W. (2007). Stigma towards people with mental illness in developing countries in Asia. *International Review of Psychiatry*, *19*(2), 157–178.

Laursen, B., and Hartl, A. C. (2013). Understanding loneliness during adolescence: Developmental changes that increase the risk of perceived social isolation. *Journal of Adolescence*, *36*(6), 1261–1268.

Lenhart, A. (2009). Teens and sexting. Pew Internet and American Life Project. Retrieved from www.pewinternet.org/-/media//Files/Reports/2009/PIP-Teens and Sexting.pdf (accessed 01/09/15).

Lenhart, A., Ling, R., Campbell, S., and Purcell, K. (2010). Teens and mobile phones: Text messaging explodes as teens embrace it as the centerpiece of their communication strategies with friends. *Pew Internet and American Life Project.*

Lenroot, R. K., and Giedd, J. N. (2010). Sex differences in the adolescent brain. *Brain and Cognition*, *72*(1), 46–55.

Levine, M. P., and Smolak, L. (2010). Cultural influences on body image and the eating disorders. *The Oxford Handbook of Eating Disorders*, 223–246.

Li, R., Polat, U., Makous, W., and Bavelier, D. (2009). Enhancing the contrast sensitivity function through action video game training. *Nature Neuroscience*, *12*(5), 549.

Litwack, S. D., Aikins, J. W., and Cillessen, A. H. (2012). The distinct roles of sociometric and perceived popularity in friendship implications for adolescent depressive affect and self-esteem. *Journal of Early Adolescence*, *32*(2): 226–251.

Livingstone, S. (2009). *Children and the Internet.* Cambridge: Polity.

Livingstone, S., Haddon, L., Vincent, J., Mascheroni, G. and Ólafsson, K. (2014). *Net Children Go Mobile: The UK report.* London: London School of Economics and Political Science.

Luna, B., Padmanabhan, A., and O'Hearn, K. (2010). What has fMRI told us about the development of cognitive control through adolescence? *Brain and Cognition*, *72*(1), 101–113.

Ma, J., Lee, K. V., and Stafford, R. S. (2005). Depression treatment during outpatient visits by US children and adolescents. *Journal of Adolescent Health*, *37*(6), 434–442.

McCabe, M. P., and Ricciardelli, A. (2004). A longitudinal study of pubertal tlming and extreme body change behaviors among adolescent boys and girls. *Adolescence*, *39*(153), 145–166.

McCrone, P., Dhanasiri, S., Patel, A., Knapp, M., and Lawton-Smith, S. (2008). *Paying the price: The cost of mental health care in England to 2026.* London: The King's Fund.

McDougall, J., Evans, J., and Baldwin, P. (2010). The importance of self-determination to perceived quality of life for youth and young adults with chronic conditions and disabilities. *Remedial and Special Education*, *31*(4), 252–260.

McLoone, J., Hudson, J. L., and Rapee, R. M. (2006). Treating anxiety disorders in a school setting. *Education and Treatment of Children, 29*(2), 219–242.

McQueeny, T., Schweinsburg, B. C., Schweinsburg, A. D., Jacobus, J., Bava, S., Frank, L. R., and Tapert, S. F. (2009). Altered white matter integrity in adolescent binge drinkers. *Alcoholism: Clinical and Experimental Research*, *33*(7), 1278–1285.

Madden, M., Lenhart, A., Cortesi, S., Gasser, U., Duggan, M., Smith, A., and Beaton, M. (2013). Teens, social media, and privacy. *Pew Internet and American Life Project*.

Madge, N., Hewitt, A., Hawton, K., Wilde, E. J. D., Corcoran, P., Fekete, S., . . . and Ystgaard, M. (2008). Deliberate self-harm within an international community sample of young people: Comparative findings from the Child and Adolescent Self-harm in Europe (CASE) Study. *Journal of Child Psychology and Psychiatry*, *49*(6), 667–677.

Mann, J. J., Apter, A., Bertolote, J., Beautrais, A., Currier, D., Haas, A., . . . and Hendin, H. (2005). Suicide prevention strategies: A systematic review. *Jama*, *294*(16), 2064–2074.

Markey, P. M., and Markey, C. N. (2010). Vulnerability to violent video games: A review and integration of personality research. *Review of General Psychology*, *14*(2), 82.

Masia-Warner, C., Nangle, D. W., and Hansen, D. J. (2006). Bringing evidence-based child mental health services to the schools: General issues and specific populations. *Education and Treatment of Children, 29*, 165–172.

Masten, C. L., Eisenberger, N. I., Borofsky, L. A., Pfeifer, J. H., McNealy, K., Mazziotta, J. C., and Dapretto, M. (2009). Neural correlates of social exclusion during adolescence: Understanding the distress of peer rejection. *Social Cognitive and Affective Neuroscience*, *4*(2), 143–157.

Masten, C. L., Eisenberger, N. I., Pfeifer, J. H., and Dapretto, M. (2010). Witnessing peer rejection during early adolescence: Neural correlates of empathy for experiences of social exclusion. *Social Neuroscience*, *5*(5–6), 496–507.

Masten, C. L., Telzer, E. H., Fuligni, A. J., Lieberman, M. D., and Eisenberger, N. I. (2012). Time spent with friends in adolescence relates to less neural sensitivity to later peer rejection. *Social Cognitive and Affective Neuroscience*, *7*(1), 106–114.

Matchock, R. L., and Susman, E. J. (2006). Family composition and menarcheal age: Anti-inbreeding strategies. *American Journal of Human Biology*, *18*(4), 481–491.

Maughan, B., and Kim-Cohen, J. (2005). Continuities between childhood and adult life. *The British Journal of Psychiatry*, *187*(4), 301–303.

Meagher, S. M., Rajan, A., Wyshak, G., and Goldstein, J. (2013). Changing trends in inpatient care for psychiatrically hospitalized youth: 1991–2008. *Psychiatric Quarterly*, *84*(2), 159–168.

Meltzer, H., Gatward, R., Goodman, R., and Ford, T. (2003). Mental health of children and adolescents in Great Britain. *International Review of Psychiatry*, *15*(1–2), 185–187.

Meltzer, L. J., Johnson, S. B., Prine, J. M., Banks, R. A., Desrosiers, P. M., and Silverstein, J. H. (2001). Disordered eating, body mass, and glycemic control in adolescents with Type 1 diabetes. *Diabetes Care*, *24*(4), 678–682.

Mental Health Foundation. (2004). *Lifetime impacts. Childhood and adolescent mental health: Understanding the lifetime impacts*. Report of a seminar organised by the Office of Health Economics and the Mental Health Foundation, April 2004.

Mental Health Foundation (2006). *Truth hurts: Report of the national inquiry into self-harm among young people*. London: Mental Health Foundation.

Merikangas, K. R., He, J. P., Burstein, M., Swendsen, J., Avenevoli, S., Case, B., . . . and Olfson, M. (2011). Service utilization for lifetime mental disorders in US adolescents: Results of the National Comorbidity Survey – Adolescent Supplement (NCS-A). *Journal of the American Academy of Child and Adolescent Psychiatry*, *50*(1), 32–45.

Merikangas, K. R., He, J. P., Rapoport, J., Vitiello, B., and Olfson, M. (2013). Medication use in US youth with mental disorders. *JAMA Pediatrics*, *167*(2), 141–148.

Merry, S. N., Hetrick, S. E., Cox, G. R., Brudevold-Iversen, T., Bir, J. J., and McDowell, H. (2012a). Cochrane Review: Psychological and educational interventions for preventing depression in children and adolescents. *Evidence-Based Child Health: A Cochrane Review Journal*, 7(5), 1409–1685.

Merry, S. N., Stasiak, K., Shepherd, M., Frampton, C., Fleming, T., and Lucassen, M. F. (2012b). The effectiveness of SPARX, a computerised self help intervention for adolescents seeking help for depression: Randomised controlled non-inferiority trial. *British Medical Journal*, 344, e2598, 1–16.

Micali, N., Hagberg, K. W., Petersen, I., and Treasure, J. L. (2013). The incidence of eating disorders in the UK in 2000–2009: Findings from the General Practice Research Database. *British Medical Journal* open, 3(5), e002646, 1–8.

Michaud, P. A., Suris, J. C., and Deppen, A. (2006). Gender-related psychological and behavioural correlates of pubertal timing in a national sample of Swiss adolescents. *Molecular and Cellular Endocrinology*, 254, 172–178.

Milne, F. H., and Judge, D. S. (2010). Brothers delay menarche and the onset of sexual activity in their sisters. *Proceedings of the Royal Society B: Biological Sciences*, rspb20101377.

Mojtabai, R. (2006). Serious emotional and behavioral problems and mental health contacts in American and British children and adolescents. *Journal of the American Academy of Child and Adolescent Psychiatry*, 45(10), 1215–1223.

Moore, S., and Rosenthal, D. (2006). *Sexuality in adolescence: Current trends*. New York: Routledge.

Moran, P., Coffey, C., Romaniuk, H., Olsson, C., Borschmann, R., Carlin, J. B., and Patton, G. C. (2012). The natural history of self-harm from adolescence to young adulthood: A population-based cohort study. *The Lancet*, 379(9812), 236–243.

Murray, J., and Cartwright-Hatton, S. (2006). NICE guidelines on treatment of depression in childhood and adolescence: Implications from a CBT perspective. *Behavioural and Cognitive Psychotherapy*, 34(02), 129–137.

Muss, R. E. (1988). *Theories of adolescence* (5th ed.). New York: Random House.

Natsuaki, M. N., Biehl, M. C., and Ge, X. (2009). Trajectories of depressed mood from early adolescence to young adulthood: The effects of pubertal timing and adolescent dating. *Journal of Research on Adolescence*, 19(1), 47–74.

Neil, A. L., and Christensen, H. (2009). Efficacy and effectiveness of school-based prevention and early intervention programs for anxiety. *Clinical Psychology Review*, 29(3), 208–215.

Ng, C. H. (1997). The stigma of mental illness in Asian cultures. *Australian and New Zealand Journal of Psychiatry*, 31(3), 382–390.

Ng, R., Ang, R. P., and Ho, M. H. R. (2012). Coping with anxiety, depression, anger and aggression: The mediational role of resilience in adolescents. In *Child and Youth Care Forum*, 41(6), 529–546.

NICE (2005). *Depression in children and young people identification and management in primary, community and secondary care*. National Clinical Practice Guideline 28. London: National Institute for Health and Care Excellence.

NICE (2011). *Alcohol-use disorders: diagnosis, assessment and management of harmful drinking and alcohol dependence*. NICE Clinical Guideline 115. London: National Institute for Health and Care Excellence.

NICE (2013). *Antisocial behaviour and conduct disorders in children and young people: recognition, intervention and management*. NICE Clinical Guideline 158. London: National Institute for Health and Care Excellence.

Ohida, T., Osaki, Y., Tanihata, T., Minowa, M., Suzuki, K., Wada, K., and Kaneita, Y. (2004). An epidemiologic study of self-reported sleep problems among Japanese adolescents. *Sleep*, 27(5), 978–985.

O'Keeffe, G. S., and Clarke-Pearson, K. (2011). The impact of social media on children, adolescents, and families. *Pediatrics*, 127(4), 800–804.

Oliver, K., Collin, P., Burns, J., and Nicholas, J. (2006). Building resilience in young people through meaningful participation. *Advances in Mental Health*, 5(1), 34–40.

ONS (2014). *Suicides in the United Kingdom, 2012 registrations*. London: Office for National Statistics.

Pagel, J. F., Forister, N., and Kwiatkowski, C. (2007). Adolescent sleep disturbance and school performance: The confounding variable of socioeconomics. *Journal of Clinical Sleep Medicine, 3*(1), 19–23.

Parry-Langdon, N. (Ed.) (2008). *Three years on: Survey of the development and emotional well-being of children and young people*. London: Office for National Statistics.

Patel, V., Flisher, A. J., Hetrick, S., and McGorry, P. (2007). Mental health of young people: A global public-health challenge. *The Lancet, 369*(9569), 1302–1313.

Patton, G. C., Coffey, C., Romaniuk, H., Mackinnon, A., Carlin, J. B., Degenhardt, L. and Moran, P. (2014). The prognosis of common mental disorders in adolescents: A 14-year prospective cohort study. *The Lancet, 383*(9926), 1404–1411.

Paus, T. (2010). Growth of white matter in the adolescent brain: Myelin or axon? *Brain and Cognition, 72*(1), 26–35.

Pelkonen, M., and Marttunen, M. (2003). Child and adolescent suicide. *Pediatric Drugs, 5*(4), 243–265.

Pempek, T. A., Yermolayeva, Y. A., and Calvert, S. L. (2009). College students' social networking experiences on Facebook. *Journal of Applied Developmental Psychology, 30*(3), 227–238.

Petersen, A. C., Compas, B. E., Brooks-Gunn, J., Stemmler, M., Ey, S., and Grant, K. E. (1993). Depression in adolescence. *American Psychologist, 48*(2), 155.

Petersen, A. C., and Crockett, L. (1985). Pubertal timing and grade effects on adjustment. *Journal of Youth and Adolescence, 14*(3), 191–206.

Pirkis, J., and Nordentoft, M. (2011). Media influences on suicide and attempted suicide. In O'Connor, R. C., Platt, S., and Gordon, J. (Eds.), *International handbook of suicide prevention: Research, policy and practice*. Chichester: Wiley (531–544).

Punamäki, R. L., Wallenius, M., Nygård, C. H., Saarni, L., and Rimpelä, A. (2007). Use of information and communication technology (ICT) and perceived health in adolescence: The role of sleeping habits and waking-time tiredness. *Journal of Adolescence, 30*(4), 569–585.

Radford, L., Corral, S., Bradley, C., Fisher, H., Bassett, C., Howat, N., and Collishaw, S. (2011). *Child abuse and neglect in the UK today*. London: NSPCC.

Rambaldo, L. R., Wilding, L. D., Goldman, M. L., McClure, J. M., and Friedberg, R. D. (2001). School-based interventions for anxious and depressed children. In VandeCreek, L., and Jackson, T. L. *Innovations in clinical practice: A source book, 19*. Sarasota, FL: Professional Resource Press (347–358).

Rapee, R. M., Kennedy, S., Ingram, M., Edwards, S., and Sweeney, L. (2005). Prevention and early intervention of anxiety disorders in inhibited preschool children. *Journal of Consulting and Clinical Psychology, 73*(3), 488.

Richardson, G., Partridge, I., and Barrett, J. (Eds.). (2010). *Child and adolescent mental health services: An operational handbook*. London: RCPsych Publications.

Richardson, T., Stallard, P., and Velleman, S. (2010). Computerised cognitive behavioural therapy for the prevention and treatment of depression and anxiety in children and adolescents: a systematic review. *Clinical Child and Family Psychology Review, 13*(3), 275–290.

Roberts, R. E., Roberts, C. R., and Duong, H. T. (2009). Sleepless in adolescence: Prospective data on sleep deprivation, health and functioning. *Journal of Adolescence, 32*(5), 1045–1057.

Rogers, A., and Pilgrim, D. (2010). *A sociology of mental health and illness*. Maidenhead: Open University Press.

Rosser, J. C., Lynch, P. J., Cuddihy, L., Gentile, D. A., Klonsky, J., and Merrell, R. (2007). The impact of video games on training surgeons in the 21st century. *Archives of Surgery, 142*(2), 181–186.

Rowe, R., Costello, E. J., Angold, A., Copeland, W. E., and Maughan, B. (2010). Developmental pathways in oppositional defiant disorder and conduct disorder. *Journal of Abnormal Psychology, 119*(4), 726.

Rushton, J. L., Forcier, M., and Schectman, R. M. (2002). Epidemiology of depressive symptoms in the National Longitudinal Study of Adolescent Health. *Journal of the American Academy of Child and Adolescent Psychiatry, 41*(2), 199–205.

Rutter, M., and Smith, D. J. (1995). *Psychosocial disorders in young people: Time trends and their causes*. Chichester: Wiley.

Sansone, R. A., Songer, D. A., and Miller, K. A. (2005). Childhood abuse, mental healthcare utilization, self-harm behavior, and multiple psychiatric diagnoses among inpatients with and without a borderline diagnosis. *Comprehensive Psychiatry, 46*(2), 117–120.

Schaffer, H. R. (2006). *Key concepts in developmental psychology*. London: Sage.

Schoenwald, S. K., Heiblum, N., Saldana, L., and Henggeler, S. W. (2008). The international implementation of multisystemic therapy. *Evaluation and the Health Professions, 31*(2), 211–225.

Scholte, R. H., and van Aken, M. (2013). Peer relations in adolescence. In Jackson, S., and Goossens, L. (Eds.), *Handbook of Adolescent Development*. New York: Psychology Press.

Selfhout, M. H., Branje, S. J., Delsing, M., ter Bogt, T. F., and Meeus, W. H. (2009). Different types of Internet use, depression, and social anxiety: The role of perceived friendship quality. *Journal of Adolescence, 32*(4), 819–833.

Siegel, J. M., Yancey, A. K., Aneshensel, C. S., and Schuler, R. (1999). Body image, perceived pubertal timing, and adolescent mental health. *Journal of Adolescent Health, 25*(2), 155–165.

Simmons, R. G., and Blyth, D. A. (1987). *Moving into adolescence: The impact of pubertal change and school context*. New York: AldineTransaction.

Singh, S. P., Paul, M., Ford, T., Kramer, T., Weaver, T., McLaren, S., . . . and White, S. (2010). Process, outcome and experience of transition from child to adult mental healthcare: Multi-perspective study. *The British Journal of Psychiatry, 197*(4), 305–312.

Skegg, K. (2005). Self-harm. *The Lancet, 366*(9495), 1471–1483.

Spear, L. P. (2000). The adolescent brain and age-related behavioral manifestations. *Neuroscience and Bio-behavioral Reviews, 24*(4), 417–463.

Spence, S. H., Donovan, C. L., March, S., Gamble, A., Anderson, R. E., Prosser, S., and Kenardy, J. (2011). A randomized controlled trial of online versus clinic-based CBT for adolescent anxiety. *Journal of Consulting and Clinical Psychology, 79*(5), 629.

Stallard, P., Sayal, K., Phillips, R., Taylor, J. A., Spears, M., Anderson, R., . . . and Montgomery, A. A. (2012). Classroom based cognitive behavioural therapy in reducing symptoms of depression in high risk adolescents: pragmatic cluster randomised controlled trial. *British Medical Journal, 345*, e6058, 1–13.

Stallard, P., Udwin, O., Goddard, M., and Hibbert, S. (2007). The availability of cognitive behaviour therapy within specialist child and adolescent mental health services (CAMHS): A national survey. *Behavioural and Cognitive Psychotherapy, 35*(04), 501–505.

Steinberg, L. (2008). A social neuroscience perspective on adolescent risk-taking. *Developmental Review, 28*(1), 78–106.

Steinberg, L. and Morris, A. S. (2001). Adolescent development. *Annual Review of Psychology, 52*, 83–110.

Stice, E., Ragan, J., and Randall, P. (2004). Prospective relations between social support and depression: Differential direction of effects for parent and peer support? *Journal of Abnormal Psychology, 113*(1), 155.

Stice, E., Shaw, H., Bohon, C., Marti, C. N., and Rohde, P. (2009). A meta-analytic review of depression prevention programs for children and adolescents: Factors that predict magnitude of intervention effects. *Journal of Consulting and Clinical Psychology, 77*(3), 486.

Striegel-Moore, R. H., and Bulik, C. M. (2007). Risk factors for eating disorders. *American Psychologist, 62*(3), 181.

Striegel-Moore, R. H., McMahon, R. P., Biro, F. M., Schreiber, G., Crawford, P. B., and Voorhees, C. (2001). Exploring the relationship between timing of menarche and eating disorder symptoms in black and white adolescent girls. *International Journal of Eating Disorders, 30*(4), 421–433.

Suler, J. (2004). The online disinhibition effect. *Cyber-psychology and Behavior, 7*(3), 321–326.

Supekar, K., Musen, M., and Menon, V. (2009). Development of large-scale functional brain networks in children. *PLoS Biology, 7*(7), e1000157.

Surgeon General's Office. (2001). *Mental Health: A Report of the Surgeon General*. U.S. Public Health Service. Department of Health and Human Services. Retrieved from http://profiles.nlm.nih.gov/ps/access/NNBBHS.pdf (accessed 01/09/15).

Susman, E. J., Dorn, L. D., and Schiefelbein, B. L. (2003). Puberty, sexuality, and health. In Lerner, R. M., and Easterbrooks, M. A. (Eds.), *Handbook of psychology: Developmental psychology*. New York: Wiley (295–324).

Svetaz, M. V., Ireland, M., and Blum, R. (2000). Adolescents with learning disabilities: Risk and protective factors associated with emotional well-being: Findings from the National Longitudinal Study of Adolescent Health. *Journal of Adolescent Health*, *27*(5), 340–348.

Swanson, S. A., and Colman, I. (2013). Association between exposure to suicide and suicidality outcomes in youth. *Canadian Medical Association Journal*, *185*(10), 870–877.

Swanson, S. A., Saito, N., Borges, G., Benjet, C., Aguilar-Gaxiola, S., Medina-Mora, M. E., and Breslau, J. (2012). Change in binge eating and binge eating disorder associated with migration from Mexico to the US. *Journal of Psychiatric Research*, *46*(1), 31–37.

Taliaferro, L. A., Hetler, J., Edwall, G., Wright, C., Edwards, A. R., and Borowsky, I. W. (2013). Depression screening and management among adolescents in primary care factors associated with best practice. *Clinical Pediatrics*, *52*(6), 557–567.

Tanner, J. M. (1981). Growth and maturation during adolescence. *Nutrition Reviews*, *39*(2), 43–55.

Taylor, D. J., Jenni, O. G., Acebo, C., and Carskadon, M. A. (2005). Sleep tendency during extended wakefulness: Insights into adolescent sleep regulation and behavior. *Journal of Sleep Research*, *14*(3), 239–244.

Tennant, R., Goens, C., Barlow, J., Day, C., and Stewart-Brown, S. (2007). A systematic review of reviews of interventions to promote mental health and prevent mental health problems in children and young people. *Journal of Public Mental Health*, *6*(1), 25–32.

Townley, M., and Williams, R. (2009). Developing mental health service for children and adolescents. In Dogra, N., and Leighton, S. (Eds.), *Nursing in child and adolescent mental health*, Milton Keynes: Open University Press (181–192).

Turp, M. (1999). Encountering self-harm in psychotherapy and counselling practice. *British Journal of Psychotherapy, 15*(3), 307–321.

U.S. Department of Health and Human Services. (1999). *Mental health: A report of the Surgeon General*. Rockville, MD: U.S. Department of Health and Human Services, Substance Abuse and Mental Health Services Administration, Center for Mental Health Services, National Institutes of Health, National Institute of Mental Health.

Valkenburg, P. M., Peter, J., and Schouten, A. P. (2006). Friend networking sites and their relationship to adolescents' well-being and social self-esteem. *CyberPsychology and Behavior*, *9*(5), 584–590.

Van den Bulck, J. (2004). Television viewing, computer game playing, and Internet use and self-reported time to bed and time out of bed in secondary-school children. *Sleep-New York Then Westchester*, *27*(1), 101–104.

Van Gastel, W. A., Tempelaar, W., Bun, C., Schubart, C. D., Kahn, R. S., Plevier, C., and Boks, M. P. M. (2013). Cannabis use as an indicator of risk for mental health problems in adolescents: A population-based study at secondary schools. *Psychological Medicine*, *43*(09), 1849–1856.

Van Geel, M., Vedder, P., and Tanilon, J. (2014). Relationship between peer victimization, cyberbullying, and suicide in children and adolescents: A meta-analysis. *JAMA Pediatrics*, *168*(5), 435–442.

Vostanis, P. (2007). Mental health and mental disorders. In Coleman, J., and Hagell, A. (Eds.), *Adolescence, risk and resilience: Against the odds*, Chichester: Wiley (89–106).

Wang, S., and Dey, S. (2009, November). Modeling and characterizing user experience in a cloud server based mobile gaming approach. In *Global Telecommunications Conference, 2009. GLOBECOM 2009. IEEE* (1–7).

Ward, C. L., Flisher, A. J., Zissis, C., Muller, M., and Lombard, C. (2001). Exposure to violence and its relationship to psychopathology in adolescents. *Injury Prevention*, *7*(4), 297–301.

Weisz, J. R., and Gray, J. S. (2008). Evidence-based psychotherapy for children and adolescents: Data from the present and a model for the future. *Child and Adolescent Mental Health*, *13*(2), 54–65.

Weisz, J. R., McCarty, C. A., and Valeri, S. M. (2006). Effects of psychotherapy for depression in children and adolescents: A meta-analysis. *Psychological Bulletin*, *132*(1), 132–149.

Wertheim, E. H., Paxton, S. J., and Blaney, S. (2009). Body image in girls. In Smolak, L., and Thompson, J. K. (Eds.), *Body image, eating disorders, and obesity in youth*. Washington, DC: American Psychological Association.

West, P., and Sweeting, H. (2003). Fifteen, female and stressed: Changing patterns of psychological distress over time. *Journal of Child Psychology and Psychiatry*, *44*(3), 399–411.

Westwood, M., and Pinzon, J. (2008). Adolescent male health. *Paediatrics and Child Health*, *13*(1), 31.

WHO. (2014). *Health for the world's adolescents. A second chance in the second decade*. Geneva: World Health Organisation.

Wiesner, M., Kim, H. K., and Capaldi, D. M. (2005). Developmental trajectories of offending: Validation and prediction to young adult alcohol use, drug use, and depressive symptoms. *Development and Psychopathology*, *17*(01), 251–270.

Wolke, D., Lereya, S. T., Fisher, H. L., Lewis, G., and Zammit, S. (2013). Bullying in elementary school and psychotic experiences at 18 years: A longitudinal, population-based cohort study. *Psychological Medicine*, *44*(10), 2199–2211.

Wood, A. (2009). Self-harm in adolescents. *Advances in Psychiatric Treatment*, 15, 434–441.

Yang, L. H., Kleinman, A., Link, B. G., Phelan, J. C., Lee, S., and Good, B. (2007). Culture and stigma: Adding moral experience to stigma theory. *Social Science and Medicine*, *64*(7), 1524–1535.

Yap, M. B. H., Pilkington, P. D., Ryan, S. M., and Jorm, A. F. (2014a). Parental factors associated with depression and anxiety in young people: A systematic review and meta-analysis. *Journal of Affective Disorders*, *156*, 8–23.

Yap, M. B., Pilkington, P. D., Ryan, S. M., Kelly, C. M., and Jorm, A. F. (2014b). Parenting strategies for reducing the risk of adolescent depression and anxiety disorders: A Delphi consensus study. *Journal of Affective Disorders*, *156*, 67–75.

Yaroslavsky, I., Pettit, J. W., Lewinsohn, P. M., Seeley, J. R., and Roberts, R. E. (2013). Heterogeneous trajectories of depressive symptoms: Adolescent predictors and adult outcomes. *Journal of Affective Disorders*, *148*(2), 391–399.

Ybarra, M. L., and Mitchell, K. J. (2004). Youth engaging in online harassment: Associations with caregiver–child relationships, Internet use, and personal characteristics. *Journal of Adolescence*, *27*(3), 319–336.

Zehr, J. L., Culbert, K. M., Sisk, C. L., and Klump, K. L. (2007). An association of early puberty with disordered eating and anxiety in a population of undergraduate women and men. *Hormones and Behavior*, *52*(4), 427–435.

7 Mental health in adult men

Steve Robertson, Mark Robinson,
Brendan Gough and Gary Raine

Introduction

It is generally recognised that there are significant sex differences in physical health. The most notable difference is men's reduced life expectancy and higher rates of premature death (European Commission, 2011), but patterns relating to sex-differences in morbidity are much more complex (Payne, 2006). This complexity is nowhere more apparent than in the mental health, wellbeing and illness arena. Women attempt suicide far more frequently than men, yet rates for male suicide are approximately three times higher than those for female suicide (ONS, 2013). Women are diagnosed with more of the common mental health problems than men (for example anxiety and depression), yet there are concerns that, for socio-cultural reasons, these problems may be underdiagnosed in men (Wilkins, 2010: 33). Following diagnosis there are gender differences in care pathways through services; for example, men are more frequently treated as inpatients and women in the community for depression and, in recent times, more men are detained under the Mental Health Act than women (Payne, 2006: 93*ff*). As if this were not complicated enough, when other aspects of identity, culture and socio-economic circumstances are taken into consideration the jigsaw becomes even more difficult to piece together; that is to say, sex-differences are often intersected by other aspects of identity in the way that mental health problems are understood and experienced. Given the complexity of understanding not only the sex-differences in mental health between men and women but also differences amongst different groups of men, it becomes clear why a chapter specifically looking at the mental health and wellbeing of men is necessary.

This chapter aims to help clarify some of this complexity, to put several pieces of this jigsaw together. It begins by outlining some of the key data available on men's mental health and wellbeing (mainly focusing on UK data but drawing on international data when necessary) and by highlighting some of the key issues and questions about men's mental health that are suggested by this data. The second section follows on directly from this and explores the role that 'masculinity' – what it is to be a man, one's sense of male identity – plays in positive and negative aspects of men's mental health and wellbeing. Men are not a homogeneous group and the section on ethnicity and age (pp. 161–165) moves the discussion forward by looking at how these other aspects of culture and identity intersect with masculinity to create different mental health and wellbeing issues for various groups of men. The final section of the chapter considers what it is like for men to live with poor mental health and explores some of the interventions that are available, using case studies to also link these with aspects of masculinity and culture to maximise learning from these projects.

The chapter makes significant use of previous research and the discussions presented are therefore underpinned throughout by empirical evidence.

This chapter will consider:

- The evidence and recognition of men's mental health and wellbeing;
- The role of masculinity and how this can influence men's mental health and wellbeing;
- How culture and socio-economic circumstances can play a role in risks to men's mental health and wellbeing;
- Some gender differences and complexities surrounding mental health care and support;
- What it is like for men to live with mental health problems and their experiences of seeking help and support.

The nature of the problem – key data on men's mental health and wellbeing

It is important to begin by trying to understand the nature and extent of the mental health and ill-health issues that impact on men. Mental health conditions are among some of the most common health problems. In England, it is estimated that one in four people are affected by a mental health problem in any one year, and the aggregate cost of mental health conditions was £105.2 billion in 2009/10 (Centre for Mental Health, 2010). For ease of reading here, we first consider complex mental health conditions before looking at suicide, then common mental disorders, issues for specific groups of men and finally more recent work on mental wellbeing measures, though we recognise that this is, in some way, an artificial distinction as mental health conditions are often a continuum of psychological states rather than discrete entities.

Complex mental health conditions

Overall, it is suggested that men and women are almost equally at risk for the most severe mental disorders, such as psychotic illnesses (Payne, 2006: 93) with previous year prevalence being 0.3 per cent in males and 0.5 per cent for females (Sadler and Bebbington, 2009). However, there are some interesting and notable differences. (Refer to Chapter 8, pp. 177–185, to understand further some gender differences) In schizophrenia, men are thought to have higher rates (though this is contested), tend to develop it earlier in life than women (around age 15–20 years) and often suffer more negative symptoms (lack of interest, emotional flatness, inability to concentrate) than women (Ochoa et al, 2012). (See Chapter 6, p. 120, for further explanation.) There are also differences in prevalence between groups of men. Black males have a prevalence of 3.1 per cent compared to 0.2 per cent amongst white males (Sadler and Bebbington, 2009) and elevated rates of psychosis amongst ethnic minority males have also been reported elsewhere (Centre for Social Justice, 2011). (See Chapter 3, pp. 47–48, for further insights into ethnic minority and risks of mental health). Prevalence of such disorders is also more common amongst divorced males at 1.5 per cent, which is 15 times higher than amongst married men, five times higher than amongst single men and 2.5 times higher than amongst cohabiting men (Sadler and Bebbington, 2009).

Further to this, gender differences are found in admission rates for complex mental health conditions. Admission rates for schizophrenia and associated disorders in the UK are 0.57 per 1000 for men compared to 0.36 per 1000 females but admission rates for bipolar affective disorder show a reverse pattern at 0.14 per 1000 for men and 0.2 per 1000 for women (HMDB, 2013). This links to wider sex-differences in hospital admissions for mental health; 8 per cent of men who accessed mental health services spent some time in hospital compared to 5.5 per cent of women and the average number of inpatient days is higher for males than females (Health and Social Care Information Centre, 2013).

Suicide and suicidal thoughts

The statistics relating to male suicide are perhaps some of the most shocking of all the mental health data. In the UK, official statistics (ONS, 2013) show that 75 per cent of all suicides were male. In 2011, 4552 men took their own life: that is over 12 men each day and an age standardised rate of 18.2 per 100,000. As shown in Figure 7.1, the highest rate amongst males is between the ages of 35 and 39 years (24.2 per 100,000) and this rate has been remarkably consistent over the last decade. Suicide in young men, age 15–29 years, declined significantly between 2001 and 2006 but has remained at a similar level (a slight but not statistically significant increase) since then.

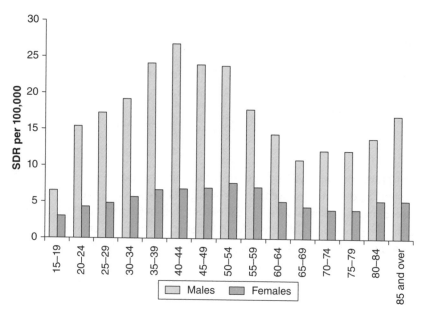

Figure 7.1 Age specific UK suicide rate by sex per 100,000

Nicholson et al. (2009) found that 19.2 per cent of females and 14 per cent of males had thought about suicide at some point in their lives (16.7 per cent of all adults). Females were more likely than males to have attempted suicide (6.9 per cent compared to 4.3 per cent). For males, the highest prevalence of suicidal thoughts and suicide attempts was in the 25–34 yr age group (it is in the 16–24 yr age group for females). There are some ethnic differences in terms of suicidal ideation and attempts, with white males having a prevalence of suicidal thoughts more than twice that of other ethnic groups, yet suicide attempts are similar for males across the ethnic groups (apart from amongst South Asian men where they are much lower). Suicidal thoughts and suicide attempts were three times higher amongst divorced men, and two times higher amongst separated men when compared to married men. Finally, both suicidal ideation and suicide attempts amongst men (and women) show a clear gradient in relation to household income, with the lower prevalence amongst those with highest income and greatest prevalence in the lowest income households.

Common mental disorders (CMD)

CMDs (also known as neurotic disorders/neuroses) are those conditions that cause distress and interfere with daily function, but do not generally impact on cognition or insight. They are the most prevalent mental health problems and comprise a number of different types of anxiety and depression disorders, including generalised anxiety disorder (GAD), panic disorders, phobias and obsessive compulsive disorder (OCD) (Deverill and King, 2009).

Overall rates of CMD are lower in males, with 13 per cent of males and 20 per cent of females reporting an episode in the last week (Deverill and King, 2009). When looked at by specific type of CMD, all are reported as more prevalent in females than males (Deverill and King, 2009). The three most frequently reported breakdown as follows (all figures relate to per cent of reported episodes in the last week):

1   Mixed anxiety and depressive disorder. This affected 6.9 per cent of males and 11 per cent of females, which is approximately 1 in 14 men and 1 in 9 women. In total 9 per cent of individuals were found to have this disorder, which represents 56 per cent of adults with a CMD.
2   Generalised anxiety disorder (GAD). This affected 3.4 per cent of males and 5.3 per cent of females (4.4 per cent of all adults).
3   Depressive episode. This affected 1.9 per cent of males and 2.8 per cent of females (2.3 per cent of all adults).

There are differences in prevalence of CMD by age, with the highest male prevalence being in the 35–44 years age range (15 per cent), followed by 25–34 years (14.6 per cent) and 45–54 years (14.5 per cent). The lowest rate was amongst men 75 year old and over at 6.3 per cent (Deverill and King, 2009). CMDs also show some interesting gendered patterns in relation to ethnicity. Figure 7.2 shows the age standardised proportion of adults reporting at least one CMD in the past week amongst four ethnic groupings. Amongst males, the highest rate of CMD was in the "Other" ethnic group (20.2 per cent), which includes Chinese and mixed ethnicities. Furthermore, the male prevalence amongst the "Other" ethnic group was almost identical to the female rate (20.6 per cent), which was not replicated for the White, Black or South Asian populations.

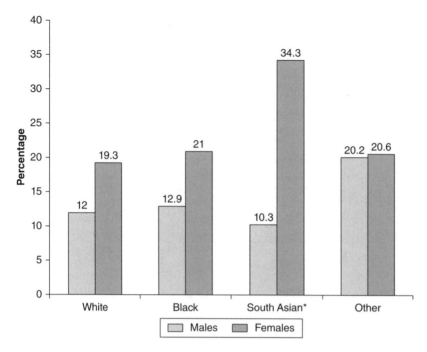

Figure 7.2 Age standardised prevalence of CMD by ethnicity and sex (per cent)

Note: *The number of South Asian women in the sample was small and consequently the age standardised rate should be treated with caution.

Prevalence of CMD also varies by marital status. Figure 7.3 shows the prevalence of CMD by marital status for both males and females. A striking feature is the much higher rate of CMD amongst divorced males than any of the other groups of men. In total, nearly 28 per cent of divorced men had experienced a CMD, which was higher than the rate for divorced women (26.6 per cent) and higher than every other group of women except those who were separated (33 per cent). Amongst other groups of males, widowed and married men had similar rates (10.4 per cent and 10.4 per cent), as did single and cohabiting men (14.8 per cent and 14 per cent).

There is also an established statistical association between prevalence of CMDs and financial strain, debt, poverty and unemployment (Deverill and King, 2009). Males with the lowest household income have prevalence rates higher than any other group and 2.7 times greater than men in the highest income group. In the case of depressive episodes, the rate was almost 35 times greater amongst males with the lowest household income compared to those men in the highest income group and rates of GAD almost six times higher.

Specific groups of men

There are a couple of specific groups of men that it is worth briefly considering in more detail in relation to mental health concerns.

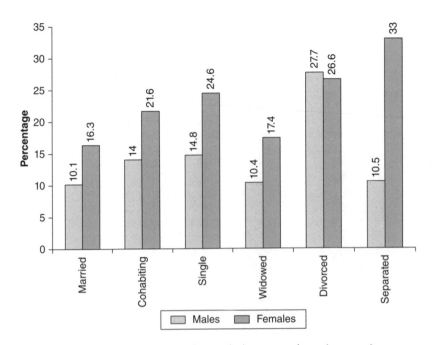

Figure 7.3 Prevalence of CMDs by marital status and sex (per cent)

The health of prisoners can be viewed as a particularly pertinent men's health issue as 95 per cent of prisoners in England and Wales are male (Ministry of Justice, 2013). They are also predominately young and socially disadvantaged (Shaw et al, 2004).

It is widely recognised that prisoners generally have both poorer mental and physical health than the general population. The Mental Health Network (2011) reported that 72 per cent of male and 70 per cent of female prisoners in England and Wales have two or more mental health problems. This compares to just 5 per cent of males and 2 per cent of females in the general population. Similarly, the proportion of male prisoners with psychosis is 14 times higher than in the general population (7 per cent vs. 0.5 per cent). Higher rates of suicide amongst prisoners have been found in many countries (Fazel and Baillargeon, 2011).

Shaw et al (2004) analysed data on self-inflicted deaths in prisons in England and Wales between 1999 and 2002. Out of the 172 deaths that occurred over the period studied, 159 (92 per cent) occurred amongst males. From the analysis, the average rate of suicide rate was calculated to be 133 per 100,000 population. This compared to a rate amongst the general population at the time of 9.4 per 100,000. Out of the 172 prisoners who died, 110 (72 per cent) had a history of mental health problems. The most common primary diagnosis was drug dependence (n=39), and 26 (18 per cent) of those who died had bipolar disorder. A third of deaths (32 per cent) occurred within one week of going into prison and 1 in 10 (11 per cent) within 24 hours.

The Ministry of Justice (2013) reported that there were 60 self-inflicted deaths amongst prisoners in England and Wales in 2012, which is 31 per cent of all deaths in custody and 3 per cent higher than in 2011. All but 1 of these 60 deaths were male prisoners and half (31) occurred in the 30–39 (16) and 40–49 years age group (15).

In addition to self-inflicted deaths, rates of self harm are also high amongst the prison population. The Ministry of Justice (2013) highlighted a contrasting trend in the rates of self harm amongst male and female prisoners in England and Wales. Statistics show that self harm amongst male prisoners is less common but increasing, whereas in females it is more prevalent but incidences are decreasing. Amongst males, the number of self-harming incidences increased by approximately 38 per cent from 146 per 1000 prisoners in 2005 to 201 in 2012. Although the rate of self harm remains significantly higher amongst females than males, in 2012, for the first time, a greater number of men committed 20 or more self harm incidents than women.

Another group of particular concern are gay men, as highlighted through a study conducted by Stonewall in 2012 (Guasp, 2012). This study gathered data from 6861 respondents across Britain and was described as the largest survey ever conducted of the health/health needs of gay and bisexual men anywhere in the world. Rates of anxiety and depression and attempted suicide were all found to be higher in gay and bisexual males than men in general. Overall, it was reported that:

- Thirteen per cent of gay and bisexual males had mixed depression and anxiety that was described as being moderate to severe.
- Four per cent of gay and bisexual males had anxiety that was described as being moderate to severe.
- Nine per cent of gay and bisexual males had depression that was described as being moderate to severe.
- Seven per cent of gay and bisexual males had committed at least one act of self harm in the last year compared to 3 per cent of men in general. Furthermore, when the results were analysed by age, 1 in 5 gay and bisexual males (21 per cent) aged 16 to 19 years and 15 per cent of 16–24 year olds self-harmed.
- Half of all the gay and bisexual men who responded said they had at some point felt that life was not worth living, and 46 per cent had done so in the last year.
- Three per cent of gay men, 5 per cent of bisexual men and 5 per cent of gay men of an ethnic minority had attempted suicide in the last year. Again, rates were related to age, with 10 per cent of 16–19 year olds and 6 per cent of 16–24 year olds indicating they had tried to kill themselves.

Mental wellbeing

Using measures of wellbeing is relatively new within the UK context, with the idea that it is important to target national wellbeing as a measure of government progress being articulated by the Prime Minister, David Cameron, soon after the last election. It is linked to both the "Foresight Report", *Mental Capital and Wellbeing* (2008), commissioned by the previous government and to the more recent public health White Paper, *Healthy Lives, Healthy People* (Department of Health, 2010). There are no specific outcome objectives for population wellbeing but the government has given responsibility for developing and publishing a set of national wellbeing measures to the Office for National Statistics (ONS). ONS began this process by organising a national consultation on the issue in 2011. The dataset itself remains a work in progress but ONS has developed a series of relevant metrics by drawing on (or adding questions to) existing national social surveys. From this, four new questions, designed to elicit subjective views of individual wellbeing, have been added to the Integrated Household Survey for the specific purpose of providing data for the National Wellbeing Measures. These questions are:

- Overall, how satisfied are you with your life nowadays?
- Overall, to what extent do you feel the things you do in your life are worthwhile?
- Overall, how happy did you feel yesterday?
- Overall, how anxious did you feel yesterday?

The ONS (2013c) subsequently reported findings on personal wellbeing in the UK from this survey:

- *Life satisfaction*: The mean rating of life satisfaction for females (7.5) and males (7.4) was similar. However, a higher proportion of females had high life satisfaction (28 per cent) than males (24 per cent).
- *Worthwhile*: On average, females rated the things they do in life as worthwhile higher than males (7.8 compared to 7.6) and once again more women (35 per cent) gave a "high" score than men (28 per cent).
- *Happy yesterday*: Females rated their level of happiness on average very slightly higher than males (7.32 compared to 7.26). One third of women (33 per cent) had high levels of happiness yesterday compared to 29 per cent of men.
- *Anxious yesterday*: The mean anxiety level of females (3.1) was higher than males (2.9), with the proportion of females with very high scores on this dimension 23 per cent as compared to 19 per cent of males.

Having considered some of the main data on men's mental health and wellbeing, we now turn to consideration of how social constructions of gender, of 'masculinities', might play a role in helping understand some of these differences.

Masculinity, 'being a man', and mental health

There are many explanations for the sex differences in mental health and wellbeing highlighted in the previous section. Biological factors, especially those linked with reproductive hormonal processes (monthly cycles, pregnancy and childbirth and menopause for example), have been implicated, usually in a negative way, for their impact on women's mental health and wellbeing. Similarly, lower levels of male hormones have been associated with poorer mental health for some conditions in men (Payne, 2006: 99). However, as Payne (2006: 99) points out, "the evidence for biology as a factor in the mental health of either women or men is relatively lacking."

This being the case, other disciplines, within the social sciences in particular, have been active in facilitating an understanding of these sex/gender differences in ways that move beyond an overly simplistic biomedical model. They have done so by identifying how 'masculinity' (what it is to 'be a man' in society) has an impact on men's lives, including their mental wellbeing. Back in the 1970s, Brannon and David (1976) identified four social rules that govern socially acceptable forms of masculinity:

1 *No Sissy Stuff*: Real men must avoid any behaviour or characteristic associated with women; any behaviour that hints of femininity runs the risk of being emasculating;
2 *Be a Big Wheel*: Masculinity is measured by success, power, and the admiration of others. Therefore, one must possess wealth, fame, and status to be considered manly;

3   *Be a Sturdy Oak*: Manliness is predicated on rationality, toughness, and self-reliance. A man must remain calm in any situation, show no emotion, and admit no weakness;

4   *Give 'em Hell*: Men must balance the 'rationality' of the sturdy oak with daring and aggression, and must be willing to take risks in order to become the big wheel.

That society expects these characteristics from men, and that men accept and invest in (to a greater or lesser degree) these 'social norms', has consequences for their mental health and wellbeing. For example, the ability to give and receive care can be seen to be feminine, yet is a crucial part of everyday life; lack of success (in jobs, in relationships etc) can be particularly damaging when success is so much expected; not being able to show weakness or emotion has significant consequence in situations that are emotionally challenging (relationship breakdown, bereavement etc); the need to be daring and take risks is often at odds with minor mental health morbidity, such as anxiety and depression, that can be characterised by lack of motivation, difficulty in decision making and lethargy.

This work on 'social rules' was expanded by Joseph Pleck (1981), who focused on how the greater acceptance of masculine sex roles by men created a greater potential for what he termed 'sex role strain' at points in men's lives when these could not be lived up to. Men face a double bind in relation to fulfilling gendered societal roles, particularly that of economic provider. To be successful in many male oriented jobs and careers relies on maintaining a presentation of oneself in line with the male norms mentioned above – strength, rationality, risk-taking and control – which can create pressure and stresses affecting mental wellbeing. However, if a man cannot fulfil this role because it is too difficult, or due to redundancy or unemployment, this then also has a significant impact on mental wellbeing. The particularly strong effect for men (Artazcoz et al, 2004) is attested to by higher rates of depression in men who are unemployed or made redundant (Wilkins, 2010: 24) and increased national male suicide rates during times of economic recession (Mind, 2009: 19). Added to this are the challenges associated with men's abilities to form and sustain supportive relationships. Whilst there may be some debate about whether men's relationships are qualitatively different from rather than 'worse' than women's, self-reported measures of social support do show that men rate their access to physical and emotional engagement with family and friends lower than women and this has a correlation with measures of mental health (Boreham et al, 2000). Again, this difficulty in developing supportive relationships has been associated with processes of gender socialisation and particularly the development of emotional restraint and fear of being perceived as gay (Bank and Hansford, 2000).

But how has this situation arisen? Victor Seidler (1991: 252*ff*) describes how, historically, within the 'post-Enlightenment period' (from around the seventeenth century), there developed a philosophical separation of the mind from the body – what has become known as the Cartesian dualist split – as a requirement for organising a pre- and then post-industrial society where particular gendered roles (man as worker in the public domain, woman as home-maker in the private domain) were necessary. In turn, there was an identification of masculinity (specifically a white, heterosexual masculinity) with the mind (and therefore reason) which was radically separated from forms of femininity associated with nature, the body and thus emotionality. This historical legacy, he argues, has left men unwilling, or unable, to give expression to their emotions, a situation technically known as 'alexithymia'. As men became identified with reason, they were expected to legislate what was best for others as well as themselves and this, in turn, has meant hiding anxieties and uncertainty; in short, suppressing emotion and feeling.

Moving away from these 'role theory' and socialisation models, work by Connell (1995) suggests that masculinity and gender are actually about sets of hierarchical relationships that don't only act at the individual level but also become embedded in social structures and institutions that then become 'gendered' in the way they (implicitly or explicitly) facilitate and restrict, condemn or condone particular individual actions for men and women. This is what is known as a 'gender relations' model of masculinity where particular forms of masculine practices become privileged and valorised – what is termed hegemonic masculinity – and other forms of practices become subordinated to these or marginalised by them. Within such models mental health concerns could be generated for certain groups of men (for example BME men, gay men, disabled men) as they are marginalised from or subordinated to hegemonic expectations that restrict their opportunities, access to resources and engagement with certain social institutions. Yet the process of living up to hegemonic norms can also be damaging to mental health even for ostensibly successful men, as shown in the high rates of suicide amongst groups such as doctors and lawyers – though this has changed over time (Roberts et al, 2012). However, as we shall discuss further (pp. 166–167), some aspects of hegemonic masculinity, particularly related to responsibility and control, can also be leveraged to promote mental health and deal with minor mental health morbidity (such as depression) and recovery from this.

These social processes are also very significant when considering how men cope, or don't cope, with situations that are emotionally demanding. Box 7.1 presents findings from a survey by the UK charity Mind (2009), which highlights some of the important gender differences in attitudes and practices to situations of stress or challenges to mental wellbeing.

Box 7.1 Results of Mind (2009) survey

Men aged 35–44 years were less than half as likely as women to seek help from their GP if they were feeling low. 45 per cent of men compared to 36 per cent of women thought they can fight off feeling down. Young men (18–24 years) were 5 times more likely than young women to take recreational drugs when worried. Twice as many men as women drank alcohol to cope when feeling down. Twice as many men as women admitted to getting angry when worried. Men aged 45–54 years were 7 times more likely than women of the same age to have suicidal thoughts when worried. Men were less likely than women to talk to friends about problems (29 per cent and 53 per cent respectively) or to family when feeling low (31 per cent and 47 per cent respectively).

What we see at work here are the different ways that many men and women express (or don't express) and cope with aspects of everyday life that can create anxiety, concern or distress. The socialisation, from a young age, of boys into the masculinity 'norms' outlined earlier can readily lead to situations where it is difficult for them to show vulnerability, to be emotionally expressive, and therefore to seek help and support when needed for fear that this will bring various social sanctions.

Brownhill et al (2005) have identified a framework showing how this process of socialisation leads men to cope with mental health concerns (particularly depression) in ways that escalate; what they call the 'big build'. They suggest that men initially begin with behaviours they term 'acting in'; which include strategies of 'avoidance' (such as overwork), 'numbing it' (through drug or alcohol use) and 'escaping it' (through increased risk-taking behaviours like excessive drugs and alcohol, gambling or extra-marital affairs). If such mechanisms are not able to ameliorate the feelings of depression they can lead to 'acting out' behaviours, which include more of the 'escaping it' behaviours outlined above which can escalate further to 'hating me, hurting you' (acts of violence, aggression and crime) and 'stepping over the line' (deliberate self harm and suicide).

That men act out depressive symptoms in this way has been said to have significance for the way that depression in men is recognised, or more accurately not recognised, using current measures i.e. it is thought that depression in men currently goes under-diagnosed/recognised as current tools are inherently 'feminised' in nature and measure different things in men and women. The processes of male socialisation discussed earlier mean that health professional questions aimed at eliciting 'care-requiring' signals as part of recognising depression are antithetical to men's experiences of having to hide or minimise showing weakness and vulnerability in order to present and sustain a socially acceptable male identity. Consequently, some have developed specific measures, such as the Gotland Scale (Martin et al, 2013), for more accurately picking up depression in men. These scales focus on recognition of what authors call 'alternative symptoms' (such as aggression, anger, substance misuse), as well as incorporating 'traditional symptoms'. When used these scales show that rates of depression are much more equal between men and women than when using traditional measures, suggesting that much male depression currently remains hidden from clinical view (Martin et al, 2013).

So far we have discussed issues of 'masculinity', being a man, in isolation from other factors and contexts that influence identity and can therefore influence men's mental health and wellbeing. We now turn to consider some of these intersections and their impact.

Intersections: ethnicity and age

Among the important contexts that influence men's identity and their mental health and wellbeing is the social environment in which they grow up and live. We can illustrate the ways in which social contexts intersect with masculinity to influence men's wellbeing and mental health with two examples: that of ethnicity and of ageing.

Black and minority ethnic (BME) men and mental health

A cluster of groups of particular concern consists of people from black and ethnic minority (BME) communities. People from BME communities are more likely to experience inequality and social exclusion, including racial discrimination, poor socio-economic status and unemployment, all of which are risk factors for poor mental health (Palmer and Kenway, 2007; Gervais, 2008). There are issues specific to particular groups and shared concerns that affect several BME groups, such as high rates of schizophrenia and psychotic disorders (Bhugra et al, 1997; Kirkbride and Jones, 2008), and low levels of confiding/emotional support for BME men with mental health difficulties (Sproston and Nazroo, 2002). Social factors have been identified as important in the onset of mental ill-health and development and recovery pathways (Kleinman et al. 2006). In particular, a relationship has been identified between perceived racism and mental ill-health (Karlsen et al. 2005), made much worse by the social disadvantages experienced by many BME men (Nazroo, 1997; Erens et al. 2001). The overrepresentation of BME men in prisons, with associated raised levels of mental health problems, has also been connected with social exclusion (Nazroo, 1997; Fazel et al 2005).

Compared to white men, BME men disproportionately come into contact with mental health services via adversarial or crisis-related routes (Sainsbury Centre for Mental Health, 2006). Rates of hospitalisation with mental health issues are higher among BME men altogether, and admissions and lengths of stay particularly high among Black Caribbean and Black African groups (Commission for Healthcare Audit and Inspection, 2005; Care Quality Commission, 2011). Similarly, once in hospital, Black Caribbean and Black African groups have been shown to receive more physical treatments (such as ECT, prescribed neuroleptics, physical restraint and seclusion) rather than talking approaches such as counselling and psychotherapy (McKeown et al, 2008). These findings have been interpreted as evidence of persistent institutional racism (McKenzie and Bhui, 2007; McKeown et al, 2008; Holland and Ousey, 2011). Evidence of pathways to care for common mental disorders (NCCMH, 2011) suggests that delayed diagnosis and referral to secondary care in non-emergency contexts are related to individual factors such as: distrust of health services and feelings of stigma and shame; practitioner factors including poor communication, racial/ethnic stereotyping, and inadequate assessments; and system factors including lack of flexibility to take account of individuals' cultural beliefs. A reluctance of BME men specifically to engage at an early stage with services (NIMHE, 2004; Galloway and Gillam, 2006;) has been viewed in terms of: mistrust of services; gender attitudes to health and expressing vulnerability, reinforced by racialised experiences of services lacking in cultural competence; the power of institutions to control and coerce people with mental health problems; and stigmatisation of mental ill-health in society (Bhui et al, 2001; Foolchand, 2006; Keating, 2007). In some community environments also, where socio-economic disadvantage poses a threat to health, ill-health of a family member puts family reputation at risk and stigma constitutes a further economic threat; care may be viewed as a family responsibility. Some BME communities are less able or willing to identify poor mental health or perhaps hold diverse concepts of ill-health, which can contribute to a lack of awareness of sources of help (Centre for Mental Health, 2013). Delay in help-seeking then contributes to low referral rates for further treatment (Begum, 2006).

While policy recognition of the complex interplay between gender and ethnicity and its importance for mental health promotion has been forthcoming (NIMHE, 2007), evidence is still rather sparse about the intersection of gender with these other factors. However, there is emerging evidence that the socialisation, from a young age, of boys into the masculinity 'norms' outlined earlier, where it is difficult for them to show vulnerability, and therefore to seek help and support, especially as health services are perceived to be feminised, can be reinforced by the stigma surrounding mental illness, which is universal and can also have community specific elements, and by the mistrust individuals and some BME communities feel for services, drawing on negative and racialised experiences.

In contexts of community marginalisation, perceptions of racialised services reinforcing gendered patterns and the stigma surrounding mental health often lead to fear, avoidance of help-seeking, and further risks for vulnerable men of isolation (Robinson et al, 2011). For some younger men in specific, highly disadvantaged BME communities, in the context of perceptions of lack of economic opportunity and marginalisation, peer norms can reinforce a hyper-masculine identity focused on strength, risk-taking and control, but this offers little support for negotiating vulnerability or coping relationally with transitions, for example from adolescence to adulthood, and around employment, family stress or bereavement. For mature men in some BME communities gendered pressures are sharpened from community cultural expectations to be economic providers for family networks, and failure to do this could lead to self-stigmatising thoughts in the context of community norms and the impact of service treatment. The intersection of factors around gender, socio-economic position and ethnicity therefore influences men's expectations concerning services, delaying their access to services, and can later lead to cycles of stalled recovery and disempowerment (Keating, 2007; Robinson et al, 2011).

Recommendations for improving service delivery and enhancing engagement include:

- development of culturally competent mainstream services and advocacy services,
- person-centred holistic practice,
- better financed support services for recovery, training staff, improved partnerships,
- resourcing non-statutory, community centred provision with user involvement (Seebohm et al, 2005; Centre for Mental Health, 2013).

To address needs of BME men around mental health in a culturally competent, person-centred way, it is important first to engage with the intersecting complexity of their formative social experiences as black or minority ethnic men; to engage with BME men's own understandings of and wishes for their own health and wellbeing, and, given the issues of trust that underpin access and engagement, to consider how partnerships including community/voluntary provision and independent advocacy can help men to break out of cycles of delayed treatment and blocked recovery (Robinson et al, 2011).

Ageing

A further important intersection which influences men's mental health and wellbeing consists of that between gender and age. We will briefly examine this by touching on some of the key contextual risk and protective factors for mental wellbeing in older age. Older men are less likely to have their mental health conditions diagnosed than younger men, less likely to receive treatments, such as psychological therapy, and more likely to commit suicide than older women (Wilkins and Kemple, 2011). This under-diagnosis and under-treatment among older men occurs despite the fact that older people are proportionately more likely to visit their GP than younger men, so that primary care services are in a better position to proactively discuss mental health with them (Wilkins and Kemple, 2011). Key risk factors for worsening mental ill-health in later life include retirement and other transitions, chronic medical illness, pain and disability, psycho-social adversity, daily stressors, life events, organic brain disease, low levels of physical activity and financial insecurity. (See Chapter 9, p. 209, for further explanation.) Key protective factors for mental wellbeing include social ties, connectedness, living in a supportive and enabling physical environment, personal factors such as self-esteem and confidence, and physical activity (Mental Health Foundation, 2013).

Of course, 'older age' covers a wide span in life-course terms. The masculine expectation which we referred to above of being an economic provider is challenged by transitions such as unemployment and retirement and a legacy of social assumptions about the 'burden' of age. Retirement, often associated with earlier older age, is one transition posing a potential threat to men's mental wellbeing. Many older men will have been in full-time employment for large parts of their adult lives, and have defined companionship largely in terms of colleagues at work, whereas many older women, despite often having also been in employment, may have a broader range of contacts developed through family and community links (Mental Health Foundation, 2010). The transition from work to retirement for older men therefore poses the double risk to mental health of loss of protective fellowship and loss of masculine identity through provider activity, role and status. While abrupt or enforced 'out-of-control' retirement poses higher risk for mental health, flexible retirement and choice over timing and process is protective (Mental Health Foundation, 2013). For some older men, with diminished social networks, existing community activities, groups and day centres can seem female-dominated, or aimed at people who are dependent (Mental Health Foundation, 2010). Older men may prefer to avoid provision which appears to position them in a passive role (Arber and Davison, 2003). Isolation then poses a particular threat to the mental health of older men after retirement. (See Chapter 9 for some further insights.)

Bereavement can pose an aggravated risk to some older men where it brings home to them their isolation or shortage of social routines and contacts; for example if their partner was the main route to social contact in later life. The most isolated older men are those who live alone, particularly if they are widowed or divorced, and are older (i.e. over 75) (Mental Health Foundation, 2013). A further source of isolation and a risk factor for depression is care-giving, with a key aspect being the loss of social networks for the care-giver, especially for men who previously relied on the partner for social networking (Godfrey, 2009).

A further main threat to mental wellbeing for men in older age consists of deterioration in physical health and mobility through chronic medical conditions which can undermine men's capacity to do physical tasks associated with traditional masculine roles (e.g. repair, heavy lifting). The effects of chronic illness and depression are interactive and can cumulatively lead to increased disability and poorer life outcomes (Godfrey, 2009). A related aspect is that with lower diagnosis of mental health issues, access to treatments such as talking therapies is lower than for younger people (Mind, 2013). Since older people present more frequently with symptoms of physical chronic conditions, this can mask identification of symptoms of mental health issues (Dixon-Woods et al, 2005; NCCMH, 2011). Older people's wariness of being referred to specialist services from GPs (Dixon-Woods et al, 2005), and difficulties for some in accessing services further from home (Mind, 2013) contribute to the challenges of identifying and treating mental health concerns. Further, men's propensity to hide or minimise showing emotional vulnerability does not necessarily vanish as they become 'older men', so reporting of physical symptoms may not always be accompanied by reporting emotional issues, especially with time-limited appointments with GPs who may not be well trained in communicating in a gender-sensitive way about mental health. The intersection of gender and age is therefore a powerful factor in delaying early intervention and recovery around mental health. This presents serious concerns, given the lower diagnosis of depression for men, and the higher levels of suicide.

A range of preventive interventions have been developed to assist older men to maintain their mental health and wellbeing and to obtain early guidance, support, and treatment where appropriate. Services can reach out older to men who are socially isolated by meeting some of the following conditions (Mental Health Foundation, 2010):

- Services should be physically accessible and visibly 'male-friendly';
- Pre-retirement planning support helps men to cope with transition;
- Volunteering opportunities can help men to retain a productive role;

- Activities away from traditional day centres (e.g. Men's Sheds) might be tailored to meet men's interests better; especially those which: relate to men's previous lives and identities; include physical activity; involve a social element and sharing of experiences.

Enhanced and positive mental wellbeing for older men and women often comes from participating in physical activity and social and community involvement (Seymour and Gale, 2004; Foresight Mental Capital and Wellbeing Project, 2008). Older people's (especially over 75) own priorities in ageing actively may, however, focus less on strenuous physical action or participation than on agency and autonomy, setting (and living by) one's own norms towards a 'lifestyle' focused on day-to-day quality, including perhaps mental, or physical and social activities (Stenner et al, 2011), while taking account of age- or health-related limitations (Boudiny, 2013).

Pleasurable work-like practical activities with social participation such as Men's Sheds and community gardens can play an important role in many older men's lives, affording self-esteem, a sense of masculinity in older age and contributing to their mental wellbeing (Golding et al, 2009; Milligan et al, 2012, 2013). However, there is no universal 'masculine' older man and alternatives are needed so diverse men may be supported to retain choice and control and sustain resilience and wellbeing at different life-course stages (Milligan et al, 2013).

Since 2008 the Improving Access to Psychological Therapies (IAPT) programme has accepted referrals of people aged over 65, but levels of take-up among older men remain low. Talk-based responses to mental health issues are also lower among socially disadvantaged men (Samaritans, 2012). Issues surrounding this low take-up need to be better understood and addressed; for example, why GPs refer fewer older people, and fewer male older people; and which forms of therapy take best account of the intersection of masculinity, social position and older age. Therapy provision needs adapting to fit the preferences of older men and women, for example: where it occurs; how long; what kind of session (Mind, 2013), considering age variation. Concerning primary care services, GPs should, it has been argued, be trained and supported to proactively discuss mental health with older men undergoing transitions or where physical problems may mask mental health concerns (Wilkins and Kemple, 2011). Outside primary health services, community activities such as Men's Sheds provide a vital preventive route to supporting and signposting men who might need further help, while social prescribing can also direct men to such activities (Friedli and Watson 2004; Scottish Development Centre for Mental Health 2007).

So far we have highlighted key (objective) statistics about men's mental health and have introduced conceptual ideas about the role of masculinities and wider culture and societal influences in generating these statistics and explaining the current state of men's mental health. We now wish to consider how men personally experience issues that impact on their mental health and wellbeing; that is, we wish to consider their own accounts: how it actually is for men to live with a mental health concern, rather than just focusing on statistics or on conceptual explanations.

Living with poor mental health

There is currently a limited amount known about men's personal experiences of mental 'disorder' or their experiences of 'distress' (Ridge et al., 2011). Within this section we outline findings from empirical work on men's experience of mental health, focusing on depression (as one of the main areas empirically researched).

Depression is one of the few areas to be empirically researched in relation to men's experience of mental illness, which is probably quite telling in itself. Drawing on 16 in-depth interviews with men experiencing depression, Emslie et al (2006) found that highlighting elements of hegemonic masculinity – particularly control, responsibility to/for others and being 'one of the boys' – was an important part of (re)establishing a sense of identity as the men attempted to survive and recover from depression. However, some of the men also emphasised the importance of creativity, sensitivity and intelligence in identity formation, specifically positioning these attributes (and therefore themselves) as being in opposition to some traditional, stereotypical aspects of masculinity and as a positive part of a redefined self as they attempted to deal with depression and its consequences. This resonates with work by Valkonen and Hänninen (2012), whose interviews with men with depression in Finland suggested that such depression could be a consequence of both achieved and unattained hegemonic masculinity, but also that men could both challenge and utilise hegemonic norms as a resource for coping with mental distress. They concluded that there is not a single type of association between masculinity and depression.

Expanding on this work, Oliffe et al (2011) interviewed 26 couples where the men self-identified as having depression. They identified three patterns of coping: 'trading places', where the couples exchanged certain stereotypical roles (such as the breadwinner role); 'business as usual', where couples strived to maintain stereotypical roles and thereby conceal any possible 'depression-induced deficits'; and 'edgy tensions', where there was disharmony and/or disagreement in relation to expected roles, leading to resentment and threats to sustaining the relationship. What was clear is that within couples, the experience of men's depression is heavily influenced by the relations with their partner and the limits of their partner's care-giving and resilience. To this extent, men's depression is obviously more than an individual experience; rather, it is influenced by a range of intersubjective encounters. In a related study, Oliffe et al (2012) interviewed 38 men to explore depression-related suicidal ideation. Here again, relationships with family and peers were seen as crucial to countering suicidal actions and dislocating depression from self harm. Recognising the importance of 'masculine protector' and fathering roles helped the men position help-seeking as the rational action and assisted with re-gaining a sense of self-control. In line with Brownhill et al.'s (2005) work mentioned earlier, an alternative pathway for the men was 'escaping', for example through excessive alcohol or drugs. This pathway was far more negative, often increasing feelings of isolation and heightening vulnerability to suicidal actions.

Finally, work by Galasiński (2008) analysing the discourses identified in interviews with men with depression provides some fascinating insights. There are two main findings of interest from his work that have resonance for this chapter. First, he suggests that the men interviewed did not really engage with medical models of depression that focus on 'low mood'. Rather, the men were more concerned with the social experience and impact. In negotiating these experiences, he suggests that the men distanced themselves from 'depression' as being associated with their self; that is, as forming part of their identity. What this means, in essence, is that to understand men's experience of depression requires understanding their social context and suffering, not just noting where they stand on a range of diagnostic criteria. Second, he outlines how the experience of depression 'is a thoroughly gendered affair' (p. 171). In line with Oliffe's work outlined above, Galasiński demonstrates how the men in his study always had to position themselves – their experiences, their possible 'recovery' – in relation to dominant models of masculinity. In ways that reflect the 'double bind', the men in his study provided stories (narratives) of depression that were underpinned by the social expectations of what it is to be a man. Again, these were presented as both 'success' stories – where elements of hegemonic masculinity were utilised within these narratives to present a positive male identity despite depression (or even in order to help defeat or control the depression) – and 'failure' stories – where the men's suffering because they could not achieve hegemonic norms loomed large in their experience.

Case studies of interventions

We now provide case study examples from four diverse project interventions that support: socially isolated/bereaved older men; men requiring anger management for domestic violence; men with depression; men with post traumatic stress disorder.

Case study 1. The men at EccyMeccy project (UK)

Aim: To provide a venue where vulnerable older men can meet informally and be encouraged and supported to join appropriate activities and groups that meet their needs. The provision was needed to help older men who have experienced life-changing events, particularly bereavement or very challenging periods of care for their partners, to overcome isolation, enhance their mental wellbeing, and build their confidence and self-esteem. The project was also intended to encourage men to volunteer and support other older people; and provide health professionals with a service to refer to for men most in need of support.

Setting: The Eccleshill Mechanics Institute building offered a community space for men to meet and take part in activities. Other groups such as: Karate club, Photography club, Silver Surfers, a Local History group and a Retirement Group use the resource.

Method/Approach: the project was funded over 18 months. A (younger male) project coordinator was recruited, supported by a steering group, which included older men. By month 18, 38 participants were engaged. Weekly drop-in sessions were held. These gave men the chance to practice domestic skills e.g. cooking, household maintenance; to socialise; and to plan for and participate in activities and excursions e.g. learning photography, remembering at Bradford Industrial Museum, researching family trees, listening to guest speakers, visiting an art gallery, Wii bowling, darts, walking, the golf driving range. Cook and eat courses were delivered by a sessional food worker. Advice sessions were delivered by a qualified worker (benefits, debt management, care allowance, winter fuel payments). Outside speakers talked on relevant issue; health MOTs were carried out. Participants were assessed at recruitment, 3 months and 6 months to gauge their initial needs and ongoing progress. Men were recruited as formal volunteers, undertaking appropriate training, to support potential new group members and less active vulnerable older men.

(continued)

(continued)

Link to masculinity: The project has strongly engaged older men partly because it is embedded in community activity, not separate or dominated by a particular service e.g. health; not confined to offering men somewhere to meet and chat. Understanding that men like to talk and will do so in the context of purposeful activity and using skills to accomplish tasks, the project gave the men appealing activities to do, and a skills focus, and the men got to trust each other through the activities, and to provide each other with emotional and practical support. Some skills were relevant to the men's immediate health and social care needs, while using skills for leisure activities and making a civic contribution enhances the men's identity and satisfaction with life.

Outcome: An independent evaluation survey found that that life satisfaction and overall feelings of wellbeing of the men were significantly higher at 6 months than at baseline. Men felt more useful, more relaxed, with gains in self-esteem and feeling connected to other people. Men enjoyed the group for the companionship, activities, and effects on their mood and wellbeing. Men enjoyed feeling useful, providing mutual self-help and building trusting relationships. They benefitted from a renewed sense of purpose. Sharing fellowship helped men to overcome isolation and sometimes depression. They welcomed learning practical domestic skills about cooking and diet, and hobbies such as fishing. Men were inspired to take new initiatives outside the project such as joining a walking group, reminiscence sessions, and a photography group. The men felt the project had transformed their lives. The project coordinator and referrers confirmed the project helped men overcome isolation through shared activities, forming social networks and becoming volunteers. Evidence of progression came as they initiated activities and volunteering away from the centre.

Special Considerations: The project's success was importantly due to the participatory, asset-based approach. It was vital that the programme is not a one-size fits all model. Project delivery required resources to fund a coordinator. Success in recruiting, retaining and supporting men was partly due to working partnerships between health and social care services. Training men towards undertaking voluntary roles can be empowering and make a contribution to sustainability. The model's sustainability could be enhanced through further embedding within the community, for example inter-generational work. The fact that the men showed improved wellbeing suggests benefits for the NHS, since these men were previously likely to be frequent attenders with long-term physical conditions and often mild or moderate mental health concerns. Improved emotional wellbeing is expected to have a positive medium term impact on older men's self-care.

Case study 2. The BRAVE Project: Reducing anger and other violent emotions (UK)

Aim: To reduce abusive behaviour.

Setting: A comfortable room, free from interruption, where one-to-one counselling or group work can take place. A men-only group. (A similar service is also available to women.)

Method/Approach: Individuals self-refer, or are referred by agencies, to address abusive behaviour; physical, psychological and/or emotional.

An initial evaluation is used to assess the most suitable method of working with the service-user. This can be one-to-one sessions, a 12–week programme of group work or a combination of both as is deemed appropriate. The subject is first accepted as a person. This facilitates the process of acknowledging behaviour and taking responsibility for this: overcoming the barriers of lying, denying, blaming and minimising. The person can then identify if they wish to behave differently. In group education sessions participants are encouraged to recognise their past experiences of triggers which led to unhelpful behaviour. Once patterns have been identified work can then focus on all the points within the pattern where the individual can, at that point forwards, be mindful about their choices and opt for less abusive ways of expressing emotion. An invitation is given to take responsibility for their actions and to consciously choose their response to future stimuli (both external and internal). Graduates of the 12–week programme are offered continued support.

Link to masculinity: The project is based on recognition that many men often have difficulty in verbalising how they are feeling and in coping with emotionally charged intimate relationships. Consequently, threatening and enacting abuse, whilst certainly not condoned, is seen as a negative but understandable way that men express fear, stress and frustration within such relationships or at times when these break down or become unstable. Cognitive approaches, which draw upon hegemonic masculine ideas of rationality and being solution-focused, are therefore utilised to identify trigger moments and to adjust how these are viewed and/or responded to; alternative, positive actions/behaviours are suggested.

Outcome: The service has been in existence for 10 years. Pre- and post-mental health questionnaire data show reliable improvement after 12–weeks in subjective wellbeing, problems/symptoms, life functioning and risk/harm to themselves or others. Men have also self-reported that the intervention has helped them to recognise and respond less violently. The service offers a non-judgemental sanctuary of support to assist the processing and the consolidation of experiences; which are few and far between in society for men.

Special Considerations: Facilitators are required to have sat through the 12–week programme and to have a counselling qualification prior to running sessions.

Case study 3. Muted: Support for men with depression

Aim: To increase understanding and encourage acceptance of depression amongst men and to reduce stigma and improve access to treatment. To help create a scalable platform providing support, understanding and knowledge to men, their families and friends who are affected by depression. Key areas to be targeted are prevention, stigma reduction via knowledge provision, and support during the patient journey from acceptance or diagnosis to recovery and wellbeing, also by improving access to treatment.

Setting: There are two routes to accessibility. One providing a trusted, responsive point of contact via a 'warm-line' (for general support as opposed to a 'crisis line' for suicide support), an online forum and face-to-face support groups. Secondly, reaching out and meeting men 'where they are' through planned initiatives at: sports supporters clubs, male-dominated workplaces and barber shops etc.

(continued)

(continued)

Method/Approach: Initiatives and services offered are based on lived experience from peers backed up with evidence-based interventions as advised by professionals. Personal narratives are used as a means of encouraging men to ask for help and to campaign to ensure it is there when they need it. Following the registration of the charity, 'traditional' methods of communication, support and awareness, such as a website, social media and networking were established. The founder publicly shared his experience and suffering of depression after he became aware that he was not alone in encountering an unmet need for support. Local media was used to publicise the charity, highlighting the support it provides and its aims.

All the trustees have either suffered from depression or experienced the effects of the illness when close friends or family members have suffered. In addition to the trustees, a team has been formed of other sufferers, medical professionals and consultants. Men are encouraged to engage in five ways to wellbeing (connecting, learning, being active, noticing and giving) by becoming involved with mutual aid indirectly through the use of appealing socially inclusive activities such as fishing, gardening and sports. Further initiatives and actions are progressing and projections from research and input of the organisations team indicate potential positive results. The aim is to have a mix of both proven methods and actions as well as promising innovations based on opinions and the ideas of all those involved.

Although relatively new, Muted is (through using the framework of social capital) already helping people by providing bonding capital (peer support), bridging capital (connecting the 'hard to reach' with services and vice versa), and eventually linking capital (providing a voice for an underserved population). This community capacity building is combined with individual resilience or 'recovery capital' as men are helped to stay well and seek help in a timely fashion.

Links to masculinity: The project challenges traditional ideas about male stoicism by presenting and offering examples of personal sharing of experiences around depression that can help 'normalise' alternative masculinity styles of coping. The focus on differing forms of social capital is based on previous evidence that men can and do provide positive peer support if a safe, trusting context can be provided in which to facilitate this. Linked to this, reaching out to men in settings where they already gather (rather than expecting them to come to existing services with which they are often not familiar) has been shown to be particularly effective in engaging men, possibly as it helps them retain a sense of (hegemonic) control.

Outcomes: Measured results of initial work are very positive with enquiries for help, information and offers of support being far greater than expected. Two main areas of stated benefit from those engaged to date are: (1) The simplicity and accessibility of information on the website has helped them recognise and understand symptoms and made it easier and more acceptable for them to contact Muted or to seek other help. (2) The peer-led nature of the work, being able to speak to someone with first-hand experience, has helped overcome barriers to engagement and has generated the trust required to facilitate opening up about a range of issues in a safe context.

Over time it is anticipated that all actions, campaigns and initiatives will be subject to formal robust evaluations to maximise their effectiveness and help steer future plans.

Case study 4. Veteran's Transition Program (VTP) (Canada)

Aim: To help veterans returning from military service to "drop the baggage" of operational stress injuries and re-integrate fully into civilian life.

Setting: Six to eight veterans meet for approximately 80 hours in a residential program. The format of the program is several weekend sessions. Consistent with military nomenclature, participants refer to the program as a ''course'' rather than a therapy group.

The leading team consists of three professional clinicians (i.e., combination of psychologists, counsellors and a physician) assisted by two paraprofessional soldiers who have previously participated in the VTP and received additional training.

Method/Approach: The VTP program focuses on: (a) creating a safe, cohesive environment wherein soldiers can experience mutual support, understanding from others who have ''been there'' and process their reactions; (b) normalising of the soldiers' military experiences overseas and the difficulties with re-entry back to civilian life; (c) offering critical knowledge to understand trauma and its origins, symptoms, impact on self and others along with provision of specific relational and self-regulation strategies for trauma symptom management; (d) reducing the symptoms of the stress-related issues arising from their military experiences; (e) teaching of interpersonal communication skills to help manage difficult interactions or enhance relationships with others (e.g. spouses, friends, co workers); (f) generating life goals and learning how to initiate career exploration; and (g) involving spouses and other family members in family awareness sessions

After establishing a solid working group, therapists begin to assist individuals to address symptoms and begin the work of trauma repair by having members share life-narratives through a group-based process. In this process participants write short autobiographical accounts on pre-selected themes (civil and military) between sessions then read these stories aloud in the group. After each story has been read, others respond to what they have heard without interpretation, letting the speaker know what they said was heard and understood. Following the telling of their individual narratives the members become ready to enact critical life events through the therapeutic enactment (TE) process through which they learn about triggers, stressors and patterns of activation, relapse and regression. Through TE they experience the process of 'dropping the baggage'; allowing the externalisation of internal processes of trauma in a structured and safe environment which helps lessen trauma symptoms over time. Having released much of the trauma stored within from the past, participants begin to shift their focus to the future, consolidating this new learning and creating clear and achievable goals and objectives.

Link to masculinity: The program recognises how military masculinities make men particularly reluctant to admit psychologically based 'weaknesses' (see also Green et al, 2010). 'Trust' for these men is particularly important and the program utilises peer-based approaches to help generate this. This peer-driven approach has proven to be particularly effective as it is anchored in the same team-based principles, language and initiatives used in the men's

(continued)

(continued)

military training, thus replicating what is familiar for these men. Developing trust in this way then creates the opportunity to challenge hegemonic norms of stoicism and facilitate openings for positive forms of emotional control and expression. The structured narrative process also helps to highlight the men's strengths and capabilities; it takes a salutogenic approach which helps promote self-esteem and decrease depressive symptoms.

Outcome: To date, close to 400 veterans have completed the program. Ongoing research has shown that over half the veterans that enter a VTP with clinical depression no longer meet that diagnosis after completing the program, and all graduates show significant reductions in depression and traumatic stress, as well as increased self-esteem [Cox et al (2014); Westwood et al (2010)].

Special Considerations: The VTP is currently being piloted with two sub-groups of non-military men – college age men and men with prostate cancer. Additional information about the work can be found at: vtncanada.org/

Conclusions

It is clear that there are gender differences in mental health experiences and outcomes for men and women and that the reasons for these differences are complex. Moreover, there are issues of difference between groups of men, as other aspects of identity apart from gender – such as ethnicity, sexuality, age – also impact positively and negatively on mental health and wellbeing and further complicate this picture. Nevertheless, one issue that persists as an area of concern is how processes of socialisation for boys seem to generate problems for many with being able to cope in positive ways with stressful life events. The societal expectations on boys and men to be strong, successful and rational, rather than appearing weak and emotional, creates pressures and also difficulties in coping and in seeking help when struggling with mental health concerns or experiencing stressful life events. However, a considerable amount of recent work also shows that certain elements of traditional (hegemonic) masculinity, particularly ideals of responsibility and self-control, can also be helpful in promoting positive coping with minor mental health concerns and stressful life events. At the same time, it is important to make provision for alternative masculinities. Finally, recent work, some of which is highlighted in the case studies presented here, has shown how an understanding of the contradictory nature of masculinity can be used to help design and deliver gender-sensitive programmes and projects of work which successfully promote and sustain the mental wellbeing of boys and men.

Reflective exercise

- Think about the men in your life: what do you think are their attitudes to mental health and why?
- Why do you think there is a high rate of CMDs amongst prisoners? Think about whether a CMD contributed to them being in prison or whether being in prison contributes to them having CMD? What is the evidence?

- How would you help men understand their masculinity? What would you deem important for them to know?
- Why are individuals with a BME background categorised as having a higher incidence of CMD? How would you increase understanding in this area? Is the mental health care system sensitive to BME needs? How or why not?

References

Arber, S. Davidson, K. (2003) *Older men: Their social worlds and healthy lifestyles.* Sheffield: Economic and Social Research Council.

Artazcoz, L. Benach, J. Borrell, C. Cortes, I. (2004) Unemployment and mental health: Understanding the interactions among gender, family roles and social class. *American Journal of Public Health* 94(1): 82–88

Bank, B. Hansford, S. (2000) Gender and friendship: Why are men's best same-sex friendships less intimate and supportive? *Personal Relationships* 7(1): 63–78.

Begum, N. (2006) *Doing it for themselves: Participation and black and minority ethnic service users.* Participation report 14, Bristol: Policy Press.

Bhugra, D. Leff, J. Mallett, R. Der, G. Corridan, B. and Rudge, S. (1997) Incidence and outcome of schizophrenia in whites, African-Caribbeans and Asians in London. *Psychological Medicine*, 27: 791–798.

Bhui, K. Chandran, M. Sathyamoorthy, G. (2001) *Asian men and mental health assessment.* London: Confederation of Indian Organisations.

Bhui, K. McKenzie, K. (2006) *Final report: Suicide prevention for BME groups in England. Report from the BME Suicide Prevention Project.* Centre for Health Improvement and Minority Ethnic Services (CHIMES).

Boreham, R. Stafford, M. Taylor, R. (2000) *Health survey for England 2000: Social capital and health.* London: Stationery Office.

Boudiny, K. (2013) 'Active ageing': From empty rhetoric to effective policy tool. *Ageing and Society* 33: 1077–1098. doi:10.1017/S0144686X1200030X.

Brannon, R. David, D. (1976) The male sex role: Our culture's blueprint for manhood and what its done for us lately. In: David, D. Brannon, R. (Eds) *The Forty-Nine Percent Majority: The Male Sex Role.* Reading, MA: Addison-Wesley.

Brownhill, S. Wilhelm, K. Barclay, L. Schmied, V. (2005) 'Big Build': Hidden depression in men. *Australian and New Zealand Journal of Psychiatry* 39(10): 921–931.

Care Quality Commission (2011) *Count me in 2010: Results of the 2010 national census of inpatients and patients on supervised community treatment in mental health and learning disability services in England and Wales.* London: Care Quality Commission.

Centre for Mental Health (2010) *The economic and social costs of mental health problems in 2009/2010.* London: Centre for Mental Health.

Centre for Mental Health (2013) *The Bradley Commission Briefing 1: Black and Minority Ethnic communities, mental health and criminal justice.* London: Centre for Mental Health.

Centre for Social Justice (2011) *Mental health: Poverty, ethnicity and family breakdown.* Interim policy breakdown. London: Centre for Social Justice. www.centreforsocialjustice.org.uk/UserStorage/pdf/Pdf%20reports/MentalHealthInterimReport.pdf (accessed 01/09/15).

Commission for Healthcare Audit and Inspection (2005) *Count me in, Results of a national census of inpatients in mental health hospitals and facilities in England and Wales.* London: Commission for Healthcare Audit and Inspection.

Cox, D.W. Westwood, M.J. Hoover, S.M. Chan, E.K.H. Kivari, C.A. Dadson, M.R. Zumbo, B.D. (2014) The evaluation of a group intervention for veterans who experienced military-related trauma. *International Journal of Group Psychotherapy* 64(3): 367–380.

Department of Health (2010) *Healthy lives, healthy people: Our Strategy for public health in England*. London: Department of Health.

Deverill, C. King, M. (2007) Common mental disorders. In: McManus, S. Meltzer, H. Brugha, T. Bebbington, P. Jenkins, R. (Eds.) (2009) *Adult psychiatric morbidity in England, 2007. Results of a household survey*. Leeds: NHS Information Centre for Health and Social Care.

Dixon-Woods, M. Kirk, D. Agarwal, S. Arthur, T. Harvey, J. Hsu, R. Katbamna, S. Olsen, R. Smith, L. Sutton, A.J. and Riley, R. (2005) *Vulnerable groups and access to health care: A critical interpretive review*. Report for the National Coordinating Centre for NHS Service Delivery and Organisation R and D (NCCSDO). London: National Co-ordinating Centre for NHS Service Delivery and Organisation. Available at: www.sdo.nihr.ac.uk/files/project/ SDO_ES_08–1210–025_V01.pdf (viewed 4 September 2014).

Emslie, C. Ridge, D. Ziebland, S. Hunt, K. (2006) Men's accounts of depression: Reconstructing or resisting hegemonic masculinity? *Social Science and Medicine* 62(9): 2246–2257.

Erens, B. Primatesta, P. Prior, G. (Eds.) (2001) *Health survey for England: The health of minority ethnic groups '99 Volume 1: Findings*. London: The Stationery Office.

European Commission (2011) *The state of men's health in Europe: Report*. Brussels: European Commission.

Fazel, S. Baillargeon, J. (2011) The health of prisoners. *Lancet*, 377(9769): 956–965.

Fazel, S. Benning, R. Danesh, J. (2005) Suicides in male prisoners in England and Wales 1978–2003. *The Lancet* 366: 1301–1302.

Foolchand, N. (2006) *The mental health of the African-Caribbean community in Britain*. London: MIND.

Foresight Mental Capital and Wellbeing Project (2008). *Final Project report*. London: Government Office for Science.

Friedli, L. Watson, S. (2004) *Social prescribing for mental health*. Durham: Northern Centre for Mental Health.

Galasiński, D. (2008) *Men's Discourses of Depression*. Basingstoke: Palgrave Macmillan.

Galloway, C. Gillam, S. (2006) *Mental health of Chinese and Vietnamese people in Britain*. London: Mind.

Gervais, M. (2008) *The drivers of Black and Asian people's perceptions of racial discrimination by public services: A qualitative study*. Paper for Communities and Local Government. London: Communities and Local Government.

Godfrey, M. (2009) Depression and anxiety in later life: Making the invisible visible. In Williamson, T. (Ed.) *Older people's mental health today*. Brighton: OLM Pavilion.

Golding, B. Foley, A. Brown, M. Harvey, J. (2009) *Senior men's learning and wellbeing through community participation in Australia*. Report to National Seniors Productive Ageing Centre. Ballarat: University of Ballarat.

Green, G. Emslie, C. O'Neill, D. Hunt, K. Walker, S. (2010) Exploring the ambiguities of masculinity in accounts of emotional distress in the military among ex-servicemen. *Social Science and Medicine* 71(8): 1480–1488.

Guasp, A. (2012) *Gay and bisexual men's health survey*. London: Stonewall. www.stonewall.org.uk/ what_we_do/research_and_policy/health_and_healthcare/4922.asp (viewed 01/09/15).

Health and Social Care Information Centre (2013) *Mental health bulletin: Annual report from MHMDS returns, England – 2012/2013*. Leeds: HSCIC. www.hscic.gov.uk/catalogue/PUB12745.

HMDB (2013) *European hospital morbidity database*. World Health Organization Regional Office for Europe. data.euro.who.int/hmdb/.

Holland, L. Ousey, K. (2011) Inclusion or exclusion – recruiting Black and Minority ethnic community individuals as simulated patients. *Ethnicity and Inequalities in Health and Social Care* 4(2): 81–90.

Karlsen, S. Nazroo, J.Y. McKenzie, K. Bhui, K. Weich, S. (2005) Racism, psychosis and common mental disorder among ethnic minority groups in England. *Psychological Medicine* Dec, 35(12): 1795–1803. 29.

Keating, F. (2007) *African and Caribbean men and mental health.* Better Health Briefing no. 5, London: Race Equality Foundation.

Kirkbride, J. Jones, P. (2008) *The mental ill-health of people who migrate, and their descendants: Risk factors, associated disability and wider consequences.* State-of-Science Review: SB13. London: Government Office for Science.

Kleinman, A. Eisenburg, L. Good, B. (2006) Culture, illness and care: Clinical Lessons from anthropologic and cross-cultural research. *Journal of Lifelong Learning in Psychiatry* 4(1): 140–149.

Martin, L.A. Neighbors, H.W. Griffith, D.M. (2013) The experience of symptoms of depression in men vs women: Analysis of the National Comorbidity Survey Replication. *JAMA Psychiatry* 70(10): 1100–1106.

McKeown, M. Robertson, S. Habte-Mariam, Z. Stowell-Smith, M. (2008) Masculinity and emasculation for black men in modern mental health care. *Ethnicity and Inequalities in Health and Social Care* 1(1): 42–51.

Mental Health Foundation (2010) *The Grouchy Old Men Project*, www.mentalhealth.org.uk (viewed 01/09/15).

Mental Health Foundation (2013) *Getting On . . . with life: Baby boomers, mental health and ageing well* (Full report) www.mentalhealth.org.uk (viewed 01/09/15).

Mental Health Network (2011) *Key facts and trends in mental health. Updated figures and statistics.* www. nhsconfed.org/Publications/Documents/Key_facts_mental_health_080911.pdf (viewed 01/09/15).

Milligan, C. Dowrick, C. Payne, S. Hanratty, B. Irwin, P. Neary, D. Richardson, D. (2013) *Men's Sheds and other gendered interventions for older men: Improving health and wellbeing through social activity. A systematic review and scoping of the evidence base.* Lancaster: Lancaster University Centre for Ageing Research.

Milligan, C. Payne, S. Bingley, A. Cockshott, Z. (2012) *Evaluation of the men in sheds pilot programme.* London: Age UK.

Mind (2009) *Men and mental health: Get it off your chest.* London: Mind.

Mind (2013) *We still need to talk. A report on access to talking therapies.* Mind.org.uk (viewed 01/09/15).

Ministry of Justice (2013) Safety in custody statistics England and Wales. Update to December 2012. www.gov.uk/government/publications/safety-in-custody (viewed 01/09/15).

National Collaborating Centre for Mental Health (NCCMH) (2011) *Common mental health disorders: Identification and pathways to care.* Leicester: British Psychological Society/Royal College of Psychiatrists (NICE Clinical Guidelines, No. 123). Available from: www. Ncbi.nlm.nih.giv/books/NBK92265/.

Nazroo, J. (1997) *Ethnicity and mental health – findings from a national community survey.* London: Policy Studies Institute.

Nicholson, S. Jenkins R. Meltzer, H. (2009) Suicidal thoughts, suicide attempts and self harm. In: McManus, S. Meltzer, H. Brugha, T. Bebbington, P. Jenkins, R. (Eds) (2009) *Adult psychiatric morbidity in England, 2007. Results of a household survey.* Leeds: NHS Information Centre for Health and Social Care.

NIMHE (National Institute for Mental Health in England) (2004) *Celebrating our cultures: Guidelines for mental health promotion with the black and minority communities.* London: Department of Health.

Ochoa, S. Usall, J. Cobo, J. Labad, X. Kulkarni, J. (2012) Gender differences in schizophrenia and first-episode psychosis: A comprehensive literature review. *Schizophrenia Research and Treatment* 2012, Article ID 916198. doi:10.1155/2012/916198.

Office for National Statistics (ONS) (2013) Suicides in the United Kingdom 2011. www.ons.gov.uk/ons/rel/subnational-health4/suicides-in-the-united-kingdom/2011/stb-suicide-bulletin.html (viewed 01/09/15).

Oliffe, J. Kelly, M.T. Bottorff, J.L. Johnson, J.L. Wong, S.T. (2011) "He's more typically female because he's not afraid to cry": Connecting heterosexual gender relations and men's depression. *Social Science and Medicine* 73(5): 775–782.

Oliffe, J. Ogrodniczuk, J.S. Bottorff, J.L. Johnson, J.L. Hoyak, K. (2012) "You feel like you can't live anymore": Suicide from the perspectives of Canadian men who experience depression. *Social Science and Medicine* 74(4): 506–514.

Palmer, G Kenway, P. (2007) *Poverty rates among ethnic groups in Great Britain.* York: Joseph Rowntree Foundation.

Payne, S. (2006) *The health of men and women.* Cambridge: Polity Press.

Pleck, J.H. (1981) *The myth of masculinity.* Cambridge, MA: MIT Press.

Ridge, D. Emslie, C. White A. (2011) Understanding how men experience, express and cope with mental distress: Where next? *Sociology of Health Illness* 33(1): 145–159.

Roberts, S.E. Jaremin, B. Lloyd, K. (2012) High-risk occupations for suicide. *Psychological Medicine* 43(6): 1231–1240.

Robinson, M., Keating, F. Robertson, S. (2011) Ethnicity, gender and mental health. *Diversity in Health and Care* 8: 81–92.

Sadler, K. Bebbington, P. (2009) Psychosis. In: McManus, S. Meltzer, H. Brugha, T. Bebbington, P. Jenkins, R. (Eds) (2009) *Adult psychiatric morbidity in England, 2007. Results of a household survey.* Leeds: NHS Information Centre for Health and Social Care.

Sainsbury Centre for Mental Health (2006) *The costs of race inequality. Policy paper 6.* London: Sainsbury Centre for Mental Health.

Samaritans (2012) *Men, Suicide and society. Research report.* www.samaritans.org (viewed 01/09/15).

Scottish Development Centre for Mental Health (2007) *Developing social prescribing and community referrals for mental health in Scotland*, a report commissioned by the Scottish Government and written in partnership with the Scottish Development Centre for Mental Health. www.sdcmh.org.uk (viewed 01/09/15).

Seebohm, P. Henderson, P. Munn-Giddings, C. Thomas, P. Yasmeen, S. (2005) *Together we will change: Community development, mental health and diversity.* Sainsbury Centre for Mental Health.

Seidler, V. (1991) *Recreating sexual politics.* London: Routledge.

Seymour, L. Gale, E. (2004) *Literature and policy review for the joint inquiry into mental health and wellbeing in later life,* For the Mental Health Foundation and Age Concern England. London: mentality.

Shaw, J. Baker, D. Hunt, I. Moloney, A. Appleby, L. (2004) Suicide by prisoners: National clinical survey. *British Journal of Psychiatry* 184: 263–267.

Sproston, K. Nazroo, J. (eds) (2002) *Ethnic minority psychiatric illness rates in the community (EMPIRIC).* London: National Centre for Social Research, TSO.

Stenner, P. McFarquhar, T. Bowling, A. (2011) Older people and 'active ageing': Subjective aspects of ageing actively, *Journal of Health Psychology* 16(3): 467–477.

Valkonen, J. Hänninen, V. (2012) Narratives of masculinity and depression. *Men and Masculinities* 16(2): 160–180.

Westwood, M.J. McLean, H. Cave, D. Borgen, W. Slakov, P. (2010) Coming home: A group-based approach for assisting military veterans in transition. *The Journal for Specialists in Group Work* 35(1): 44–68.

Wilkins, D. (2010) *Untold problems: A review of the essential issues in the mental health of men and boys.* London: Men's Health Forum.

Wilkins, D. and Kemple, M. (2011) *Delivering male. Effective practice in male mental health.* Men's Health Forum and Mind. www.menshealthforum.org.uk/ (viewed 01/09/15).

8 Mental health in adult women

Mandy Drake, Elizabeth Newnham and Mary Steen

Introduction

Women have distinctive life experiences that are unique to their gender and all of which have their own potential psychological ramifications and may lead to either adaptation or mental illness, for instance: menarche, pregnancy, miscarriage, abortion, childbirth, stillbirth, uterine and ovarian cancers, and menopause. Similarly, women are statistically more likely to undergo inter-partner violence and childhood sexual abuse, both of which increase their subsequent vulnerability to depression and post-traumatic stress disorder. Relationships between gender and health have been debated since the 1970s and there have been some contradictory trends. See Chapter 7 for further insights, but overall women appears to have higher rates of mental ill health at most stages of their lives. It is only over the last few decades that we have started to look at patterns rather than just counting incidences, which has assisted us to begin to understand the specific risks to women in terms of conditions they are most susceptible to. This more insightful approach has helped to develop knowledge and understanding of mental health in vulnerable women and learn how to recognise these women in clinical practice and in society. Some disguised real life case scenarios have been included to give an insight into some women's experiences of mental health problems and how a practitioner can help and offer support.

This chapter will consider

- The risks to women of poor mental health, including specific conditions to which they are more susceptible;
- How to recognise these conditions and the treatments and support that are available;
- Living with a mental health condition and the role of the family;
- The influences of physical, social and cultural effects of a woman's sex (biological characteristics) upon her mental health;
- How gender, 'what it means to be a woman', can impact on her identity and mental health status.

Adult women and mental health

That women are overrepresented in mental health diagnoses is a fact that is no longer disputed, but that alone takes us no closer to understanding this finding. Indeed, the focus that has been placed on overall numbers of women with diagnoses has detracted from the detail of such diagnoses, but, recently, Rogers and Pilgrim (2014) have broken this down. In moving away from overall numbers to types of diagnosis they have identified an evident gendered pattern, with conditions being classified as either inevitably limited to women, overwhelmingly female or more likely in women. Those inevitably limited to women (mainly related to pregnancy) have been covered in Chapter 4 but the other classifications will be explored below.

Conditions that are overwhelmingly female

Anorexia nervosa (AN)

More than 90 per cent of diagnosed cases of AN are female with less than 10 per cent of clinical diagnoses being given to men (Walsh and Cameron 2005). Around 1 per cent of women are thought to be affected by the condition (Walsh and Cameron 2005) though the secrecy associated with AN makes this a very conservative estimate. There are three essential features of AN (American Psychiatric Association 2013), which can be found in Figure 8.1.

Controlling a low body weight is desirable in AN with weight loss being commonly induced by avoiding 'fattening food'. This is often accompanied by excessive exercise and/or self-induced purging by vomiting or laxative misuse. AN is in fact often precipitated by a period of dieting with positive comments and a sense of achievement acting as reinforcers for continuing this behaviour. Those who do not develop AN this way have often experienced weight loss due to illness, with positive comments and self-perception again acting as reinforcers (NICE 2004).

When thinking about risk factors for the development of AN cultural norms are still held as central. The association between attractiveness and thinness are widely believed to play a part in the development of the disorder with media reporting and the beauty, fashion and health industries influencing an individual's already poor self-perception (Thomas 2013a). The role of sexual abuse in the development of AN has also drawn interest. McGowen and colleagues (2009) found evidence to support the impact of early childhood experiences on AN, particularly childhood abuse. Green (2009) suggests that up to 50 per cent of young people with AN have been sexually abused and suggests that anorexia may be a means of trying to forestall puberty and emerging adult sexuality; a view supported by Zimmerman (2008).The dominant view, however, is that the condition arises

---

1   Refusal to maintain body weight *despite being underweight*

2   Intense fear of gaining weight

3   Marked disturbance in self-image, particularly body shape and size

---

Figure 8.1 Essential features of anorexia nervosa

due to a complex interaction between genetics, family dynamics, culture, trauma and personality (Thomas 2013a).

Anorexia nervosa can be found among younger and older people but the typical onset is in adolescence, between ages 14 and 18. The course of the condition is highly individual with some recovering fully, others fluctuating through periods of remission and relapse and some experiencing a chronic course of deterioration (Thomas 2013a). It is, however, very difficult to maintain AN and many people will change their behaviour from restricting to bingeing and purging. In time this may change to bulimia nervosa. For those who maintain the disorder mortality rates are high with death occurring in over 10 per cent of people (APA 2013) perhaps even as high as 20 per cent (Green 2009) with starvation, suicide and electrolyte imbalance as the main causes (APA 2013).

There are a range of interventions available to those with AN but given the seriousness of the condition these would generally be provided by specialist mental health services where a psychological approach would aim to look at the attitudes and beliefs underlying the condition. Medication may also be considered though results of its use have been disappointing (NICE 2004). As a complex problem, an integrated medical, dietary and psychological approach is often taken (Gilbert 2005).

However, for a person to receive treatment their condition needs to be recognised and unfortunately detection rates for AN are poor (NICE 2004) so, consequently, NICE promote the development of a therapeutic rapport as a first line priority, irrespective of setting. Being supportive and empathic can encourage an individual to engage in an open discussion about their difficulties and potentially disclose symptoms. Although treatment should take place in mental health services, assessment can begin anywhere and an empathetic and supportive response should always be routinely adopted for an individual suspected of experiencing AN.

Bulimia nervosa (BN)

There is considerable overlap between BN and AN, not least in that BN is also a condition with an overwhelming gender bias towards women. 90 per cent of all diagnoses are female and it is still considered unusual for males to have this (Thomas 2013b). Amongst the female population up to 2 per cent experience BN (Cooper, Todd and Wells 2000). A higher prevalence among professions such as dancing, modelling, acting and athletics has been noted where a focus on weight and body shape is present (Thomas 2013b), but the secrecy of the condition makes estimates difficult.

The essential features of BN are binge eating and compensatory behaviour aimed at preventing weight gain (APA 2013) and these are further explained in Figure 8.2. As with AN, body shape and weight are central to an individual's self-evaluation and thoughts around these will often dominate a person's life. Emotional consequences of BN are high with feelings of guilt and shame being associated with a person's behaviour. Symptoms of anxiety are common, as is self-harm. Additionally, life can become dominated by shopping, eating and purging and avoidance of situations or places where food may be consumed can be quite marked. Physically fatigue, lethargy, bloatedness, constipation and erosion of dental enamel are all common (NICE 2004).

As with AN risk factors for the development of this condition are not well understood and there is a similar consensus that a combination of biological, psychological and social factors often underlies the development of BN. Feminist theorists favour the argument that it is the social ideal of thinness that puts pressure on women to conform with a resulting impact on an already poor self-perception (Malson and Burns 2009). The impact of early childhood experiences is evident

Binge eating	Compensatory behaviour
Eating in a discrete period of time (usually less than 2 hours) amounts of food larger than would be considered normal Can occur in one setting (e.g. home) or across settings (e.g. starts at work, continues on journey home and ends at home)	Vomiting Laxative use Excessive exercise Fasting

Figure 8.2 Explanations of binge eating and compensatory behaviour

(McGowen, Sasaki, D'Alessio, Dymov, Labonte, Szyf et al 2009) and there is some support for the dietary restraint theory (that calorie restriction led to BN), though this is far less conclusive than with AN (NICE 2004).

Onset of BN tends to be slightly older, at age 18–19. It can lead on from AN or can be precipitated by similar events: namely a period of dieting. Unlike AN, an individual with BN maintains a body weight within normal range, sometimes falling slightly under or overweight. It can be a serious condition and whilst some people will recover many will experience a lifelong course with periods of remission being broken by relapses during stressful times.

Cognitive behavioural therapy (CBT) is the treatment of choice for BN and this can be delivered in primary or secondary care settings. The aim of therapy would be to address core attitudes and beliefs that underlie the condition and NICE (2004) advocate the use of specifically adapted CBT over a 4–5 month period. The first option they advocate though is self-management, specifically using self-help packages with the assistance of a support person. This person could be from outside mental health services as long as they have an awareness of the self-help materials available. Medication can also be used in the treatment of BN as some antidepressants can contribute to the cessation of binge and purging behaviours. However, this is best used alongside self-help programmes and only if this approach has failed should it be considered as an option on its own (NICE 2004).

As with AN, detection rates for BN are poor and NICE (2004) again advocate the development of an empathetic and supportive relationship with any individual suspected of experiencing BN as, if symptoms are to be revealed, a non-judgemental approach is essential.

Conditions that are more likely in women

Depression

Depression is the leading cause of disability worldwide and is a major contributor to the global burden of disease (World Health Organization (WHO) 2012). There is wide agreement that women are at significantly increased risk of developing depression with estimates of prevalence commonly being cited as double that of men (APA 2013; Larkin 2011; NICE 2011a). In the United Kingdom [UK] alone it is estimated that 7–8 per cent of women will experience moderate to severe depression each year, as opposed to 3–4 per cent of men (NICE 2011a), which reflects the gender bias more globally (Seedat, Scott, Angermeyer, Berglund, Bromet, Brugha et al 2009).

Depression is best considered as being on a continuum with symptoms ranging from mild to severe with no defined cut off point between what is clinical and what is 'normal'. An episode of depression can be mild, moderate or severe, the milder end being characterised by difficulties with day to day activities and the more severe end as an inability to function in such activities. Depression is most commonly recognised when individuals report a decline in their mood which is accompanied by a loss of interest and enjoyment in their daily lives. However, there are a range of associated emotional, cognitive, behavioural and physical symptoms too and whilst these will vary from person to person, Figure 8.3 can be used as a guide for recognising the more common presentations.

As with most mental health conditions, the cause of depression is complex and it is often the result of an interaction between several factors. Some will be longer term background factors that increase an individual's susceptibility to the condition (predisposing risk factors) whilst others will be more recent incidents that have triggered the condition (precipitating factors) (Ross 2012).

As well as being female other predisposing risk factors include being of a younger age, having lower educational achievements and a family member with depression (King, Walker, Levy, Bottomley, Royston, Weich et al 2008). Early life experiences often play a part in increasing risk with sexual and physical abuse, neglect and poor parental relationships all increasing an individual's vulnerability to depression in later life (NICE 2011a).

In relation to precipitators, life events are key. In the UK an influential study conducted in the 1970s found a number of social factors for depression in women. These included not having confiding relationships, no role outside of the home and having three or more children under 14 at home (Brown and Harris 1978). Contemporary studies reflect a similar picture with key precipitators rooted in daily life,

Emotional	• Can remain low throughout the day with no reaction to daily events • For those who do react maintaining any positivity is difficult • For some, their mood will gradually increase throughout the day but return to being low by the next morning
Cognitive	• Concentration is poor • Attention reduced • Outlook is pessimistic • Thoughts tend to be negative in style and have a theme of guilt • Ruminating thoughts are common • Thoughts of worthlessness are common • Self-esteem is low • Loss of confidence apparent • Suicidal thoughts may be present
Behavioural	• Social withdrawal • Stop engaging in things of interest and which give them enjoyment (e.g. hobbies) • Lack of self-care (in women this may be stopping wearing make-up or styling their hair) • Self-harming may be present, as may suicidal attempts
Physical	• Tearfulness • Fatigue/loss of energy • Reduced sleep • Loss of appetite • Loss of weight • Agitation • Loss of libido

Figure 8.3 Common symptoms of depression

particularly difficulties in relationships or adapting to changes in roles (e.g. being a full time mother) (NICE 2011a). A substantial proportion of people with depression will experience their first episode of depression in childhood or adolescence (Fava and Kendler 2000). Unfortunately, earlier onset is generally associated with poorer outcomes although it is unclear whether this is due to the delay in individuals presenting to services or in services identifying the depression; either way, early recognition is key.

Treatment for depression involves numerous approaches that have proven effective, though WHO (2012) estimate that these are only provided for fewer than half of the worldwide population with depression. Widespread barriers include a lack of resources, a lack of willingness on the part of the individual to come forward and a lack of recognition of the condition. To aid the latter NICE (2011a) recommend the use of two screening questions for those in a clinical role which can be used when some of the symptoms outlined earlier have been noted. These are:

1   During the last month have you often been bothered by feeling down, depressed or hopeless?
2   During the last month have you often been bothered by having little interest or pleasure doing things?

A positive answer to either would support the potential presence of depression, indicating that a fuller assessment should be completed by a competent mental health practitioner. Psychological therapies, potentially with antidepressants, are central to mental health interventions where symptoms are persistent or more severe. If access to mental health care is restricted then providing information about depression, supporting individuals to use self-help materials and encouraging them to become more physically active are all crucial and effective interventions to be considered (NICE 2011a).

Generalised anxiety disorder (GAD)

As with previous conditions GAD is more prevalent in women, with estimates of 55–60 per cent of those diagnosed with the condition (APA 2013). However, this is a conservative estimate with accurate diagnoses known to be problematic, particularly in the primary care setting where most individuals with GAD will initially present (NICE 2011b).

The main features of GAD are excessive worry and anxiety. From a diagnostic perspective these have to have occurred on more days than not, for a period of at least six months and be about a number of events or activities (not just one). The anxiety and worry needs to be excessive, intrusive and difficult to control and, in accordance with APA (2013) guidelines, must be accompanied by at least three of the following:

• Restlessness
• Fatigue
• Difficulty concentrating
• Irritability
• Muscle tension
• Sleep disturbance.

The reasons for the development of GAD are unclear but several risk factors have been identified. As with depression, having a family member with a history of anxiety, being from a low socio-economic background and having a history of childhood abuse may all act as predisposing factors. A high intolerance of uncertainty is also increasingly seen as significant with many people reporting having felt anxious and nervous all of their lives (APA 2013).

Without recognition and appropriate assessment GAD will inevitably become a chronic condition which will have a significant impact on the individual (Henning, Turk, Mennin, Fresco and Heimberg 2007), and so the initial focus of any treatment approach should always be on early recognition.

As with depression, NICE (2011a) have developed two screening questions that can assist in this process and they advocate that all those in a clinical role should adopt these where any form of anxiety is suspected:

1   Do you find yourself avoiding places or activities?
2   Does this cause you problems?

Whilst not specific to GAD a positive answer to either question indicates a potential presence of anxiety which can then be used to support a referral to specialist services. Offering information on GAD and supporting the individual with self-help materials are effective approaches. More specific questioning regarding GAD is usually carried out by those experienced in mental health care and include assessing the individual's abilities to control their worries. If the condition worsens then referral to mental health services would normally be needed to provide a combination of psychological therapies such as CBT, medication and self-help groups (NICE 2011b).

Post-traumatic stress disorder

Post-traumatic stress disorder (PTSD) is not a particularly well understood disorder and why it is more likely to develop in women is unclear. International studies have found that men actually experience more traumatic events than women but women are more likely to develop PTSD in response to such events (NICE 2005). Whilst the type of events experienced between genders has been found to be different (women experience higher-impact events which are those most likely to lead to PTSD) the higher incidence among women is felt to be related to more than just this, though data to support this is limited.

PTSD essentially develops as a response to one or more traumatic events, examples of which include military combat, violent assault, sexual abuse, road traffic collision and observing serious injury or death of others. Traumatic childbirth is also becoming recognised as a precipitator for PTSD, thus increasing the risk for women further (Foa, Keane, Friedman and Cohen 2009).

There are a number of symptoms characteristic of PTSD including re-experiencing, avoidance and numbing. Re-experiencing is where people have nightmares, intrusive thoughts and see distressing images of the traumatic event, or experience sensory reminders such as noises, smells and tastes from the event. Flashbacks are a common re-experiencing symptom. Avoidance can take the form of avoiding places associated with the event, thoughts about the event and even talking about it. Numbing tends to be an inability to have any feelings with the individual often reporting feeling detached from others. It can also result from amnesia. Other symptoms include sleep disturbance, irritability, outbursts of anger and hyper vigilance (APA 2013).

A common difficulty in identifying PTSD is what can be considered 'normal' in the face of such traumatic incidents. Indeed, all of the above could in fact constitute a normal reaction under such circumstances and so a key consideration is whether the symptoms have been present for more than one month and if so whether they still cause significant distress and impairment. If the answer to those is yes than PTSD is a possibility.

Risk factors for developing PTSD are similar to those of other common mental health disorders, these being a family history, history of previous trauma and being female (Ozer Best, Lipsey and Weiss 2003).

An initial step when intervening with PTSD is accurate identification and assessment. As with GAD, all clinicians should be alert to the possibility of anxiety disorders but a particular consideration for PTSD is a recent traumatic event. The use of the anxiety screening questions identified earlier is again proposed alongside education about the condition. Referral to mental health services is the most appropriate ongoing intervention though as specific trauma-focussed interventions are often required (NICE 2005).

Recognising PTSD: Laura's experience

Laura, 54, presents at her GP practice for a routine health check. The practitioner notices that she looks tired and a little irritable and asks her if she has been sleeping okay. Laura says that she hasn't and on further prompting discloses that she witnessed a traffic collision on her way to work, where a man died. Though Laura is clearly reluctant to talk about it the practitioner continues to prompt her, suspecting by her increased agitation that the incident has had a negative impact. Laura tells the practitioner that she can't stop re-playing in her mind the moment the man's body was pulled from the car and that she can even smell the fuel that had leaked from the engine and hear the sirens of the emergency vehicles. She is clearly on edge talking about this and so, assuming the incident was very recent, the practitioner tells Laura that her reaction is understandable and will ease with time. Laura then discloses that it actually occurred 3 months ago and the practitioner begins to wonder if the response Laura is experiencing is related to anxiety.

The practitioner asks Laura the 2 screening questions that help to identify anxiety and finds that she has avoided taking the same route to work since the accident occurred. She is also avoiding all busy roads and has more recently started to take the bus, rather than drive. This is causing her problems as it is taking her much longer to get to work and on a number of occasions she has been late, resulting in a warning from her employer. Both responses indicate the presence of anxiety and with the recent traumatic incident the practitioner begins to suspect this is a case of PTSD. Laura, however, is sceptical stating that PTSD is a condition that affects people who have been to war.

The practitioner downloads a fact sheet on PTSD and goes through this with her. Laura confirms that she experiences a number of the symptoms and begins to re-consider the potential that she may have the condition. The practitioner offers her a more detailed leaflet on PTSD, which talks about the treatment options available, and she accepts this. They agree to meet again in 1 week to discuss this further, at which point Laura seems brighter. She states that knowing that her response is part of a recognised condition has helped her to accept it and that she has been more open with her family as a result. Her avoidance is still problematic though, as is her sleep, and what she now knows are flashbacks are still very distressing. With this in mind the practitioner offers to refer Laura to the mental health service for treatment, which she accepts.

Social anxiety

Social anxiety, or social phobia, is a prevalent disorder with up to 13 per cent of the general population experiencing this at some point in their lives. Whilst there is no clear consensus as to gender bias there is growing support for the theory that women experience this disorder the most (Wittchen, Stein and Kessler 1999, NICE 2011, APA 2013).

The central characteristic of social anxiety is an intense fear of social or performance situations in which the individual is open to scrutiny by others. In these situations it is negative judgement of others that is feared, alongside a belief that this will result from them having behaved in a manner that is unacceptable, embarrassing or humiliating. Ultimately, the individual fears rejection (Drake 2013). The fear is evident in everyday life with an inability to talk to new people, reluctance to eat in public, excessive blushing, stuttering and trembling being common symptoms. Feelings of nausea and palpitations are often described as are panic attacks as a result of exposure to the feared situations, which, not surprisingly, are avoided (Drake 2013).

There is a high risk of comorbid conditions, most commonly other anxiety disorders, but also depression (Kendall, Stafford, Flannery-Schroeder and Webb 2004). The use of alcohol and or drugs is not uncommon as people use these as an attempt to cope with the symptoms.

There is a paucity of research into the potential reasons for an individual developing social anxiety resulting in a lack of evidence for any cause. What is known is that there is a relatively clear age of onset (15–25), that the condition develops slowly over months and even years and that there is often no clear precipitator. There is, however, an alternative pattern with abrupt onset tending to follow a stressful or humiliating experience (APA 2013).

In terms of outcome age of onset and timely access to support are key determinants as, if social anxiety is not caught when the person is younger, normal social learning can be interrupted. Chronicity is also linked to a lack of help seeking behaviour.

The need for clinicians to increase their ability to recognise the condition is clear and, again, the anxiety screening questions can help with this. In addition, there are two questions specific to social anxiety (NICE 2011a):

1   Do you find yourself avoiding social situations or activities?
2   Are you fearful or embarrassed in social situations?

A positive response to either requires referral for a comprehensive assessment.

Unlike some of the other conditions interventions for social anxiety should be delivered by clinicians who are competent in psychological interventions. First-line treatment is specifically adapted CBT and for those who decline this, or fail to respond, a CBT-based self-help package should be offered. Medication is a second-line treatment but tends to be used where individuals have declined CBT.

Gender: cultural and societal influences

Whether a person is male or female will influence their health risks and health outcomes. This section will look at some of the underlying influences of possible mental health problems related to the physical, social and cultural effects of a woman's sex (biological characteristics) and gender (the social construct of what it means to be a 'woman').

The impact of gender on the identity and physical and mental health of women has been widely discussed, largely due to the focus of Western feminism on women's oppression. Feminist scholars have shown how gender roles after the industrial revolution impacted on women's economic autonomy. Prior to industrialisation, women played a large role in economic and social life, which afforded them the ability to be involved in primary income production in areas such as textiles, brewing and agriculture (Rich, 1986; Miles 1989). With the changes brought about by the move to a capitalist economy and increasing reliance on industry, gender roles became more dichotomised and women were seen as belonging in the 'private' sphere of the home, and were increasingly aligned with qualities such as passivity, irrationality and unpredictability. Men became associated with the 'public' sphere, and were therefore free to participate in politics, education and professional occupation. Men were aligned with activity, rationality and mastery (Merchant 1980; Martin 1989).

Box 8.1 The female disease

Ehrenreich and English (1979) in their classic text *For her own Good* give an excellent overview of how women's position in society came to influence their health. They use the example of the nature of the 'invalid' middle and upper class women during the nineteenth century, whose role in life had dwindled to complete economic dependence, expected idleness, unfailing virtue and intellectual inferiority. Women suffering from these nervous disorders were weak and prone to headaches, depression, listlessness and 'hysteria'. In one case, Charlotte Gilman described how her symptoms disappeared when she was away from her home and family, and reappeared on her return. Her doctor, dismissing her obvious distress at complete domesticity, prescribed that she live 'as domestic a life as possible', and advised her to shy any intellectual stimulation; that she 'never touch pen, brush or pencil' (Gilman, in Ehrenreich and English 1979, p. 92). Nineteenth-century female invalidism is deconstructed and understood by these authors as a way in which women both reacted to and resisted their oppressive circumstances. As with other socially situated diseases, the cause and the symptoms were difficult to separate, although its origin was often located in the uterus, reaffirming the notion that women were incompetent to enter the world of men. Working class women, viewed as robust by the medical profession, were exempt from the invalidism epidemic, although suffered from many other health risks due to overwork, overcrowding and poverty. As a disease of the wealthy, the 'invalid' woman became an idealised form, one associated with beauty and immortalised in the paintings of the Romantic period (Ehrenreich and English 1979).

The way that society began to view women was also shaped by science and medicine. Influenced by the social norms of the day, science began to 'construct' a view of women as weak. Women's bodies, held against the standard of the male body, were seen as defective. The female body undergoes many more changes: the onset of menstruation and the cyclical menstrual cycle; pregnancy; birth and breastfeeding; and menopause. As science and medicine came to be influenced by the metaphor of 'machine', popular in the seventeenth and eighteenth centuries, women's normal, physiological functions began to be interpreted as medical problems to be fixed. This is evident to this day, with many of these processes (childbirth and menopause in particular) still being subject to medical scrutiny as though they were illnesses (Martin 1989,1997; Lock and Nguyen 2010, p. 50). Although this cannot be linked in a direct way to specific mental health diagnoses, women continuously need to reconcile their own experience with the medicalisation of female bodily processes, which can be detrimental to the process itself, or to the woman's experience of it.

As first and second wave feminism made inroads into attaining basic rights for women, the focus has shifted somewhat. Women – in the West at least– can participate in voting, get an education and be gainfully employed. However, there are problems still remaining. For example, women are still paid approximately two thirds less than men, are more likely to occupy casual positions in the workforce and undertake the majority of unpaid caregiving roles such as looking after children, sick or disabled relatives and elderly parents (WHO n.d). As a result, women are more likely than men to live in poverty. Women are also more likely to experience domestic violence and sexual assault, which increases their risk of mental health problems (WHO 2015). The physical and mental health and living conditions of women in developing countries are much worse; more women live in poverty, gender roles are more pronounced, education and health care are lacking or inaccessible and maternal and infant mortality is significantly higher (World Bank 2012).

More recently, third wave feminism seeks to address the continuing inequitable status of women in society, identifying that each woman's experience is unique, and that gender is not the sole origin of categorisations and stereotypes. It also recognises that some of the discourses of second wave feminism, such as women's choice and empowerment, far from overturning patriarchal inequity, have been appropriated by mainstream neoliberal discourse – which emphasises individualism and consumerism – to create the woman as 'consumer' of her own identity (Budgeon 2011). This paradox is visible in the discussion of the Dove® Campaign for Real Beauty, discussed below. New ways of conceptualising feminism must allow for the ambiguous, contradictory nature of the postmodern world if it is to keep identifying, critiquing and exposing social beliefs and practices that contribute to mental health disorders in women.

Box 8.2 Standards of femininity

In her essay on femininity, Sandra Lee Bartky remarks the following about the pressure women are under to maintain bodily ideals:

> Under the current 'tyranny of slenderness' women are forbidden to become large or massive; they must take up as little space as possible. The very contours a woman's body takes on as she matures – the fuller breasts and rounded hips – have become distasteful. The body by which a woman feels herself judged and which by rigorous discipline she must try to assume is the body of early adolescence, slight and unformed, a body lacking flesh or substance, a body in whose very contours the image of immaturity has been inscribed. The requirement that a woman maintain a smooth and hairless skin carries further the theme of inexperience, for an infantalized face must accompany her infantalized body, a face that never ages or furrows its brow in thought. The face of the ideally feminine woman must never display the marks of character, wisdom and experience that we so admire in men.
>
> (Bartky 1997, p. 141)

Although Bartky wrote this some time ago, it could be said that these standards of femininity remain, if they have not, actually, become more pronounced.

Gender roles and femininity: being a woman

Women's reproductive life needs to be considered in a discussion of gender and health. As discussed in Chapter 4, women are at increased risk of several mental health issues, or exacerbation of existing mental health issues in the perinatal period. Throughout their life, women are also at risk of reproductive health problems such as sexually transmitted diseases, childbirth-related problems and lack of access to reproductive rights issues such as unwanted pregnancy due to lack of contraception or termination (WHO 2009). These in turn can instigate mental health problems.

The reproductive lifespan of women is under constant regulation and scrutiny. The right to contraception and abortion is still a struggle in many countries where access is lacking or the practice is illegal. Reproductive autonomy, and the choice about when and where to start a family, including limiting the number of children, is crucial to women's physical and mental health. There is increasing surveillance on pregnant women, and a concerning trend in the United States where women are being prosecuted for taking alcohol or drugs in pregnancy. Knowing that addictive behaviours are a co-morbidity of mental health issues, it can be argued that these women are being criminalised for behaviour that actually requires support and rehabilitation. Additionally, it is far more likely that the women who are prosecuted for such behaviours are young, poor or black, reinforcing the problem of intersectionality and creating further sub-classes of women and children.

Women are also subject to the ideals of motherhood. Think of television advertisements for nappies or baby food where 'beautiful' white women in big clean houses reflect the image of the perfect mother, and the fascination of the popular media with celebrities who have 'bounced back' from their 'baby belly'. Ideals of motherhood include invoking women's 'natural' femininity; it is a discourse of selflessness, of serene joy and everlasting patience. In fact, the reality of motherhood is far different for most women; the joys of motherhood are often interspersed with despair or at least bewilderment as women struggle to come to terms with such things as lack of independence, decrease in income, sleep deprivation and simply the overwhelming sense of responsibility that comes with raising a child. This reality, far from glamorous, can then be guilt-inducing as women strive to fit an unattainable ideal (see Budgeon 2011). Women who are childless, whether by accident or by design, can be made to feel inferior by the close association of motherhood with what it means to be a woman (Yeo 2005). Ideals of essential motherhood and fatherhood roles are also used in the objections against homosexual couples raising children.

These social ideals, such as normalised standards of beauty or unrealistic standards of motherhood, can influence women's self-image and contribute to mental health problems such as eating disorders or postnatal depression. The next section will explore some recent campaigns aimed at improving women's body image.

Body image campaigns

As discussed above, women's bodies have been subject to a variety of imagery and stereotypes which continue into the present day. In an increasingly visual society, the media is replete with images of the perfect body ideal, which can affect women's self-image and may affect self-esteem.

This in turn can lead to harmful practices such as fad dieting or excessive exercise, which can in turn lead to more generalised eating disorders. Even if not affected in this way, many women are dissatisfied with their appearance and this takes time and energy away from more positive life experiences. The ideal of women's body image has been the subject of several media campaigns, three of which are discussed below.

The Dove® Campaign for Real Beauty

In 2004 Unilever, the parent company of Dove (body products), commissioned a report on women's self-image (Etcoff, Orbach, Scott and D'Agostino 2004). The report showed that only 2 per cent of women considered themselves 'beautiful', leading to the Dove® Campaign for Real Beauty, which included images of 'real' women of differing sizes, shapes, shades and ages (www.dove.us/ Social-Mission/campaign-for-real-beauty.aspx). The campaign has had mixed reviews, with critics claiming that as a for-profit company there is an inevitable exploitative aspect, as well as noting that focussing on women's beauty (even if 'real' not 'ideal') reinforces the idea that women's happiness is dependent on looking beautiful, rather than on other determining factors (Johnston and Taylor 2008; Celebre and Denton 2014). Nevertheless, it does provide women with more 'real' standards of beauty than the airbrushed, over-thin fantasy ideal of the fashion industry. Interestingly, in the Introduction to the report, Dr. Susie Orbach claims that women's ideas of self were not in fact tied to their looks, and that:

> women want to be physically attractive and they want to be perceived as such. Their looks are important to how they feel about themselves, how they regard beauty in themselves and in others. But at the heart of this study is a result which is highly significant: Women regard being beautiful as the result of qualities and circumstance: being loved, being engaged in activities that one wants to do, having a close relationship, being happy, being kind, having confidence, exuding dignity and humor. Women, who are like this, look beautiful. They are beautiful.
>
> (Orbach, in Etcoff et al 2004, p. 5)

This quote highlights the importance that life circumstances such as social support and relationships, environment, self-esteem and mental health have on women's images of their physical selves. If more women were able to fulfil these areas of life, then perhaps the focus on physical appearance would decrease.

The 4th Trimester Bodies Project

The 4th Trimester Bodies Project is 'dedicated to embracing the beauty inherent in the changes brought to our bodies by motherhood, childbirth and breastfeeding'. The founder, Ashlee Wells Jackson, is a mother of three, a son Xavier and twin daughters Nova and Aurora who suffered from twin to twin transfusion syndrome. The syndrome caused Aurora to be stillborn, and Nova was born premature. Five months after bringing her surviving daughter home from the NICU, Ashlee, a photographer, founded the Project, taking photographs of postnatal women in a celebration of the individual journeys and hidden markings of motherhood.

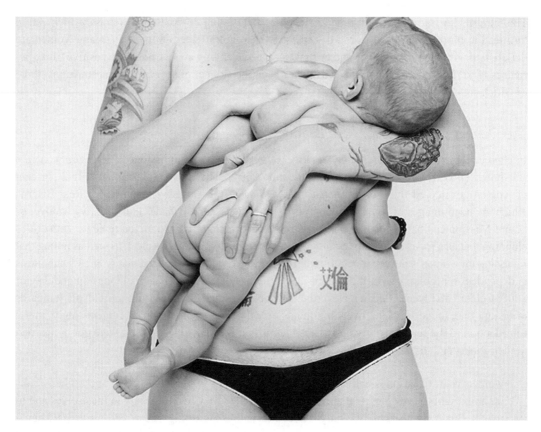

Figure 8.4 Breastfeeding mother and baby

Source: Ashlee Wells Jackson, 4th Trimester Bodies Project, used with permission. 4thtrimesterbodies.com.

The Great Wall of Vagina

Despite these campaigns to raise positive body image awareness in women, an increasing percentage of young women are undergoing the relatively new surgical procedure of labiaplasty. The aim of labiaplasty is to decrease the size of the labia minora (inner labia) to within the margins of the labia majora (outer labia) (Gress 2013, p. 675). This anatomical form is unlikely in most adult women, and more closely resembles the anatomy of a prepubescent girl. The growing emphasis on the appearance of genitalia has been attributed to the popularity of vulval shaving or waxing, which makes the labia visible, and increased access to pornography (see Navarro, 2004; Williams 2013), which, like so many industries, airbrushes out the inconsistencies and irregularities of women's bodies – the uniqueness of real life. In individual women, surgically adjusting the labia might help to improve their self-esteem and so improve their general mental health, however the subtle effects of normalising women's bodies to represented artificial social ideals cannot be understated.

Artist Jamie McCartney set out to alleviate the anxiety felt by some women about the appearance of their genital area. Over the space of five years, Jamie took 400 plaster casts of women's vulvas – each one different from the next. Set out in 10 panels, the artwork contains casts from women aged

18 to 76, and includes before and after casts of women who have had labiaplasty, and given birth, casts of mothers and daughters, twins, and transgendered men and women. This work was completed in 2011. There are more works in the pipeline, focussing on areas of body image and raising awareness of the unique nature of bodily structures.

What these campaigns have in common is to change and broaden the imagery by which women compare themselves, in an attempt to surround women with the huge variety of body shapes and forms that exist. In seeing these images, it is hoped that women begin to feel better about their bodies, rather than trying to fit to a narrow ideal perpetuated in the media and other industries, and to decrease the anxiety, and sometimes guilt or self-loathing, that trying to fit to an 'idealised' self can instigate. They are also a celebration of women's bodies, women's individuality and women's experiences.

Social determinants of health

As seen in Chapter 2, there are various social determinants of health (SDH) that impact on the health and wellbeing of individuals and communities. These can vary widely between countries, and also compare differently when looking at differing sectors within the one country.

However, while gender is a significant SDH, it is important to note that being a woman is a different experience for each woman. Other parts of life play a part, such as social cohesion, social capital, geographical location and socio-economic status. This has been noted by women who have

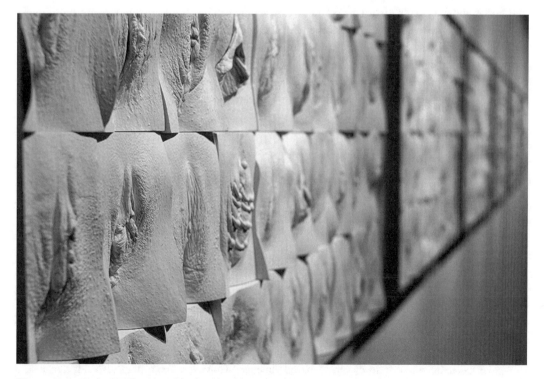

Figure 8.5 Great Wall of Vagina, used with permission.

questioned Western feminism as being blind to its own prejudices and assumptions. Therefore, women of colour, women of differing ability or sexuality than the 'norm' of the white, able-bodied, heterosexual, middle-class feminist, have argued that this adds another layer of complexity to the concern of gender, and this has been termed 'intersectionality' (Chanter 2006, p. 10). With respect to mental health, women who experience intersectionality are at higher risk again, due to the negative impact of other kinds of inequality or oppression. These can include social isolation and discrimination, poverty, racism or religious oppression, and becoming victims of war.

The problem of gender in women's health led the World Health Organization (WHO) to list it as one of the 'Millennium Development Goals' (MDGs): a list of eight of goals set in 2010 aimed at reducing the inequities and disparities in health. Millennium development goal 3 'Gender equality and empowerment for women' is therefore a global health priority. The global statistics of the impact of gender and health include:

- 30 per cent of women have experienced intimate partner violence
- 39 per cent of all female murders are by intimate partners
- More than 11 million women and girls are forced into labour or sex work (trafficking)
- Approximately 20 per cent of women report being sexually abused as children
- Approximately 800 women a day die in childbirth, 99 per cent of these are in developing countries.

(Garcia-Moreno et al 2014; WHO 2014).

This puts women at greater risk of associated mental health problems such as depression, anxiety and post-traumatic stress disorder (WHO 2015). Women in developing countries are more likely to experience these events, as well as other detrimental practices such as child or teenage marriage and childbearing and female genital cutting (Garcia-Moreno et al 2014; WHO 2015). In addition, long term health sequelae include increased alcohol and drug abuse, chronic stress and self-harm (Garcia-Moreno et al 2014). These consequences may alter the other social determinants for these women's health, such as employability and social capital, causing further deterioration in their health circumstances.

Box 8.3 Female genital cutting

Female Genital Cutting (FGC, also known as Female Genital Mutilation – FGM) is a practice that occurs throughout parts of Africa, the Middle East and Asia, and includes partial or total excision of the clitoral hood and/or the clitoris, the labia minora, and labia majora. The sewing together of remaining labial tissue (either minora or majora) is called infibulation. An estimated 130 million women worldwide have undergone FGC. The practice is thought to be based on cultural ideas of cleanliness, increasing sexual satisfaction in men, and reducing the sexual drive of women leading her to be virtuous and monogamous (Bjälkander et al, 2012; Sauer and Neubauer 2014). Sauer and Neubauer (2014, p. 237) suggest that 'As FGM does not provide any advantage for the girl involved and, in contrast, causes tremendous harm, it can only be regarded as a manifestation of sexual inequality and a form of gender-based violence.' However, one of the reasons it remains is that it perpetuates deeply held cultural values of what it is to be a woman. Therefore, although performed mainly by women in the community, it is not an isolated decision; not to perform FGC on a young girl puts her at risk of becoming a social outcast.

Health problems associated with FGC include haemorrhage, tissue damage, infection, difficulty with urination, dyspareunia, decreased sexual desire and satisfaction, infertility, childbirth complications such as prolonged labour and foetal death (Berg and Denison 2011; Bjälkander et al, 2012). Women who have experienced FGC are at increased risk of post-traumatic stress disorder (PTSD) and other psychiatric disorders (Behrendt and Moritz 2005). The United Nations Populations Fund (UNFPA) and the World Health Organization (WHO) recognise FGC as a human rights violation and are campaigning to eradicate it. In February 2015, the UNFPA, UNICEF, the International Confederation of Midwives and the International Federation of Gynecology and Obstetrics issued a 'call to action for health workers around the world to mobilize against FGM' (UNFPA 2015).

Despite continuing stark differences between the lives of women in developing vs. developed nations, the last sixty years have seen a vast improvement in the achievements of rights, autonomy and self-determination across the globe. Triumphs for women in Western countries have been slowly implemented in the developing world and there have been global forums and charters which attempt to change government policy in favour of these rights for all women, as rights to vote, to bodily autonomy, to get an education, to own property and to earn an equal wage are slowly being realised (World Bank 2012). However, one perceives the theoretical aspects of the gender divide, it is important to acknowledge the actual lived differences in women's lives as compared to men. Notwithstanding the fact that other determinants – such as economic status – also affect mental health, for reasons such as those discussed above, the health – including mental health – of the world's women is determined in part by their gender. This provides some explanation for the increased prevalence of mental health disorder diagnosis in women as compared to men (factors such as the fact that women access medical treatment more readily, or that practitioners are also influenced by cultural gender beliefs may also play a part in this). The next section will discuss various specific mental health disorders as they relate to women.

Living with poor mental health

Living with a mental health condition is a major focus of contemporary mental health services. The view that mental illness automatically confines an individual is one that is changing, and in its place is a more optimistic recognition that individuals can live a fulfilling life, irrespective of mental health status. For some years those involved in mental health care have been moving towards this position, the culmination of their work being the current emphasis on the recovery approach. This approach underpins modern mental health services but could not operate without other key initiatives. These include a return to a more values-based way of working, the introduction of self-management, a more focussed approach to public health for mental health and the involvement of family and carers. Whilst an in-depth discussion of these initiatives is beyond the remit of this chapter, an overview of each is provided below, with the references used being excellent sources for additional reading.

The recovery approach

The term recovery has been adopted to represent what is essentially a move away from an illness model to one of wellbeing. Yet recovery in this context is not to be understood in the conventional sense. It is not about symptom removal or a cure from illness but rather a move towards a life where illness does not define the individual or prevent them from pursuing their interests and goals. The concept of recovery is captured well in Perkins and Repper's (2009) statement that recovery is not about cure; it is about recovering what has been lost, a meaningful and valued life.

Despite such clarification, recovery remains a confusing and often misunderstood concept, with common interpretations being that it is a model, an approach, a philosophy and even an ideal. Whatever the interpretation there are core principles emerging that are common to most, the first being that even those individuals with symptoms of mental illness can recover. This links very much to the second principle that recovery is about the individual discovering their own identity that is separate from the illness. Thirdly, recovery is about enabling an individual to have those things that give life meaning, such as friends, work and a comfortable home. Finally, the individual needs to develop self-belief in order for them to manage their illness with optimism and hope.

Assisting an individual in their recovery can be difficult given that it is a highly personal journey that will be different for everyone. Helping the person to identify their strengths and goals can be a good starting point as using the former to achieve the latter is often a primary focus of the recovery approach. Perhaps a more practical suggestion, though, comes from Shepherd, Boardman and Slade (2008) who advise those practitioners who want to adopt a more recovery-based approach to working to measure their success by asking themselves the following questions:

'Did I . . . '
- Actively listen to help the person make sense of their problems?
- Help them to identify and prioritise their goals?
- Demonstrate belief in their existing strengths and resources?
- Encourage them to adopt helpful strategies they could use themselves?
- Support them to achieve their goals?
- Believe in them?

Not only do the questions enable a practitioner to measure the development of their approach but they offer a practical framework on which they can base this.

As a conclusion to a very brief introduction, recovery is best summarised by Collier (2010) as a journey of personal growth and change. Those practitioners who want to enable this journey can do so by adopting the principles and guidance above and in doing so will find themselves embracing a more values-based approach to mental health care.

Values-based practice

Values-based practice (VBP) has been growing in mental health care for the past 10–15 years, partly as a response to the heavy focus on evidence-based practice, where patient choice lost its value (Woodbridge and Fulford, 2004). VBP aims to put the individual back at the centre of the care process and in doing so espouses the idealism of the recovery approach, namely the development of a culture that values and respects people's choices (Cooper 2009). Indeed, partnership working is at the very core of VBP, which promotes a move away from the professional vs. patient relationship to one where the views and perspectives of the individual are actively sought by the professional and thus integrated into clinical decisions (Woodbridge and Fulford 2004).

The uniqueness of each person is also central to VBP with a recognition that everybody's recovery journey will be different and that goals will be set that will assist the individual to achieve their own valued lifestyle (Cooper 2009). Such goals and values may not be shared by the professional, and may even go against best practice, but the importance of the individual making their own choices should remain central. In Brown's 2008 study it was this individual approach and the encouragement of choice that participants felt increased their self-esteem and their hope for the future, both of which are essential for an individual to achieve recovery.

VBP therefore creates the conditions needed for recovery to be achieved and any practitioner wishing to adopt these conditions needs to focus on true partnership working. A practitioner sharing their expertise and knowledge can be very valuable to this process but actively seeking and valuing the individual's knowledge and expertise can provide them with a real sense of empowerment. Similarly, for shared decision making to be a reality the wants and needs of the individual need to be central to the care that is agreed, the result being an increased sense of control for the individual over their life.

In summary, VBP signals a shift in the relationship between professional and patient with a move away from professional expertise towards the individual being a valued partner. With this though comes a need to enable individuals to develop their own expertise, which leads on to the strong focus on self-management in contemporary mental health care.

Self-management

Whilst there are many developing strategies within health care today that aim to increase individual expertise, self-management is one that fits well with the concept of recovery. Davidson (2005) states that self-management is in fact an excellent means of translating the concept of recovery into a practical approach and for practitioners wishing to adopt a recovery focus, promoting and facilitating self-management is an effective method.

Self-management is something we all do to manage our daily lives and many will recognise the sense of empowerment and control this offers. From a recovery perspective both empowerment and control can foster the self-belief needed for an individual to begin to influence their own life (Davidson 2005) resulting in a more proactive approach to their health and wellbeing (Lovell and Gellatly 2009).

Again, there is no agreed definition of what constitutes self-management, or even what it should be called (it is often called self-help) but general consensus is that it should guide and encourage a person to make changes. There are two key features of self-management: that it should contain information to encourage its users to develop skills to cope and to manage their difficulties and it should require only minimal involvement from a professional, usually an initial explanation then brief follow up appointments to identify progress.

Self-management resources usually come in the form of leaflets and books, though there are some self-help computer programmes. These tend to take a cognitive behavioural approach where individuals are encouraged to identify their unhelpful thoughts, feelings and behaviours. Though these can be given to an individual without any further support there is good evidence for the guided nature, where an initial rationale is provided and brief follow up appointments (10–15 minutes) made (Lovell and Gellatly 2009). The general consensus is that self-management should guide and encourage the individual to make changes, focussing on methods that can be used to sustain change over time and hence reach wellbeing. There are many resources available for practitioners to use in a self-management approach but two excellent resources that are free to access can be found in Box 8.4.

Box 8.4 Self-help resources

Get self-help (www.getselfhelp.com) a website that offers self-help guides, information and resources for both practitioners and individuals experiencing mental health problems
   Northumberland, Tyne and Wear NHS Foundation Trust UK (www.ntw.nhs.uk/pic/selfhelp) who provide detailed self-help workbooks for the facilitation of self-help.

Public health

The move towards a recovery approach takes us into the field of wellbeing, a term often associated with public health and prevention of disorders. In recovery wellbeing is seen as something can be achieved alongside an existing disorder but knowing that women are at greatly increased risk of mental health conditions would also enable us to target women to prevent such conditions.

Health promotion has become an essential component of a comprehensive health service, with numerous lifestyle initiatives being promoted at any one time. The latest campaign for better mental health is the Five Ways to Wellbeing programme, which is based on the work of the UK Government's 2008 Foresight mental capability and wellbeing project. This project drew on research from around the world to consider how both mental health and wellbeing could be enhanced. The results suggested that the two were linked, with even small improvements in wellbeing decreasing the impact of mental health problems. The New Economics Foundation's (NEF) Centre for Wellbeing was consequently commissioned to develop a set of five evidence based actions for improving mental wellbeing, an overview of which can be found in Figure 8.6.

One of the most developed of the five actions is physical activity, which is now internationally recognised as a key prevention and self-management health strategy (WHO 2007). From a mental health perspective physical activity can contribute to relaxation, enhanced mood states and reduced depressive symptoms (Strohle 2009). It also has a general calming effect (Callaghan 2004), can increase self-esteem and reduce stress (Daley 2002) can reduce sensitivity to anxiety (Smits et al 2008) and decrease feelings of isolation (Craft 2005). Adding to this the individual enjoys it and thus exercise is often a patient's choice when it comes to mental health interventions (Crone 2007).

All of the actions can be promoted by practitioners, who in doing so would be helping an individual to achieve recovery. Not only would engagement in self-management provide a sense of

Connect . . .	With family, friends, colleagues and neighbours and even those around you. Connect at home, at work, at school or in your local community. Invest time in developing these connections as building them will support and enrich your life daily.
Be active . . .	Go for a walk, a run, a cycle. Step outside, play a game, garden, dance. Exercise makes you feel good. Find a physical activity that suits you and most importantly that you enjoy.
Take notice . . .	Be curious! See the beautiful, remark on the unusual. Notice the changing seasons. Savour the moment, be it talking with friends, walking to work or eating your lunch. Be aware of the world around you and notice what you are feeling. Be mindful and reflective; appreciate what matters to you.
Keep learning . . .	Try something new, rediscover an old interest. Go and sign up for that course. Take on new responsibilities at work. Fix that bike, learn to cook, start playing an instrument. Set yourself a challenge. Have fun while learning new things, increasing your confidence along the way.
Give . . .	Do something nice for a friend, or even a stranger. Thank somebody. Smile. Volunteer, join a community group. Look out, as well as in. Seeing yourself, and your happiness, linked to the wider community can be incredibly rewarding and can create connections with people around you.

Figure 8.6 Five ways to wellbeing

empowerment and control but the five actions outlined could contribute to the development of the individual's identity, meaning and self-belief.

Accordingly, NICE (2013) offers guidelines for practitioners who are in the position of offering lifestyle advice (they include mental health practitioners, midwives and practice nurses, among others), suggesting that any brief advice that is given be followed up within a self-management approach.

Involvement of the family and friends

Finally, to enable recovery, family and friends have a crucial supporting role in the individual's journey (Perkins and Repper 2009). Though the role of the professional has been emphasised so far, the participants of Brown's 2008 study were very clear that these are just people they meet along the route where those closest to them walk beside them. The same study found that positive belief and support from personal relationships along with a listening ear facilitated the recovery process, and yet professional engagement with families is often poor.

A large scale study conducted by the Department of Health (DH) in 2002 found that many family members reported feeling excluded from their relatives' care. Whilst most recognised that confidentiality limited their involvement to an extent, they stated that they also felt that they were not listened to and that they were given little opportunity to express their views. Stjernsward and Ostman (2008) remind us that it is the family that provides the bulk of care and support to the individual and they urge professionals to involve them in the care process. Simpson and Brennan (2009) support this view, stating that the VBP principle of working in partnership should extend to the family members too. Sharing knowledge and expertise of conditions and treatments is not prevented by confidentiality rules, thus there is growing support for the notion that professionals could work more closely with families, considering their needs whilst still maintaining confidentiality. Providing education on conditions, treatments and potential services available is widely advocated as is listening, allowing the family members to ask questions, informing them of signs and symptoms of the relevant conditions and discussing strategies they could adopt to help with these (DH 2002; NICE 2004; Simpson and Brennan 2009).

In addition to sharing expertise and knowledge more freely, the professional should consider the impact of the individual's condition on family members, as many will experience their own distress (Stjernsward and Ostman 2008). Physical and emotional health can be affected when living or caring for somebody with a mental health condition as can the family members' social life, education and employment (DH 2002). Being alert to this will enable early detection and intervention, where the professional's role would be to signpost the family member to an appropriate support service.

In summary, family involvement in the care of individuals with mental health problems is crucial to their recovery and professionals should aim to involve them in this process as fully as possible. In the true spirit of values-based practice they should work in partnership with the family providing them with the information and support they need to fulfil what can be a very challenging role.

A recovery focussed approach: Sara's story

Sara, aged 28, has suffered from depression from an early age. Despite several attempts at engaging in mental health support she has found the services to be too prescriptive, often telling her what she needs rather than asking her what she wants. However, a lack of improvement in her symptoms has left her isolated and withdrawn and so she has reluctantly agreed to see another mental health practitioner, Jo.

Upon meeting Jo, Sara re-tells her historical story but is surprised to find that Jo is more interested in her current life and where she sees her future. When she asks Sara what goal she is working towards she seems genuinely surprised that the answer is none. Jo listens as Sara talks about her lack of hope for the future and when she realises that Jo is not going to interrupt she starts to talk about the goals she used to have, in particular her ambition of being a writer. Jo encourages Sara to think about how it would feel to achieve this ambition and Sara is surprised to find that she feels some excitement when discussing it. Jo asks why this can't be a goal to work towards now, to which Sara repeats other peoples responses; that it is not realistic or achievable. Instead of agreeing, Jo asks Sara what strengths she has that would help her to achieve such a goal and Sara tells her that she has a degree in English literature, has won a short story prize and used to write a column for a local newspaper. When Jo asks again why this can't be a goal to work towards Sara starts to think that Jo may actually believe she could be a writer, which in turn makes her start to believe this too. They consequently agree that this will be one of Sara's goals before turning their attention to how she can begin to work towards this.

Sara states that she would like to enrol for a creative writing group but she needs to increase her confidence first. She also has a poor sleep pattern and lacks energy and so increasing each of these are agreed as shorter terms goals. Jo says that she has suggestions for how Sara can begin to work on these but asks first if Sara has any ideas. Sara says that she had been wondering about starting some kind of exercise and Jo says that this would be a good idea. In addition, Jo states that a sleep plan can be helpful and provides Sara with information on this.

In further sessions Jo shares her knowledge and experience of a number of useful strategies and a self-management approach is facilitated. Self-help guides are used as the basis for this, with Sara and Jo agreeing the strategies to try collaboratively and brief review meetings enabling these to be reviewed. Improvement in Sara's sleep and fitness start to be noted with a consequent increase in her energy, self-confidence and optimism. At this point they agree that Sara should enrol on the creative writing course, though, she starts to feel anxious, saying she doesn't think she can do it.

Jo asks if there is anybody who could go along to enrol with her and Sara says that her mum has offered but she finds her too smothering. Upon further discussion it seems Sara's mum is always saying she wants to help but doesn't know how and this annoys Sara. Jo asks if some information on depression would increase her mum's knowledge and maybe ease her anxiety but Sara is sceptical. Despite this she agrees to take some and is surprised to find that her mum had felt genuinely at a loss as to how to help. After reading the information through her mum was more relaxed and so Sara shared her self-help guides with her. At a later appointment Sara reports that she has accepted her mum's offer to attend enrolment with her and that earlier that week her mum had brought home a leaflet on the Five Ways to Mental Wellbeing, suggesting they take a mindfulness class together. Sara reports that she is giving this serious consideration.

Conclusions

This chapter has reviewed the risks to women for mental health issues and looked specifically at mental health problems associated with being a woman. The female body undergoes many physical and emotional changes during the lifespan, such as the onset of menstruation, the cyclical menstrual cycle, pregnancy, birth, breastfeeding and menopause; this needs to be taken into consideration when exploring susceptibility, as well as the social determinants, of health. It is well recognised that women are overrepresented in mental health diagnoses. Evidence to support that women are more susceptible to some mental health conditions that are unique to their gender throughout the lifespan has been included and discussed. Insights into how to recognise these conditions and the treatment, care and support that are available have been described and discussed. The case scenarios have helped to demonstrate some real life experiences, and how the influences of physical, social and cultural aspects can affect a woman's mental health and wellbeing have been considered.

What it means to be a woman can impact on personal identity and mental health status and, therefore, it is essential to have knowledge and understanding of how gender can play an important role. Gender is linked significantly to social determinants of health (SDH) and vulnerability to mental health problems, but it is important to recognise that being a woman is a different experience for each woman. Other factors in life play a part, such as social cohesion, social capital, geographical location and socio-economic status. These factors can vary widely throughout the world and between countries and they also compare differently when looking at differing sectors within a country.

It is vitally important to acknowledge that the whole family is affected when a female family member is prone to or suffering from a mental health problem. It is, therefore, important to include family members when offering care and support and be aware that they can also be at risk.

Reflective exercises

- When engaging with women with mental health problems do you focus on the Recovery approach? Take a look at the questions posed earlier (p. 194) by Shepherd, Boardman and Slade (2008) and ask yourself 'Do I . . . ?'
- Look at the Five Ways to Wellbeing in Figure 8.6. Discuss with your friends whether they engage in these and ask them which they think are most important for their wellbeing. Think about how you can incorporate this into your own approach to mental health.
- Reflect on the reasons for those mental health problems outlined being more prevalent amongst women. Do the suggestions match your own experiences and how can you use this knowledge in your approach to supporting women?
- How do social constructs of gender have the potential to influence women's mental health throughout their lifespan?
- Outline the primary differences that might impact on a woman's mental health in a developing country compared to a woman in a developed country.

References

American Psychiatric Association (2013) *Diagnostic and statistical manual of mental disorders* (5th edn). Washington DC: APA.

Bartky, S (1997) Foucault, femininity, and the modernization of patriarchal power, in K Conboy, K Medina, N and Stanbury, S (eds), *Writing on the body: Female embodiment and feminist theory*. New York: Columbia University Press.

Behrendt, A and Moritz, S (2005) Posttraumatic stress disorder and memory problems after female genital mutilation. *American Journal of Psychiatry* 162: 1000–1002.

Berg, R and Denison, E (2011) Does female genital mutilation/cutting (FGM/C) affect women's sexual functioning? A systematic review of the sexual consequences of FGM/C. *Sexuality Research and Social Policy* 9(1): 41–56.

Bjälkander, O Bangura, L Leigh, B Berggren, V Bergström, S and Almroth, L (2012) Health complications of female genital mutilation in Sierra Leone. *International Journal of Women's Health* 4: 321–331. doi:10.2147/IJWH.S32670.

Brown, G and Harris, T (1978) *The social origins of depression: A study of psychiatric disorder in women*. London: Tavistock Publications.

Brown, W (2008) Narratives of mental health recovery. *Social Alternatives* 27(4): 42–48.

Budgeon, S (2011) The contradictions of successful femininity: Third-wave feminism, postfeminism and 'new' femininities, in Gill, R and Scharff, C (eds), *New femininities: Postfeminism, neoliberalism and subjectivity*. Basingstoke: Palgrave Macmillan.

Callaghan, P (2004) Exercise: A neglected intervention in mental health care? *Journal of Psychiatric and Mental Health Nursing* 11: 476–483.

Celebre, A and Denton, A (2014) The good, the bad, and the ugly of the Dove Campaign for Real Beauty. *In-mind Magazine* 2(19). www.in-mind.org/article/the-good-the-bad-and-the-ugly-of-the-dove-campaign-for-real-beauty (viewed 21/3/15).

Chanter, T (2006) *Gender: Key concepts in philosophy*. London: Continuum International.

Collier, E (2010) Confusion of recovery. *International Journal of Mental Health Nursing* 19(1): 16–21.

Cooper, L (2009) Values-based mental health nursing, in Callaghan, P Playle, J and Cooper, L (eds), *Mental health nursing skills*. Oxford: Oxford University Press.

Cooper, M Todd, G and Wells, A (2000) *Bulimia nervosa: A cognitive therapy programme for clients*. London: Jessica Kingsley.

Craft, L (2005) Exercise and clinical depression: Examining two psychological mechanisms. *Psychology of Sport and Exercise* 6: 151–171.

Crone, D (2007) Walking back to health: A qualitative investigation into service users' experiences of a walking project. *Issues in Mental Health Nursing* 28: 167–183.

Daley, AJ (2002) Exercise therapy and mental health in clinical populations: Is exercise therapy a worthwhile intervention? *Advances in Psychiatric Treatment* 8: 262–270.

Davidson, L (2005) Recovery, self-management and the expert patient: Changing the culture of mental health from a UK perspective. *Journal of Mental Health* (Feb) 14(1): 25–35.

Department of Health (2002) *Developing services for carers and families of people with mental illness*. London: DH.

Drake, M (2013) Client presenting with social phobia, in Thomas, M and Drake, M (eds), *Cognitive behavioural case studies*. London: Sage.

Ehrenreich, B and English, D (1979) *For her own good: 150 years of the experts' advice to women*. London: Pluto Press.

Etcoff, N Orbach, S Scott, J and D'Agostino, H (2004,) *The real truth about beauty: A global report*. Unilever (viewed 21/3/15).

Fava, M and Kendler, K (2000) Major depressive disorder. *Neuron* 28: 335–341.

Foa, EB Keane, TM Friedman, MJ and Cohen, J (2009) *Effective treatments for PTSD: Practice guidelines from the International Society for Traumatic Stress Studies*. New York: Guilford Press.

Foresight Mental Capital and Wellbeing Project (2008) *Final project report*. London: Government Office for Science.

Garcia-Moreno, C Zimmerman, C Morris-Gehring, M Heise, L Amin, A Abrahams, N Montoya, O Bhate-Deosthali, P Kilonzo, N and Watts, C (2014) Addressing violence against women: A call to action. *The Lancet* 385(9978): 1685–1695, 25 April 2015. www.thelancet.com/journals/lancet/issue/vol385no9978/PIIS0140–6736(15)X6138-1

Gilbert, S (2005) *Counselling for eating disorders* (2nd edn). London: Sage.

Green, B (2009) *Problem based psychiatry* (2nd edn). Oxford: Radcliffe Publishing.

Gress, S (2013) Composite reduction labiaplasty. *Aesthetic Plast Surg* 37: 674–683.

Henning, ER Turk, CL Mennin, DS Fresco, DM and Heimberg, RG (2007) Impairment and quality of life in individuals with generalised anxiety disorder. *Depression and Anxiety* 24: 342–349.

Johnston, J and Taylor, J (2008) Feminist consumerism and fat activists: A comparative study of grassroots activism and the Dove Real Beauty Campaign. *Signs* 33(4): 941–966.

Kendall, PC Stafford, S Flannery-Schroeder, E and Webb, A (2004) Child anxiety treatment: Outcomes in adolescence and impact on substance use and depression at 7 year follow up. *Journal of Consulting and Clinical Psychology* 72: 276–287.

King, M Walker, C Levy, G Bottomly, C Royston, P Weich, S et al (2008) Development and validation of an international risk prediction algorithm for episodes of major depression in general practice attendees. *Archives of General Psychiatry* 65(12): 1368–1376.

Larkin, M (2011) Social aspects of health, illness and healthcare. Maidenhead: Open University Press.

Lock, M and Nguyen, V (2010) *An anthropology of biomedicine*. Oxford: Wiley-Blackwell.

Lovell, K and Gellatly, J (2009) Self-help, in Norman, I and Ryrie, I (eds), *The art and science of mental health nursing* (2nd edn). Maidenhead: Open University Press, McGraw Hill.

Malson, H and Burns, M (2009) *Critical feminist approaches to eating dis/orders*. London and New York: Routledge.

McGowen, PO Sasaki, A D'Alessio, AC Dymov, S Labonte, B Szyf, M Turecki, G and Meaney, MJ. (2009) Epigenetic regulation of the glucocorticoid receptor in human brain associates with childhood abuse. *Nature Neuroscience* 12(3): 342–348.

Miles, R (1989) *The women's history of the world*. Topsfield, MA: Salem House.

National Institute for Health and Clinical Excellence (2013) *Physical activity: Brief advice for adults in primary care*. London: National Collaborating Centre for Mental Health.

National Institute for Health and Clinical Excellence (2011a) *Common mental health disorders*. Clinical guideline 123. London: National Collaborating Centre for Mental Health.

National Institute for Health and Clinical Excellence (2011b) *Generalised anxiety disorder and panic disorder (with or without agoraphobia) in adults. Management in primary, secondary and community care*. London: National Collaborating Centre for Mental Health.

National Institute for Health and Clinical Excellence (2005) *The management of PTSD in adults and children in primary and secondary care*. London: National Collaborating Centre for Mental Health.

National Institute for Health and Clinical Excellence (2004) *Eating disorders: Core interventions in the treatment and management of anorexia nervosa, bulimia nervosa and related eating disorders*. London: National Collaborating Centre for Mental Health.

Navarro, M (2004) The most private of makeovers, *New York Times*, November 28.

Ozer, EJ Best, SR Lipsey, TL and Weiss, DS (2003) Predictors of PTSD and symptoms in adults: A meta-analysis. *Psychological Bulletin* 129: 52–73.

Perkins, R and Repper, J (2009) Recovery and social inclusion, in Norman, I and Ryrie, I (eds), *The art and science of mental health nursing* (2nd edn). Maidenhead: Open University Press, McGraw Hill.

Rogers, A and Pilgrim, D (2014) *A sociology of mental illness* (5th edn). Maidenhead: Open University Press.

Ross, I (2012) Client presenting with depression, in Thomas, M and Drake, M (eds), *Cognitive behavioural case studies*. London: Sage.

Sauer, P and Neubauer, D (2014) Female genital mutilation: A hidden epidemic. *European Journal of Pediatrics* 173(2): 237–238.

Seedat, S Scott, KM Angermeyer, MC Berglund, P Bromet, EJ Brugha, TS et al (2009) Cross national associations between gender and mental disorder in the World Health Organization's World Mental Health Surveys. *Archives of General Psychiatry* 66(7) 785–795.

Shepherd, G Boardman, J and Slade, M (2008) *Making recovery a reality*. London: Sainsbury Centre for Mental Health.

Simpson, A and Brennan, G (2009) Working in partnership, in Callaghan, P Playle, J and Cooper, L (eds), *Mental health nursing skills*. Oxford: Oxford University Press.

Smits, J Berry, A Rosenfield, D Powers, M Behar, E and Otto, M (2008) Reducing anxiety sensitivity with exercise. *Depression and Anxiety*, 25: 689–699.

Stjernsward, S and Ostman, M (2008) Whose life am I living? Relatives listening in the shadow of depression. *International Journal of Social Psychiatry* 54: 358–369.

Strohle, A (2009) Physical activity, exercise, depression and anxiety disorders. *Journal of Neural Transmission* 116(6): 777–784.

Thomas, M. (2013a) Client presenting with anorexia nervosa, in Thomas, M and Drake, M (eds), *Cognitive behavioural case studies*. London: Sage.

Thomas, M. (2013b) Client presenting with chronic bulimia nervosa, in Thomas, M and Drake, M (eds), *Cognitive behavioural case studies*. London: Sage.

UNFPA (2015) Joint Statement on International Day of Zero Tolerance for Female Genital Mutilation (FGM). www.unfpa.org/news/joint-statement-international-day-zero-tolerance-female-genital-mutilation-fgm (viewed 21/4/15).

Walsh, BT and Cameron, VL (2005) *If your adolescent has an eating disorder*. New York: Oxford University Press.

WHO (World Health Organization) (2015) *Gender and women's mental health,* WHO: Geneva. www.who.int/mental_health/prevention/genderwomen/en/ (viewed 16/3/15).

WHO (2014) *Maternal mortality*. Fact sheet No. 348. Geneva: WHO.

WHO (2012) *Depression*. Fact sheet No. 369. Geneva: WHO (retrieved from www.who.int/mediacentrere/factsheets/fs369/en/).

WHO (2009) *Women and health: Today's evidence, tomorrow's agenda*. Geneva: WHO.

WHO (2007) *A guide for population based approaches to increasing levels of physical activity. Implementation of the WHO global strategy on diet, physical activity and health*. Geneva: WHO.

WHO (n.d) *Gender disparities in mental health*. Geneva: WHO. www.who.int/mental_health/media/en/242.pdf?ua=1 (viewed 01/09/15).

Williams, J (2013) *Reading lips: Exploring emotive responses to labiaplasty*. Ottawa: Carleton University.

Wittchen, H-U Stein, MB and Kessler, RC (1999) Social fears and social phobia in a community sample of adolescents and young adults: Prevalence, risk factors and co-morbidity. *Psychological Medicine* 29: 309–323.

Woodbridge, K and Fulford, B (2004) *Whose values? A workbook for values-based practice in mental health care*. London: The Sainsbury Centre for Mental Health.

World Bank (2012) *World development report: Gender equality and development*, Washington DC: World Bank.

Yeo, E (2005) Constructing motherhood, 1750–1950, *Hecate* 31(2): 4–20.

Zimmerman, ML (2008) The client with an eating disorder, in Antai-Otong, D (ed), *Psychiatric nursing: Biological and behavioural concepts* (2nd edn). New York: Delmar/Thomson.

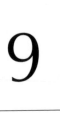

9 Mental health in the aged population

Andrew Lovell and Thomas Moncur

Introduction

This final chapter will focus on mental health in the aged population. Many older people have a positive outlook when approaching the final stage of their life cycle but some are at risk of developing mental health problems due to several health and social stressors.

One of the most common mental health problems the aged population are at risk of is depression, which often goes unrecognised. Coming to the end of one's life and coping with health, social and financial issues can have an impact on mental health status. The death of a partner, family members and friends can also take their toll. Health professionals and support workers can play an important role and offer support and care. The sense of hopelessness and abandonment that many older people are susceptible to can have a negative impact on their mental health and wellbeing in general.

Mental health problems in an older person can vary in severity and may be obvious or subtle. A depressive state, sudden changes in attitude or lack of concern in addressing daily living activities may well be signs of an older person experiencing poor mental health. Insomnia, disturbed sleep patterns, poor eating habits, decline in personal appearance or hygiene and withdrawal from social contact may alert family members to seek help and advice from a health professional and local support networks. A reflective practitioner account and two case scenarios are included to gain an insight into some of the mental health problems an older person can encounter and the challenges a health professional can face when providing care and compassion.

This chapter will consider

- Mental health issues that are associated with the aged population;
- The mental health care and support needs of the aged population;
- What mental health challenges can face the aged population upon retiring;
- The mental health needs of the aged population when approaching end of life;
- How bereavement can affect an older person's mental health status;
- Mental health problems when an aged person is suffering from dementia.

The aged population and mental health

The need to promote positive mental health as people grow older is increasingly becoming an issue that societies across Europe in particular, though also the world, are taking into account as they develop strategies for facing societal concerns of the future. The demographic changes affecting Europe mean that over the course of the next few years, there will be fewer younger people and younger adults, and a considerable increase in the number of older workers, people beyond pensionable age and very old people. This has been referred to as the 'grey tsunami', though changing circumstances also mean that there are many more older people living healthier and productive lives well into later life, so the portrayal of impending disaster is far from accurate. Nevertheless, the proportion of the population living beyond the age of 65 by the year 2050 is likely to be in the region of 30 per cent of the population, and 11 per cent of this group will be over the age of 80 years old (Jané-Llopis and Gabilondo, 2008). There are no agreed definitions of old age and the term has different connotations and meanings across cultures and societies. Most countries have selected the retiring age of 60 or 65 years as the definition of an older person (WHO, 2007), but retirement ages are currently being renegotiated according to issues of geography and economy. The European Commission has divided older people into three groups: older workers (55–64 years), older people (65–79 years) and frail old people (80+ years) (Jané-Llopis and Gabilondo, 2008). The primary consideration revolves around the significant variance in the mental health and functional ability of people older than 65 years of age, particularly since older age groups tend toward greater heterogeneity in terms of attitudes, social background, preferences, hobbies, political allegiance, education and family background.

More than 40 per cent of the UK population will be over 50 years old and 20 per cent over 65 by 2020, with those over 85, the fastest growing segment of the population, increasing by almost a third (to 2.7 per cent); this is set, furthermore, in the context of the more pronounced ageing of the European population, which has a significantly different population structure than other continents, such as Africa and South America (Office of National Statistics, 2009). The consequences for society are considerable, both in relation to family structure and role expectations and also the economic dimensions of work contribution and care costs: in effect, one of the most significant challenges of the twenty-first century (Goldie, 2010). Such societal vicissitudes bring with them an increased level of deteriorating mental health amongst older people, particularly depression and dementia, and for a significant number (60 per cent), suffering over a prolonged period of time the outlook is poor (Healthcare Commission, 2009). As many as one in five of those aged between 65 and 70 are afflicted with depression, though this is half the number of those over 85, and frequently the condition is erroneously regarded as an inevitable part of getting older (Beekman, Copeland and Prince, 1999). Less than one tenth of older people with a diagnosis of depression receive a referral to specialist mental health services, compared with nearly half of younger adults; sometimes the issue surrounds criteria for exclusion on the basis of age by GPs so that 80 per cent of older people suffering with depression fail to be treated (Age Concern, 2007). Explanations are difficult to accurately ascertain but it is at least partially connected with professional interpretation, in effect professional stigmatisation, an issue of seemingly increasing importance and one to which a section of this chapter is devoted. There is, furthermore, a wide spectrum of older people, who, though not specifically diagnosed as being mentally ill, don't enjoy good mental health as they grow older, with social isolation or loneliness constituting the key factor, with as many as 12 per cent feeling trapped in their own homes (Age Concern, 2011). Changing societal demographics mean that many older people don't have large families or relatives living close enough for regular visits or for facilitating more general contact with the wider community (Mental Health Foundation, 2010). Loneliness, therefore, is a major factor in triggering depression, compounded by issues of a diminished social network, diminishing quality of life and frequently neglected or inadequately treated illness (WHO, 2002). This issue fails to get the attention it deserves, probably because of service and professional concerns about being unable to provide the necessary support to people to make them feel less isolated and more involved

As documented in the Mental Health Foundation's report on loneliness, demographic changes mean that many older people do not have large families or families that live close enough to be able to visit regularly and who are able to help them retain their contact with wider society (Mental Health Foundation, 2010). The marginalisation of older people, particularly when compounded by disability or mental health difficulties, is exacerbated by prevailing attitudes, stigma, environmental issues, accessing services, and lack of voice and participation, which, in combination, can render people 'invisible' (Cain, 2012). These disadvantages can be diverse, sometimes overlapping, and with an absence of underpinning policy to provide relief from additional factors of gender, geographical isolation or ethnicity. The international definition of older people relates to over the age of 60 (UNDESA, 2004), which currently accounts for 11 per cent of the population and is set to double over the next 35 years (UNFPA and HelpAge International, 2012). This changing demographic also means that there are already more older people than children under the age of five, which will increase to fifteen years by 2050. The consequences of these changes are not fully understood and may differ between the developed and developing world. The phenomenon of significant numbers of people living longer and maintaining good health, for example, is altering the way that developed economies are grappling with issues of delayed retirement, payment of pensions for several decades, and retaining participation in all areas of society. The concerns of the developing world are more directly related to low income, continued working in physically demanding jobs well into old age, and the much reduced availability of pensions (Hagemejer and Behrendt, 2009). 340 million people live without any secure income and, under current conditions, this is likely to triple over the next three decades (Meissner, 2010).

Mental health disorders, according to the World Health Organization (WHO, 2008), account for 13 per cent of the world's Global Burden of Disease, affecting 450 million people, over 6 per cent of the population, with depression, currently affecting nearly 100 million, rising significantly year after year and suicide a leading cause of death in some countries (Suvedi et al., 2009). Evidence of the relationship between mental ill-health and poverty is more tenuous (Das et al., 2007) but is associated with lack of education, poor housing and low income, all factors linked to social exclusion (Lund et al., 2010). Physical and mental health conditions are often linked: depression, for example, has been related to heart problems and diabetes, and schizophrenia linked to both suicide and infectious disease (Sartorius, 2007).

Ageism, age discrimination and stigma

The terms ageism and age discrimination are frequently used interchangeably, though they are actually different in nature and this difference is often given insufficient credence. Ageism refers to an attitude of mind, which may result in age discrimination, whereas age discrimination relates to action that may be observed; it is, perhaps, inherent in the human condition (Butler, 1969). The term ageism is often used to identify stereotypes and prejudices that people hold on the basis of a person's age, whilst the process of discrimination describes behaviour designed to treat people unequally, whether directly or indirectly, simply because of their age (Ray, Sharp and Abrams, 2006). In general terms, ageism is wider than age discrimination, referring to quite deeply entrenched negative beliefs about the relationship between older people and society, with the eventual consequence of age discrimination (McGlone and Fitzgerald, 2005). Some argue that ageism is different to age-differentiated behaviour, since the former is based on stereotypes and prejudice whereas the latter requires a mature and thoughtful understanding of age differences (Hagestad and Uhlenberg, 2005). Age discrimination reflects a never-justifiable differentiation in treatment, which is based entirely on age, and may apply directly, such as exclusion from a service for age-related reasons alone, or indirectly when what appears to be a neutral provision or practice has harmful consequences for a person. Poor quality dementia provision, for example, available across a whole community, will indirectly discriminate against older people, who are likely to be the largest group utilising such services. Direct age discrimination will take place if people with needs very similar to others are treated differently because of their age, whilst indirect discrimination will occur if people from varying age groups with clearly different needs are treated exactly the same with the consequence that a particular group, the elderly, do not have their needs met. The National Service Framework for Older People interim report on age discrimination examined written policies, protocols and procedures within the health system and found age-related criteria applying to mental health, rehabilitation, psychology and alcohol services, in effect a case of explicit and direct age discrimination (Department of Health, 2002).

The issue of stigma is a complex one likely to affect older people far more potently than any other group with mental ill-health, influencing the thinking underpinning recognition and subsequent planning of services, with many professional groups, including, critically, general practitioners, being complicit in the process frequently because of casual dismissal of real need (Glassman, 2004). There is ample evidence to suggest that older people with mental health difficulties are amongst the most socially excluded in society, the stigma of old age exacerbated by the additional stigma of having a mental health issue, which in turn may be compounded by physical ill-health and temporary or permanent disability (Department of Health, 2009). There are a number of extremely powerful associations relating to mental health surrounding older people which have a marked effect on older people's psychological and emotional wellbeing. This not only means that people are affected at an individual level but also influences how mental health is regarded in later life within society, with profound consequences for those caring for older people, the professional community and general support services available. This includes fears around loss of cognitive functioning, loss of control over one's life, becoming a burden on relatives, anxiety related to which significantly influences people's decision to access services. Secondly, ignorance and reduced understanding about the relationship between ageing and mental health is further compounded by a lack of high quality information and a reluctance to talk openly about the whole subject. Thirdly, guilt and shame arise because of becoming or being emotionally unwell, feeling stressed, vulnerable or physically unwell as a result of caring for someone over a lengthy period of time (Bowers et al., 2006).

A study conducted in the United States determined that younger patients were likely to receive a more positive prognosis than older people, concluding that the likely explanation related to prejudicial attitudes, in effect ageism, towards the older group. Professionals were identified as being subject to generational prejudice, fearful of discussing ageing, with the study authors arguing that innovations in service delivery, particularly collaborative medical/psychological care, are likely to be the most effective determinants of improved access to mental health services than attempts to combat ageism (Robb, Chen and Haley, 2002). A survey conducted in the UK ascertained that 45 per cent of psychology personnel believed that the service (clinical psychology) had little to offer those of advancing years, and the responses, furthermore, reflected fears of the ageing process, a preoccupation with dying and evidence of ageism (Lee, Volans and Gregory, 2003). Concerns about stigma and ageism are further compounded by evidence that older people may be subject to abuse, with one survey of family carers of older people revealing some abusive behaviour being reported by as many as half of those surveyed (Crown and Lee, 2007). An increasing number of studies suggest that people with Alzheimer's disease are affected by the reactions to the effects of the condition, by environmental circumstances and by the impact of how they are treated. Negative self-stereotypes, both consciously and unconsciously, appear to have detrimental effects on how healthy older people perform in tasks relating to memory, and the possibility of being negatively stereotyped can have disastrous effects on how people perform in tests of recall and recollection (Scholl and Sabat, 2008).

Similarities and differences within the male and female elderly population

Older people are often considered vulnerable simply because of their advancing years, yet they are self-evidently not a homogeneous group; some live healthily and actively well into their later years, whilst the decline of others may come quickly and early in life. Older women are afflicted with more chronic health conditions, disability and depression than men (Das et al., 2007), though health policies rarely reflect these sometimes very different experiences (Stevens, Mathers and Beard, 2013). Women, especially those living alone, have increased susceptibility to mental health issues because of social isolation, reduced educational opportunities earlier in life, and subsequent lower pensions and income in later life. This is exacerbated further by the increased likelihood of continuing responsibilities as carers late into old age, and the likely consequences for the neglect of their own health. Many of the issues affecting men and women in later life are of course the same, with the differences often revolving around cultural, gender-based factors, which are also often problematic in relation to some of the assumptions made. Women's more social nature, for example, with its emphasis on extended family network and the more involved nature of female relationships is frequently much more complex, exaggerating male dependency in later years and perpetuating stigma. It is possible that many people of the current older generation who fulfilled traditional gender roles as young adults will encounter difficulties in later life, which services and professionals might be able to anticipate. Vicissitudes, however, suggest that many of the issues previously afflicting one gender more than the other will in the not too distant future become much more equally distributed, with social isolation, for example, likely to affect women as much as men.

The main health conditions afflicting older men and women are exactly the same: cardiovascular diseases, cancers, musculoskeletal difficulties, diabetes, sensory impairments and incontinence, though rates, trends and specific types of these conditions vary according to gender. Mental ill-health can not only be added to the list of physical diseases but also is likely to reflect the incidence of physical illness at least to some extent. Prostate cancer, for example, adversely affects men more than women and has a significant impact on mental health, primarily in terms of the devastating effect on self-confidence, increased anxiety, feelings of depression and loss of masculinity. The gender structure of a particular society, the complex pattern of roles, responsibilities, norms, values, limitations and attitudes, which define what we associate with notions of masculinity and femininity and varies according to time and place, has a considerable impact on the health of older people (ProMenPol, 2009). Perceived or actual gender differences might significantly affect mental health, loss of work-related status, for example, or value as carer, grandparent or dominant role within a social network. All such factors might have a gender-related component, though the evidence increasingly suggests, and this seems likely to be perpetuated over coming decades, that similar experiences of mental health around loss, exclusion, grief, depression are much more likely to be the case. Retirement can have a massive impact, financially, in terms of status, reduced role, fewer social relationships, and increasingly affects men and women to the same extent (Cattan, 2009), with further issues around sense of belonging exacerbated by changing environment and dealing with a whole set of issues for which working life provides little if any preparation (Lehtinen, 2008).

Mental health and dementia

Dementia is projected to rise as populations age and will affect an estimated 115.4 million people by 2050 (WHO and Alzheimer's Disease International, 2012). Dementia constitutes a national challenge in relation to its scale and impact. Research demonstrates that in 2014 there are 835,000 people in the UK living with dementia (Alzheimer's Society, 2014a), which includes over 700,000 people in England, more than 45,000 in Wales, 20,000 in Northern Ireland and 70,000 in Scotland. There are 40,000 younger people, under the age of 65, living with the condition. Since the population is ageing, the numbers of people with dementia are increasing, and, consequently, so are the costs of caring for this group, to the extent that dementia now costs the economy £26 billion annually. In addition to this, an estimated 670,000 people in the UK act as primary carers for people with dementia, which in effect saves the state more than £11 billion per year. The situation, therefore, is not a simple one, with unpaid care an issue frequently neglected during discussions around the increased burden of caring for those with dementia. Two-thirds of people with dementia live in the community (Alzheimer's Society, 2007), a third of whom live alone in their own homes (Mirando-Costillo et al., 2010), with one-third living in care homes, though 70 per cent of care home residents have dementia or significant memory difficulties.

The increase in diagnosis rates is important, though many people continue to live without a formal diagnosis and variation in diagnosis rates between nations remains extreme, ranging from little more than a third to as high as three-quarters (Alzheimer's Society, 2014b). Furthermore, waiting times for specialist assessment vary according to geographical area, the availability of support following diagnosis is not automatically forthcoming and there is no mandatory minimum. This constitutes a complex and difficult issue, since many people do not have family and other support available, and this is a particularly traumatic time for an afflicted individual, with subsequent feelings of fear, anxiety and depression. There is some confusion, to compound an already complicated issue, with regard to whether the responsibility for the provision of services should lie with the NHS or fall within the social care arena. This too often means that access to a diagnosis and appropriate follow-up support is dependent upon the geographical area and the options for support available within that area.

People with dementia have cause to use health and social care services on a frequent basis, with more than a quarter of hospital beds (Alzheimer's Society, 2009) and as many as 70 per cent of care home places being occupied by this population, and with over 60 per cent of people receiving homecare services having dementia (UKHCA, 2013). The last few years have witnessed unprecedented cuts to the care system and many argue that reforms to the system are leaving many people without access to vital support services; this situation is further exacerbated by simultaneous increased demand for services at the same time as social care spending is decreasing in many parts of the country (ADASS, 2014). It is abundantly clear that people with dementia and family carers can lead fruitful lives if they have access to good quality, integrated, affordable care, and if they live in an area and in environmental circumstances where their needs are fulfilled. The continually increasing costs of dementia to society can, to a great extent, be attributed to the failure of contemporary health and social care services to deliver services to the standard necessary to meet these requirements. According to a recent survey, fewer than two out of ten people believed that they received enough support from the state, and that the deficit in such care needs are consequently being met by unpaid carers who, in effect, are keeping the system going (Alzheimer's Society, 2014a).

The first key priority in relation to dementia concerns the question of ensuring a swift yet accurate diagnosis; at present, many people are receiving a diagnosis too late or sometimes not at all, to the extent that diagnosis rates in the UK vary from below 40 per cent to above 75 per cent. A second, closely related priority relates to a comprehensive assessment of the individual's needs once a diagnosis has been made. This means that the person and their carers can subsequently access the care and support required so that they can continue to live well in the present whilst also planning for the future. People who have received a diagnosis are therefore better informed and their lives are able to improve accordingly. Health and other care professionals, whether working in hospital or community settings, can significantly affect care delivery simply through recognition of the importance of accurate diagnosis and subsequently being able to support people with dementia from the onset of the condition through to the later stages. Improved understanding and awareness of dementia coupled with those with the power to make decisions prioritising the condition, and underpinned by high quality data, significantly influences the extent of diagnosis. There is a strong argument for sustained commitment to transformational change within the health and social care system, with the goal being to identify and subsequently provide support for all people afflicted with dementia.

Good quality of life for someone living with dementia is clearly related to the receipt of an early diagnosis, one which enables the person to access services and, sometimes, medication, which can retard the progress of the condition. This may, furthermore, allow the person valuable time to make important decisions about their current and future health and welfare whilst they have the capacity to engage in discussion, articulate their views and, crucially, provide informed consent (All-Party

Parliamentary Group [APPG] on Dementia 2012). Accurate diagnosis is, without doubt, the most significant initial step (Dementia Action Alliance, 2010), and for it to be given timely requires that it take place at the point when the symptoms of dementia are beginning to have an impact on daily life (Brooker et al., 2013). Once a diagnosis has been made quickly and accurately, a number of directly related issues can be effectively addressed. These include access to good quality information and advice with regard to living well with the condition, access to potential support and appropriate treatment, enhanced management of other health conditions which might be affected by the dementia, the opportunity to plan in advance and make informed decisions about future needs and personal finances. The health and social system itself is also likely to benefit from timely diagnosis through more effective use of local resources, population-based future planning, avoidance of crisis admissions, and improvement of clinical management of multiple, complex conditions.

There are a number of important barriers to effective diagnosis of dementia, comprising the absence of a strategic approach at a local level, continuing poor public awareness, frequently insufficient understanding of dementia by health and social care professionals, the reduced likelihood of diagnosis in areas lacking in the availability of services, and limited collaborative relationships between health and social care providers (APPG on Dementia, 2012). One of the most important issues confronting services is the lack of data about dementia amongst black, Asian and minority ethnic communities, so that services are frequently not designed to deliver care with a specialist ethnic dimension. There is evidence to suggest that many people from these groups are much less likely to use existing services, sometimes because of language problems, but also because of mistaken perceptions and poor knowledge with regard to the availability and structure of existing services. Consequently, many people from minority groups fail to receive a timely diagnosis or are diagnosed at a much later stage of illness than the white British population (Moriarty, Sharif and Robinson, 2011). There is some evidence of diminished levels of awareness of dementia amongst some minority groups, diagnosis consequently taking place far too late, and reduced cultural sensitivity amongst those services that are available (APPG on Dementia, 2013). The consequences are increased difficulty for people from these communities in getting the support they require, which is, of course, contextualised by the fact that the proportion of black, Asian and minority population beyond the age of 65 is increasing at a rapid rate. This means that the need for culturally appropriate services should be regarded as a priority. There have been considerable efforts over the last few years to raise awareness of dementia, particularly amongst health and social care professionals, though, as yet, this has seen limited success in engaging the professional workforce in relation to the design of a comprehensive pathway for dementia diagnosis. The development of a system-wide improvement on the right scale warrants a need to change the way that health and social care professionals think about caring for people with dementia. Transformational change necessitates the need to penetrate commissioning guidance to the extent that systems are effectively redesigned and the necessary commitment is made to investment, particularly around workforce development. This is the key factor: recognition that improvement in diagnostic rates involves more than just improving numbers. A diagnostic pathway that begins with the first appointment with the general practitioner and follows through to account for the support received in the years following diagnosis requires investment, joint working between all involved agencies, and leadership, locally, regionally, nationally and internationally.

Case study - Gillian

Gillian is a 78 year old woman with a diagnosis of vascular dementia. She used to live in a dementia registered nursing home; however, they were unable to manage her behaviours and she became unhappy. The risks she posed to herself and other residents meant that she was admitted to the ward under section 2 of the Mental Health Act for the safety of herself and other people. Gillian is at risk of self neglect, she can be uninterested in food and fluids and often has to eat and drink 'on the go' until she is able to be encouraged to sit and eat a meal. Gillian is a small slender individual.

Gillian is disorientated to time, place and person and the ward staff ward have been unable to help her to accept that she is in hospital and she is confused. Gillian remains at risk of retaliation from fellow confused peers; she will mistake them for her husband Des and she will try and get them to follow her and encourage them out of their chairs and pull them around with her and want them to go with her.

Gillian is unable to elaborate on where she wants them to go and sometimes it is "down town" or nonspecific places that she cannot explain in a way that staff understand. Gillian is mostly calm and content when her husband (Des) visits the ward. She does recognise him and will sit with him for long periods and converse. Des visits most days and telephones the ward to check on his wife's progress every day. He has had to come to terms with his wife's continual confused state of mind and says that she is almost another person now.

Gillian is very tactile and enjoys hugs and kisses from Des. There have been times when Gillian has been unable to be convinced that Des is not visiting and she attempts to engage other patients in hugs and kisses as she would her husband. This obviously places her at risk and numerous strategies were employed to try and reduce these behaviours – for example, she was given photos of her husband to demonstrate he was not there. But this wasn't helpful for Gillian who remained distressed and agitated, and we found that simply taking her arm, walking around with her or sitting with her and chatting was the only approach that works.

Gillian will talk about needing to "get up and on" and "go down the town". She is able to go for walks with staff escorted on occasions, particularly if she is giving all of her attention to that individual and therefore following them around, unable to sit calmly without their presence, trying to get them to go with her.

When out for a walk Gillian has said "lets go back to the hotel" before to staff and seemed to feel she is on holiday with her husband. When returning to the ward, staff are able to simulate a hotel environment and wait on her and the member of staff with her.

Mental health as end of life approaches

Davie (2006) points out that those with pre-existing mental health difficulties, such as bipolar disorder or clinical depression, who subsequently become terminally ill constitute some of the least represented people within society. There is little research, furthermore, so little knowledge is available, and those having undertaken such research often tend to accentuate the desperate need for more studies (e.g. Henderson, 2004; McCasland, 2007;). The predominant mental health considerations, however, in relation to terminal illness and end of life care, relate to the exaggeration of the feelings of distress that everyone in such circumstances is likely to some extent to experience rather than the effects on those with severe and enduring mental illness.

There are a number of areas to take into account when contemplating mental health issues in the context of end of life, some of which relate to the changes in life circumstances that a marked deterioration in health brings. One concern revolves around the physical location, whether in one's own home, hospital ward, nursing home, inpatient setting, hospice or residential home; each area is likely to bring its own challenges for the individual to negotiate, with professional awareness, experience and knowledge critical to successful promotion of positive mental health. An important, perhaps the most important, question is the extent to which one can retain one's dignity as the final stages of life unfold. This question is coupled with the professional and family pre-occupation with doing the best for the individual, gaining a balance between individual and family needs. The imperative of capacity contextualises mental health needs in relation to end of life, with concerns by the individual, so wise in many areas of their life, frequently desperate not to become a burden, and mental health, particularly anxiety, confusion and acute sadness becoming more pronounced. It is very difficult and complicated to successfully place the individual at the centre of the care process as the end of life approaches; promoting advocacy and ensuring the person's voice is heard are clearly important, but making it happen can be extremely hard. In essence, the primary concern is for the older person coming to terms with impending death, and negotiating the varied effects on his or her mental health, to continue to have a voice, to feel respected, essentially to die with dignity. Professionals and care staff are sometimes insufficiently skilled in helping people to retain (or gain) a voice in such circumstances: their wisdom is not always accessed, their views not always sought. This is, perhaps, one of the most pressing issues as we grapple with the ageing population, renegotiating the boundaries between life and death, truly addressing mental health and facilitating a dignified end. The needs of the individual moving towards the end of life and the needs of the family, of course, are entirely inter-related, though negotiating a path that fully accounts for all involved is more complicated than might initially appear. An effective end of life pathway inevitably needs to negotiate such complexity around mental health, somehow establishing clear communication channels, ensuring legal concerns have been addressed, and somehow facilitating a degree of emotional honesty.

The notion of 'acceptance' has become increasingly influential over recent years, encouraging people to fully comprehend and process the fact not only that they are, of course, mortal, but also that they may have very limited time left because of terminal illness. Carers, care staff and professionals are all involved in supporting the individual towards such acceptance, ascertaining the amount of insight someone has into their condition, whether they are properly aware of the prognosis, how much they might understand. All such concerns cannot be detached from the individual's mental health, since confronting one's mortality is interwoven with psychological frailty, anxiety, fear and sadness. This requires 'real' communication in order to overcome the inevitable communication barriers and, as was discussed earlier in the chapter, professionals in positions of great responsibility are implicated in the relative success or failure of such complex human negotiations. Creating a comprehensive end of life strategy across the NHS has been considered for a number of years now (DH, 2008), but understanding and reacting to the complexities presented by the challenge of mental health is difficult to bring successfully to fruition.

Case study - Cliff

Cliff is a man who is 68 and used to live at home with his wife May. He has a diagnosis of Alzheimer's disease and is a retired Army Officer. He occasionally seems to think he is still a soldier and is disorientated to time and place and person and still thinks he has to go and fight the enemy, as he puts it, "sort people out". Cliff became anxious and frustrated with his family when they were trying to orientate him and get him to realise that he had retired and was no longer required to do his Army duties. They were struggling to cope and he would become verbally and physically threatening towards his wife May when she was trying to assist him with his activities of daily living. Cliff became more and more frustrated and was neglecting himself and this was a cause for concern for his wife who was no longer able to look after him. They had a care package put in place and carers would come to the house to encourage Cliff to take medication, wash and dress and help him and his wife. Cliff would refuse help from the carers and become angry with them also. Cliff was neglecting his needs and also being aggressive to anyone who tried to help him. Cliff was admitted to the ward under section 2 of the Mental Health act. The police had to escort him on to the ward as he would not leave his home. He was deemed too unwell to reside in a nursing home and the family were at crisis point.

There have been several incidents involving Cliff since his admission to the ward where he has gone to confront fellow peers and staff have had to intervene. On one occasion Cliff attacked a member of staff cleaning and mopping the floor. Both people ended up on the floor in a scuffle. I was first on the scene and able to guide Cliff away. A calm and friendly approach worked on this occasion. I went up to the pair and said "what's happened here then mate?" and had to ensure Cliff had seen that I was taking his side during the altercation even though he was the instigator. The person cleaning was then able to quickly leave the area and get his belongings and get to a place of safety. Cliff looked at me and stood up and we walked very closely together side by side and he said "I don't like him he needed sorting out". Cliff instantly calmed whilst walking and I said "it's okay he has gone now . . . are you ok?" and he said "yes now he has gone". There were no triggers to the attack and Cliff was unable to justify his actions and why he hit and pushed the staff member causing him to fall. By knowing Cliff well and knowing that he had misidentified the staff member and misread a situation, this violent attack was defused and both parties came out unharmed.

The art of the therapeutic lie (James et al., 2006) worked on this occasion and by saying "it's ok he has gone now". Additionally, talking in a calm friendly non-threatening manner seemed to help prevent further escalation and continued violence. Cliff seems to think I am a colleague and fellow soldier, he has never attacked me and will sit and converse with me about the old days in barracks and during the war. He cannot always be orientated to place and person and will not always accept he is in hospital and his wife is at home.

Cliff is a sociable individual and does sit and converse to both staff and peers on the ward. Cliff can be distracted from his previous frustrations and anxieties. He has no insight into his mental illness. He cannot express when he is hungry and in pain. Cliff is at risk of retaliation from peers as he does mistake situations and people. Cliff can confront people and states that they "need sorting" or "look at him there" in a derogatory tone.

At these times staff have had to move peers away for the safety of all parties and create an area where a staff member and Cliff can sit alone. This has been the only way to calm Cliff. By making it feel like his home and by going along with it as opposed to trying to orientate Cliff and tell him where he is and why he is there. Cliff will at times still think he is at work and by ensuring there are minimal patients in the vicinity and in his eye line, he can then be encouraged to talk about work and tell old stories.

Medication has not helped control these thoughts. Cliff sometimes settles when he sees his wife; he does remember her but is not always nice to her during her visits. They sit and chat and talk about the old days and family and holidays. Cliff will talk about bird spotting with his wife and they will listen to music together.

Staff try and encourage Cliff to areas of the ward where there are people he likes and trusts at all times. Cliff's wife telephones the ward every day and visits him a few times a week; she struggles to accept his presentation at times and will say "that's not my Cliff . . . that's not the man I married". Cliff's wife has her visits monitored as she is at risk of Cliff attacking her and being physically and verbally aggressive to her. Staff observe the visits but try and ensure Cliff cannot see that they are doing so to respect the couple's privacy and dignity.

Conclusions

The overall picture of the relationship between older people, mental health, informal support and service provision is a complicated one, frequently defying the stereotypes of a burdensome group absorbing more than their fair share of care. The evidence suggests that older people make few demands for support and are acutely aware of their tenuous relationship with society, which frequently focuses on their current lack of productivity rather than what has been achieved over the life course; the consequence is that their needs are often overlooked by service providers because of this tendency not to demand. Many appear to lack visibility, trapped in their own homes, having difficulty connecting with and influencing service developments. One of the key issues of the coming decades is that of ensuring older people have a voice, that this voice is listened to and receives a response.

There continues to be debate amongst policy makers and service providers about the challenges of the ageing population, yet it is fairly rare to hear the contributions of older people themselves, diminished visibility making a subtle addition to the layers of disadvantage experienced by this group. It is a little worrying and problematic that older people, particularly the very old, are frequently associated with a degree of generational stoicism, knowing how to make do, yet are simultaneously associated with dependency, financially and emotionally burdensome to their families and to the state. This contradiction seems to get to the heart of many of the difficulties characterising the relationship of the elderly to society: the fact that they are viewed in such a way, often portrayed so in the media, yet acutely aware of the image and having much to contribute to family and community life. Unfortunately, later life continues to be viewed by society as a period of loss and transition from being economically productive to being passively retired, when new opportunities and experiences are unlikely to occur. Current service structures for older people, therefore, focus in the main on deficits rather than assets. This appears to be a deeply entrenched situation exacerbated by stereotypes perpetuated by professionals and services, with stigmatised processes built into systems, protocols and policies, poor understanding at every level of the effects of stigma, and prejudice and isolation felt by the individuals concerned. The focus within service provision is ordinarily on meeting the practical support and health needs of older people rather than trying to make them less isolated, a situation which appears to be underpinned by powerful discriminatory forces operating both within services and across the wider society. There are, of course, many losses to encounter during the process of ageing, exposure to repeated bereavement, disengagement from productive work, changing relationships with family members, all of which bring a reduction in income and loss of structure, status and identity.

It is possible, though, to challenge many of these assumptions and, over a period of time, to alter professional discriminatory practice, develop services reflective of real rather than perceived need, accentuate the complexity of social isolation and, in effect, develop a different system based on a changed ideology. Services that work alongside people in their own homes, supporting them at their own pace, promote a better more mature understanding of good mental health in later life. The area of mental health when associated with older age appears to be dominated by the issue of dementia and imbued with many of the fears that characterise this condition. Dementia does, of course, present significant challenges to society but there are many other mental health issues that require consideration. Depression and anxiety, for example, can be so debilitating and yet are frequently associated with the stigma and prejudice discussed earlier in the chapter. Positive mental health requires a different approach from professionals, services and society, more generally, recognising and responding to social isolation and working with older people in a more empathic way, one which involves listening carefully and developing services to respond to real rather than perceived need.

Reflective practitioner account (by Thomas Moncur)

When I qualified as an Registered Mental Nurse (RMN) back in 2009 I was offered a position as a staff nurse in a nursing home, a place that I had previously worked as a healthcare assistant for four years both before and during my nurse training with Plymouth University (Dip HE Mental Health Nursing 2006–2009). The home has four different units that I have worked in as a healthcare assistant and a nurse and I worked as a nurse at the home for nearly three years. I have worked with residents with many different types of care needs and diagnoses, such as Palliative Care, Learning Disabilities, Huntingdon's Disease, Physical Disabilities, Multiple Sclerosis, Personality Disorder, Bipolar Affective Disorder, Spinal Injuries, Epilepsy, Organic Brain Injuries, Supranuclear Palsy, Cognitive Impairment, Elderly

(continued)

(continued)

Frailty, and people with different types of Dementia including Alzheimer's Disease, Vascular Dementia, Frontal Lobe Dementia and Dementia with Lewy Bodies.

During my time working for the NHS on the complex care and dementia inpatient wards since 2012, I have been involved in the assessment and treatment of older adults with organic mental health issues. I see a big part of my role as a staff nurse is having the ability to try and get into the mind set of every patient on the ward. It is about learning where they think they are, what they are trying to do, trying to work out what they are thinking and how they are feeling and why they are behaving in the way they are. It is almost like role play and when, on shift walking around the ward engaging and observing what the patients are doing, it is essential to try and learn what each individual is thinking, and it is not often possible to orientate a patient and prevent them from behaving in certain ways.

Communication with individuals has its limitations; it can be a challenge to gain their trust and understand why they are doing what they are doing. I feel that trying to get patients to do things they do not understand is a difficult thing. For example, if a patient is pushing a chair or carrying a table around it is best to try and offer help with this and say things like "can I help?" "don't do that on your own . . . you'll hurt your back", "where are we going with this?" or encouraging and helping them to move the item of furniture and then saying "that's great there . . . thanks for your help" as opposed to negative conversation such as "stop that, it goes there" or "put that down please" or "you'll damage the furniture".

It seems and has been said by friends, carers and relatives that some patients have never been questioned in life and have always been 'in control'; that they have led their lives as the role model or leader or bread winner. Therefore, my approach to defusing a situation and preventing an individual from doing something hazardous is to make it seem like it was their own idea and a decision that was led by them.

A patient is admitted to an inpatient unit in order to carry out a full assessment of their presentation and identified needs, to maintain safety and to stabilise their mental health. The majority of patients I have worked with and cared for have come into hospital detained under section 2 of the Mental Health Act 2007 (MHA). They have become mentally unwell and assessed to be unable to safely remain living within their home environment, be it a care setting, or in the community, due to risks that they pose to themselves, or to others. They are also considered to lack the capacity (due their condition) required to agree to an admission to hospital.

The MHA is used to detaining patients when they have been diagnosed as having a mental disorder that requires them to be assessed and potentially treated in the interests of their health or safety, or for protection of others, in a safe environment. Section 2 MHA is detention for a maximum period of 28 days for the purposes of assessment. Section 3 of the Act allows someone to be detained in hospital for treatment, initially for up to six months. After this time, the section may be renewed for a further six months, and then for a year at a time. Patients on the ward can also be residing there under section 3 as well as section 2 and have the right to appeal their detention.

(continued)

(continued)

Patients are also in hospital under the legal framework of the Mental Capacity Act 2005 and within this there has to be Deprivation of Liberty Safeguards (DoLS). For all patients on the ward we have to be aware that any deprivation of liberty is only lawful if there are safeguards in place such as those surrounding detention under the Mental Health Act or DOLS and ensure that if a patient's admission amounts to a deprivation of liberty it is justified and appropriate. We have to be making decisions on behalf of people who lack the capacity to make decisions for themselves. A deprivation of liberty for such a person must be authorised in accordance with one of the following legal regimes: a deprivation of liberty authorisation or Court of Protection order under the Deprivation of Liberty Safeguards (DoLS) in the Mental Capacity Act 2005, or (if applicable) under the Mental Health Act 1983 (parts of the Act were amended in 2007).

A big part of my role as a staff nurse has been providing innovative care and treatment and most patients I have worked with on the ward lack mental capacity, have a type of dementia and need things doing that are within their best interests all the time.

This role does differ from my role on wards where I have previously worked, as in the nursing home environment, ordinarily, this is to be the individual's permanent home, and more attention is given to ensuring that longer term needs are identified and met including social and spiritual needs, as well as obviously physical and health needs.

That's not to say the inpatient setting does not consider holistic needs of the patient, we do, but the emphasis is on the assessment and the treatment of the individual with a view to helping them to move out of the inpatient setting into a suitable long term place to live as quickly as possible.

On the ward where I work there are patients who are vulnerable and at risk of getting into altercations with other patients who are not accountable for their actions. To reduce risk, every patient is on a certain level of observations – for example hourly observations, 10 minute checks, line of sight x1 staff member or x2 staff members. The level of observation required is assessed depending on a patient's previous history and current presentation; this is reviewed daily and can be increased or reduced as considered appropriate. Ward staff are allocated to carry out observations on an hourly basis, and documentation is signed to demonstrate who is responsible for the observation, where the patient is on the ward and their mental state at the time.

Risks are also reduced by the design of the ward, for example the patients' doors to their bedrooms are accessed by a key, therefore locking once shut and being unable to be opened by others from the outside unless they have a key. The patients can get out and do not need a key to exit their bed space as there is a handle on the inside. This prevents fellow patients getting in to others rooms.

Often, when staff are assisting patients with their needs, patients can be unaware and unable to comprehend that the team of staff are working in their best interests, and frequently become uncooperative and aggressive towards the staff member assisting them. This is when

(continued)

(continued)

a calm skilled approach is necessary. Patients are not always in control of their actions and are not accountable for how they behave; the safety of the patient and that of staff working with them has to be paramount on these occasions.

Incidents and accidents that occur have to be documented and discussed within the ward team, with family members and carers, and the wider multidisciplinary team, and we try and learn from each incident. Members of staff need to be trained in techniques to protect themselves and the patients, and are kept regularly updated with such techniques.

I try to be a good role model to my peers, more junior members of staff and learners when patients may be inappropriate, aggressive, unhappy or elated and becoming angry or violent, by maintaining my composure but acting quickly and skilfully to ensure the safety of all is maintained.

Risks and interventions to prevent altercations are put in place with regards to personal care. For example, one patient may layer their clothing and then become too hot throughout the day. Therefore just enough items of clothing can be left in the person's room and the rest kept safe in the laundry room to prevent this happening when the person awakes and they get dressed independently.

Many of the patients on the ward are severely cognitively impaired and have both expressive and receptive dysphasia. They cannot be guided or directed or understand staff or other patients. As already described, communication can be difficult and non-verbal communication such as physical prompts are required with lots of the patients.

One particular strategy I use to promote adequate hydration in patients who are declining fluids is to stand in the communal area with a jug of juice and some beakers – when said patient walks by I exclaim "cheers!" and have a sip of my drink. I find that more often than not, patients will pick up a beaker and have drink with me, perhaps triggered by a memory of social cues and traditions.

The ward tries to provide the social stimuli that the patients require to keep them happy whilst residing there. I try to implement progressive, innovative and socially inclusive care plans with emphasis on user involvement where possible. It is crucial in the development of innovative and individual care plans to include a patient's carers and relatives in the formulation stage. This allows us to gain real insight into a patient's likes and dislikes, which can assist us in caring for a patient, who may not be able to communicate why they are distressed, or to verbalise their own needs.

I believe in positive risk taking for the good of people and I nurse in a person centred way so that every individual is able to be recognised as one whose personality, life history, choices and preferences are taken into consideration by the people who are caring for them. I try and ensure that key relationships to the individual are maintained and I am committed to delivering high standards of care to the people I nurse, *always* ensuring that all aspects of privacy and dignity are maintained when delivering care, including where appropriate end of life wishes.

Reflective exercise

- What mental health issues are associated with the aged population?
- Reflect and think about what mental health care and support an elderly person needs.
- Then consider other issues such as gender, a physical or learning disability, financial problems, being from a minority ethnic background and the importance of these being addressed.
- What mental health challenges can face the aged population upon retiring?
- Reflect and think about the mental health needs of the aged population when approaching end of life.
- Consider how bereavement can affect an older person's mental health status.

References

ADASS (Association of Directors of Adult Social Care) (2014). *ADASS budget survey report 2014: Final.* [online] Available at: www.adass.org.uk/adass-budget-survey-2014/ [viewed 1 February 2015].

Age Concern (2007) *Improving services and support for older people with mental health problems: The second report from the UK Inquiry into Mental Health and Well-Being in Later Life* [online]. Available at: www.its-services.org.uk/silo/files/inquiry-full-report.pdf [viewed 01/09/15].

Age UK (2011) *Safeguarding the convoy.* Abingdon: Age UK Oxfordshire.[online]. Available at: www. counselandcare.org.uk/UserFiles/Safeguarding%20the%20convoy%20-%20a%20call%20to%20 action%20from%20the%20Campaign%20to%20End%20Loneliness.pdf [viewed 01/09/15].

All-Party Parliamentary Group (APPG) on Dementia (2012) *Unlocking diagnosis.* London: Alzheimer's Society.

All-Party Parliamentary Group (APPG) on Dementia (2013) *Dementia does not discriminate.* London: Alzheimer's Society.

Alzheimer's Society (2007) *Dementia UK.* London: Alzheimer's Society.

Alzheimer's Society (2009) *Counting the cost: Caring for people with dementia on hospital wards.* London: Alzheimer's Society

Alzheimer's Society (2014a) *Dementia UK* (2nd edition). London: Alzheimer's Society.

Alzheimer's Society (2014b) *Dementia 2014: Opportunities for change.* London: Alzheimer's Society.

Beekman AT, Copeland JR and Prince, MJ (1999) Review of community prevalence of depression in later life, *British Journal of Psychiatry* 174: 307–311.

Bowers, H Maclean, M Patel, M Smith, C Macadam, A Crosby, G Clark, A and Bright, L (2006) *Disregarded and overlooked: report from the 'Learning from Experience' research into the needs, experiences, aspirations and voices of older people with mental health needs, and carers, across the UK.* Older People's Programme and UK Inquiry into Mental Health and Wellbeing in Later Life. Bournemouth: Older People's Programme.

Brooker, D La Fontaine, J Evans, S Bray, J and Saad, K (2013) *Timely diagnosis of dementia: Alzheimer co-operative valuation in Europe synthesis report (WP5).* Worcester: Association for Dementia Studies.

Butler, RN (1969) Age-ism: Another form of bigotry. *Gerontologist* 9: 243–246.

Butler, RN (2009) Combating ageism: Guest editorial, *International Psychogeriatrics* 21 (4): 211.

Cain, E (2012) Voices of the marginalized: Persons with disabilities, older people, people with mental health issues. Paper presented for the *Global Thematic Consultation on Addressing Inequalities. The heart of the post-2015 development agenda and the future we want for all.* New York: UN Women and UNICEF.

Cattan, M (2009) Introduction. In Cattan, M (ed), *Mental health and well-being in later life.* Glasgow: Open University Press, pp. 1–8.

Crown, J and Lee, M (2007) *UK Inquiry into Mental Health and Well-Being in Later Life. Age Concern England and Mental Health Foundation: Improving services and support for older people with mental health problems: The second report from the UK Inquiry into Mental Health and Well-being in Later Life.* London: Age Concern, Mental Health Foundation.

Das, J Do, Q-T Friedman, J McKenzie, D and Scott, K (2007) Mental health and poverty in developing countries: Revisiting the relationship, *Social Science and Medicine* 65: 467–480.

Davie, E (2006) A social work perspective on palliative care for people with mental health problems, *European Journal of Palliative Care* 13 (1:) 26–28.

Dementia Action Alliance (2010) *National dementia declaration.* London: Dementia Action Alliance.

Department of Health (2002) *National service framework for older people: Interim report on age discrimination,* www.dh.gov.uk/prod_consum_dh/groups/dh_digitalassets/@dh/@en/documents/digitalasset/dh_4019556.pdf [viewed 01/09/15].

Department of Health (2005) *Mental Capacity Act.* London: HMSO.

Department of Health (2007) *Mental Health Act.* London: DH.

Department of Health (2008) *End of life care strategy: Promoting high quality care for all adults at the end of life.* London: DH.

Department of Health (2009) *New horizons: Towards a shared vision for mental health.* Mental Health Division. www.dh.gov.uk/en/Consultations/Liveconsultations/DH_103144 [viewed 01/09/15].

Glassman, J (2004) Gross neglect, *Care and Health Magazine* 69 (8 June): 14–16.

Goldie, I (ed) (2010) *Public mental health today: A handbook.* Brighton: Pavilion Publishing.

Hagemejer, K and Behrendt, C (2009) Can low-income countries afford basic social security? In OECD, *Promoting pro-poor growth: Social protection.* Available at: bit.ly/BNESLR9 [viewed 01/09/15].

Hagestad, GO and Uhlenberg, P (2005) The social separation of old and young: A root of ageism, *Journal of Social Issues* 61 (2): 343–360.

Healthcare Commission (2009) *Equalities in Later life: A national study of older people's mental health services* [online]. Available at: www.scie-socialcareonline.org.uk/profile.asp?guid=2fb986e7-138e-4b9e-97af-3633a99fef58 [viewed 01/09/15].

Henderson, M (2004) Mental health needs. In Oliviere, D and Monroe, B (2004) *Death, dying and social differences.* Oxford: Oxford University Press, Chapter 6, pp. 79–95.

James, IA Wood-Mitchell, AJ Waterworth, AM Mackenzie, LE and Cunningham, J (2006) Lying to people with dementia: Developing ethical guidelines for care settings, *International Journal of Geriatric Psychiatry* 21 (8): 800–801.

Jané-Llopis, E and Gabilondo, A (eds) (2008) *Mental health in older people. Consensus paper.* Luxembourg: European Communities.

Lee, K Volans, PJ and Gregory, N (2003) Trainee clinical psychologists' views on recruitment to work with older people, *Ageing and Society* 23(1): 83–97.

Lehtinen, V (2008) *Building up good mental health.* Jyväskylä: Stakes.

Lund, C Breen, A Flisher, AJ Kakuma, R Corrigall, J Joska, JA Swartz, L and Patel, V (2010) Poverty and common mental disorders in low and middle income countries: A systematic review. *SocSci Med* 71(3): 517–528.

McCasland, L (2007) Providing hospice and palliative care to the seriously and persistently mentally ill, *Journal of Hospice and Palliative Nursing* 9(6): 305–313.

McGlone, E and Fitzgerald, F (2005) *Perceptions of ageism in health and social services in Ireland: Report based on research undertaken by Eileen McGlone and Fiona Fitzgerald, QE5,* Dublin: National Council on Ageing and Older People.

Meissner, M (2010) *Ways out of old-age poverty.* Available at: bit.ly/BNESLR10 [viewed 01/09/15].

Mental Health Foundation (2010) *The lonely society. London: Mental Health Foundation* [online]. Available at: www.mentalhealth.org.uk/ publications/the-lonely-society/ [viewed 01/09/15].

Mirando-Costillo, C et al. (2010) People with dementia living alone: What are their needs and what kind of support are they receiving? *International Psychogeriatics* 22 (4): 607–617.

Moriarty, J Sharif, N and Robinson, J (2011) *Black and minority ethnic people with dementia and their access to support and services. Research Briefing 35.* [online] available at: www.scie.org.uk/publications/briefings/files/briefing35.pdf [viewed 4 February 2015].

Office of National Statistics (2009) *The mental health of older people* [online]. Available at: www.statistics.gov.uk/downloads/theme_health/PMA-MentalOlder.pdf.

ProMenPol (2009) A manual for promoting mental health and wellbeing: Older people's residences. www.mentalhealthpromotion.net/?i=promenpol [viewed 20 February 2015].

Ray, S Sharp, E and Abrams, D (2006) *Ageism: A benchmark of public attitudes in Britain.* London: Age Concern England; Canterbury: University of Kent, Centre for the Study of Group Processes.

Robb, C Chen, H and Haley, WE (2002) Ageism in mental health and health care: A critical review, *Journal of Clinical Geropsychology* 8(1): 1–12.

Sartorius, N (2007) Physical illness in people with mental disorders, *World Psychiatry* 6(1): 3–4. Available at: bit.ly/BNESLR14 [viewed 01/09/15].

Scholl, JM and Sabat, SR (2008) Stereotypes, stereotype threat and ageing: implications for the understanding and treatment of people with Alzheimer's disease, *Ageing and Society* 28(1): 103–130.

Stevens, GA Mathers, CD and Beard, JR (2013) Global mortality trends and patterns in older women. *Bulletin of the World Health Organization* 91: 630–639 doi: dx.doi.org/10.2471/BLT.12.109710.

Suvedi, BK Pradhan, A Barnett, S Puri, M Chitrakar, S.R Poudel, P Sharma, S and Hulton, L (2009) *Nepal maternal mortality and morbidity study 2008/2009: Summary of preliminary findings.* Kathmandu: Family Health Division, Department of Health Services, Ministry of Health, Government of Nepal.

UK Homecare Association (2013) *UKHCA dementia strategy and plan*, February 2013. Wallington: UK Homecare Association.

UNDESA (2004) *United Nations Demographic Yearbook review. National reporting of age and sex-specific data. Implications for international recommendations.* Available at: bit.ly/BNESLR16 [viewed 01/09/15].

UNFPA and HelpAge International (2012) *Ageing in the 21st century: A celebration and a challenge.* New York and London: UNFPA and HelpAge International. Available at: bit.ly/BNESLR17 [viewed 01/09/15].

WHO (World Health Organization) (2002) *Fifty-fifth World Health Assembly A55/17. Ageing and health. Report by the Secretariat* [online]. Geneva: WHO. Available at: apps.who.int/gb/archive/files/WHA55/ea5517.pdf [viewed 01/09/15].

WHO (2007) *Definition of an older or elderly person.* Available at: www.who.int/healthinfo/survey/ageingdefnolder/en/index.html [viewed 7 December 2014].

WHO (2008) *Global burden of disease, 2004 update.* Geneva: WHO. Available at: bit.ly/BNESLR18 [viewed 01/09/15].

WHO and Alzheimer›s Disease International (2012) *Dementia: A public health priority.* Geneva: WHO.

Index

eBooks
from Taylor & Francis

Helping you to choose the right eBooks for your Library

Add to your library's digital collection today with Taylor & Francis eBooks. We have over 50,000 eBooks in the Humanities, Social Sciences, Behavioural Sciences, Built Environment and Law, from leading imprints, including Routledge, Focal Press and Psychology Press.

Choose from a range of subject packages or create your own!

Benefits for you

- Free MARC records
- COUNTER-compliant usage statistics
- Flexible purchase and pricing options
- All titles DRM-free.

Benefits for your user

- Off-site, anytime access via Athens or referring URL
- Print or copy pages or chapters
- Full content search
- Bookmark, highlight and annotate text
- Access to thousands of pages of quality research at the click of a button.

REQUEST YOUR **FREE** INSTITUTIONAL TRIAL TODAY

Free Trials Available
We offer free trials to qualifying academic, corporate and government customers.

eCollections

Choose from over 30 subject eCollections, including:

Archaeology	Language Learning
Architecture	Law
Asian Studies	Literature
Business & Management	Media & Communication
Classical Studies	Middle East Studies
Construction	Music
Creative & Media Arts	Philosophy
Criminology & Criminal Justice	Planning
Economics	Politics
Education	Psychology & Mental Health
Energy	Religion
Engineering	Security
English Language & Linguistics	Social Work
Environment & Sustainability	Sociology
Geography	Sport
Health Studies	Theatre & Performance
History	Tourism, Hospitality & Events

For more information, pricing enquiries or to order a free trial, please contact your local sales team:
www.tandfebooks.com/page/sales

www.tandfebooks.com